The Embryology of Domestic Animals

Developmental Mechanisms and Malformations

Comparative Fetal Growth Rates

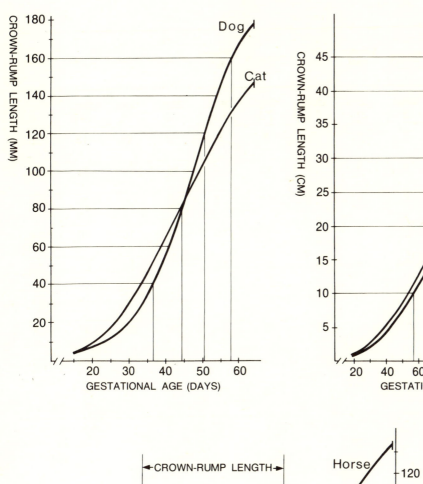

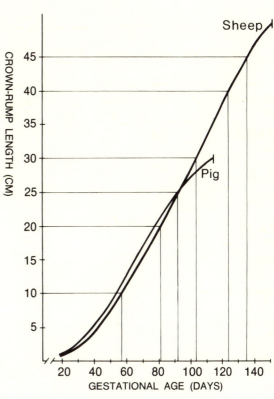

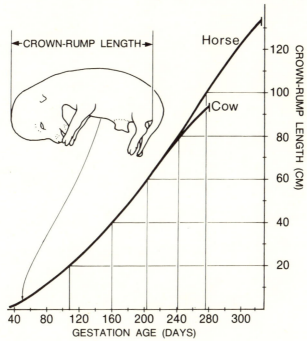

The Embryology of Domestic Animals

Developmental Mechanisms and Malformations

Drew M. Noden
Associate Professor, Department of Anatomy
New York State College of Veterinary Medicine
Cornell University
Ithaca, New York

Alexander de Lahunta
Professor, Department of Anatomy
Chairman, Department of Clinical Sciences
New York State College of Veterinary Medicine
Cornell University
Ithaca, New York

Illustrated by Drew M. Noden
with assistance by William Hamilton and Michael Simmons

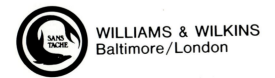

WILLIAMS & WILKINS
Baltimore/London

Editor: George Stamathis
Associate Editor: Victoria M. Vaughn
Copy Editor: Caral Shields Nolley
Design: JoAnne Janowiak
Illustration Planning: Reginald R. Stanley
Production: Anne G. Seitz

Accurate indications, adverse reactions, and dosage schedules for drugs are provided in this book, but it is possible that they may change. The reader is urged to review the package information data of the manufacturers of the mediations mentioned.

Made in the United States of America

Library of Congress Cataloging in Publication Data

Main entry under title:

Noden, Drew M.
  The embryology of domestic animals.

  Includes index.
  1. Veterinary embryology. I. DeLahunta, Alexander, 1932– . II. Title.
SF767.5.N63 1985   636.089′264   84-3597
ISBN 0-683-06545-9

Composed and printed at the
Waverly Press, Inc.

Foreword

Time devoted to the study of development in the veterinary curriculum is well spent. The veterinary practitioner is frequently asked to explain malformations in the newborn and comment upon the possible etiology or consequences. I believe this text provides the student, teacher, and practitioner with enough facts, principles, and references to allow for reasoned interpretations of the most frequently encountered developmental syndromes as seen in the dissecting room, necropsy or clinic. Hopefully, it will provide insight for understanding bizarre, or as yet undescribed, malformations as well. The number of new illustrations and clinical citations is impressive.

Although good texts for human development are available, they are not suited for veterinary teaching or research. There is great need for a text with specific information on the development of domestic animals. Each species of animal has characteristics of its own as regards blastocyst formation, implantation and placentation, and organogenesis. Domestic animal embryos show great variations in developmental rates which may result in species-specific or even breed-specific malformations. This text reviews normal development and introduces the reader to genetic and induced congenital defects in domestic animals.

Embryology is most meaningful in the professional curriculum, particularly in the first year, when it helps to explain the morphology and interrelationships of structures encountered in gross anatomy. Teachers of veterinary anatomy have long recognized the need for a student-oriented text on the development of domestic animals and should welcome this effort by their colleagues, Drew Noden and Alexander de Lahunta.

The orientation of this book is a reflection of the intellectual sincerity, passion for research, and devotion to teaching of the authors. Drew Noden is an experimental embryologist with classical training (Ph.D., 1973, Washington University, St. Louis). His primary research concerns craniofacial development, particularly the neural crest and head placodes, and is supported by the National Institutes of Health. He has taught a variety of courses in zoology at the University of Massachusetts, and since 1979 has taught developmental and gross anatomy to first-year veterinary students at Cornell. Alexander de Lahunta (D.V.M., 1958; Ph.D., 1963, Cornell) is a veterinary anatomist with past clinical experience in private practice and in the teaching hospital. He holds a joint appointment as Professor of Anatomy and Chairman of the Department of Clinical Sciences at Cornell. He formerly taught developmental anatomy and presently teaches gross and applied anatomy, neuroanatomy and clinical neurology, and neuropathology. His previous *Laboratory Guide to the Study of Embryology* was the foundation for this present work. Dr. de Lahunta is the author of *Veterinary Neuroanatomy and Clinical Neurology* and a coauthor of *Miller's Guide to the Dissection of the Dog*.

I have enjoyed teaching with both of these colleagues and have watched the materials for this text take form, first as lecture handouts primitively illustrated and reproduced, and later as elegant copy prepared for publication. The contents of the chapters steadily improved as new information became available from a plethora of new techniques. Throughout the text the authors have incorporated the results of experiments designed to provide an understanding of developmental mechanisms.

A teacher's contribution to progress is dependent upon a perception of student needs and the ability to convey essential information in useable form. I believe the authors have succeeded in their task by providing succinct, yet understandable, explanations of normal development along with clinical examples of abnormal development. I thank these busy authors for the time they have taken to produce this teaching aid, which makes veterinary gross anatomy more meaningful and thought provoking.

June, 1984

Howard E. Evans, Ph.D.
Professor and Chairman
Department of Anatomy
New York State College of
Veterinary Medicine
Cornell University
Ithaca, New York

Preface

This text is designed to provide a concise overview of animal development suitable for use by veterinary and animal science students and professionals. While the principal aspects of development are similar in all domestic animals, each species has many unique features that affect placentation, organogenesis, susceptibility to teratogenic agents, and incidence of inherited malformations. To enhance understanding of both normal development and congenital defects, we have included frequent discussions of the mechanisms controlling embryonic processes to supplement descriptive material.

It is not possible to fully describe every developing organ system in each species, or to list all reported congenital anomalies found in domestic animals. Rather, the goal of this text is to present an account of comparative and clinical embryology that conveys our excitement and enthusiasm for the subject in a format that recognizes the practical needs of the student, practitioner and researcher.

As this text evolved, first as class notes then chapter drafts, many of our colleagues and students generously provided invaluable criticisms and suggestions. We especially appreciate the scholarly advice of members of the Department of Anatomy, whose collective knowledge of mammalian development exceeds our ability to transcribe into text. In particular we thank Prof. Howard Evans, Chairman of the Anatomy Department, for his enthusiastic encouragement and continued support during the preparation of this book.

Completion of this text would not have been possible without the tireless assistance of Barbara Burton, Muriel Keller and Mary Lay. Also, we are grateful to the editors and staff at Williams & Wilkins for their support of this project and their patience and guidance during its completion.

We dedicate this book to our mentors in embryology, Professors J. Robert Harrison, Florence Moog, and especially Viktor Hamburger and Peter de Boom, who taught us about both the ways and the mysteries of animal development, and to our students, some of whom will, we hope, carry on this tradition.

Contents

Embryology in the Veterinary Curriculum

Embryology is the study of developing organisms. The subject includes descriptive examinations and comparisons of various species at different stages as well as experimental analyses of the mechanisms controlling and coordinating development. The purpose of this introduction is to illustrate how knowledge of the basic principles of development will assist the student in understanding relationships taught in gross anatomy, histology, and pathology courses, and will later serve the clinician in diagnosing certain conditions and in counseling owners of animals that have congenital malformations. The specific examples and terms used in this section will all be explained in greater detail later in the text.

EMBRYOLOGY AS AN AID TO UNDERSTANDING ANATOMY

The study of animal development provides a dynamic perspective on gross anatomy by presenting an historical view of tissue and organ relationships. Tracing complex tissue relationships back to fetal and embryonic stages often reveals a simplified pattern, knowledge of which helps clarify the more complex anatomy of the adult.

This is especially helpful in understanding systems whose components drastically change their relative positions during embryogenesis, such as the face, heart, viscera, and urogenital structures. The following examples illustrate the insights provided by an appreciation of developmental events.

Formation of the Recurrent Laryngeal Nerves

In dissecting the arteries emerging from the heart you will encounter a pair of nerves, the recurrent laryngeal nerves, which branch from the left and right vagus nerves in the cranial part of the thoracic cavity. These nerves travel caudally from the base of the skull into the thorax then turn around and pass cranially to innervate parts of the esophagus and larynx. Thus, the courses they take between their origins and terminations are long and tortuous. Moreover, their pathways are very different on each side of the thorax, as shown schematically in Fig. I.1D. In contrast the pathways of these nerves are straight and symmetrical in the young embryo (Fig. I.1B).

The explanation for the emergence of this asymmetry rests on the basic arrangement of arteries and nerves in the head of the embryo and on changes that occur during embryonic development.

On the ventrolateral aspect of the head of the embryo are a series of tissue masses called visceral arches. As shown in Figure I.1A each has an artery called an aortic arch coursing through it carrying blood from the ventrally located heart to the paired dorsal aortae. This general arrangement is retained in lower vertebrates and is similar to that

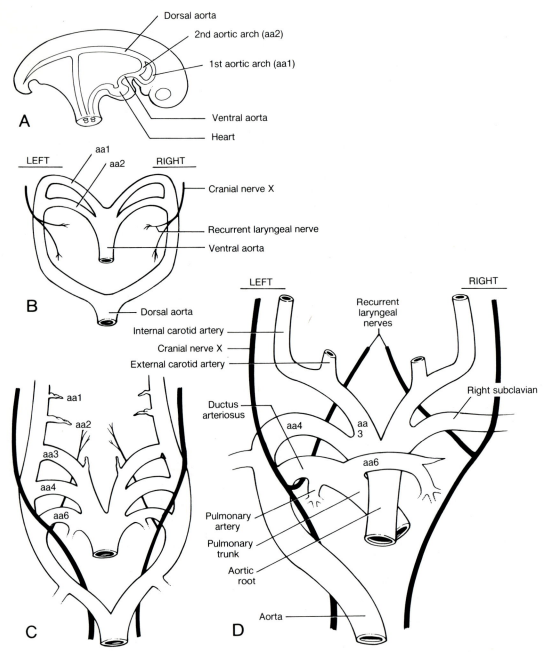

Figure I.1. Development of aortic arches and recurrent laryngeal nerve. *A,* lateral view of embryo at approximately 20-somite stage. *B,* dorsal view of same stage. *C* and *D,* show later stages in the transformation of these arches. Note how the left recurrent laryngeal nerve is caught behind the left 6th aortic arch (ductus arteriosus), which degenerates early on the right side.

seen in adult fishes. In addition, each visceral arch is innervated by a specific cranial nerve. These nerves emerge from the brain stem and enter the visceral arch lateral to the dorsal aorta immediately behind each aortic arch. Although the embryonic arterial sys-tem is initially symmetrical, certain vessels degenerate either early in embryogenesis or at the time of birth (see Chapter 11). Also, soon after their formation the heart and associated vessels shift caudally relative to other head and neck structures.

The asymmetrical degeneration of the 4th and 6th aortic arches is shown in Figures I.1C and D. The RIGHT 6th aortic arch degenerates early, while the LEFT 6th aortic arch is retained. Thus, when the caudal shift of the heart occurs, the left recurrent laryngeal nerve is pulled back by the 6th aortic arch, but the right nerve can slip forward. As we shall see later, failure of any of these events to occur in normal sequence, especially aortic arch formation or degeneration and the shift in cardiac position, can result in serious, often lethal, cardiovascular anomalies.

Innervation of the Trapezius Muscle

The perspective gained by the study of embryology often illuminates morphological relationships between structures in different animals. For example, in the dissec-tion of the dog's neck you will encounter cranial nerve XI, the accessory nerve, which projects caudally from beneath the base of the ear and innervates the trapezius muscle located at the level of the scapula (Fig. I.2C). Along its course it crosses the paths of several segmental cervical nerves. This unusual relationship results from the fact that the trapezius is thought to be homologous to gill levator muscles in fishes (Fig. I.2A).

Gills are derived from visceral arches, the muscles of which are, as previously described, innervated by different cranial motor nerves. The embryonic nerve-muscle relation is retained throughout ontogeny and phylogeny, even though the attachments of the muscle have changed dramatically in the evolution from fishes to reptiles and mammals.

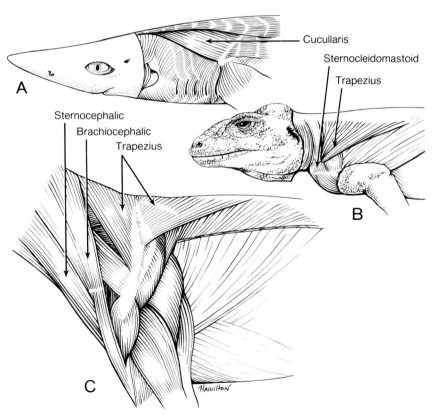

Figure I.2. Location of the trapezius (cucullaris) muscle in the *A*, shark, *B*, lizard and *C*, dog. These muscles are considered to be homologues based on their embryonic origin and similar innervation (cranial nerve XI).

EVALUATING AND UNDERSTANDING CONGENITAL MALFORMATIONS

Knowledge of the features and principles of development is essential to understanding **congenital malformations**, which include all abnormalities arising during prenatal development, regardless of the cause (inherited, induced, or spontaneous). In clinical practice you will encounter many anatomical and physiological anomalies whose pathogenesis (causative mechanism) occurs during development. Sometimes these conditions are not manifest at birth, but emerge later as the animal becomes ambulatory and more active or at sexual maturity. Your responsibilities include not only identification, diagnosis, and treatment, but also ap-

preciation of possible causes of such conditions, the risk of heritability in the particular species and breed, possible **teratogenic** (abnormality-inducing) environmental agents or medications which might be harmful to the fetus, or susceptibility to selective nutritional deficiencies or excesses. Only by knowing the changing, emerging structures and physiology of the embryo and fetus, and by understanding the mechanisms by which these developmental processes are controlled, will you be able to evaluate completely each clinical situation and advise the client accurately. The following two examples illustrate these points. The first is presented in some detail to demonstrate the method of problem solving in veterinary medicine that will be part of your training.

Examine again the development of the 6th

Every diagnosis is a process of deliberate evaluation of facts in the context of broader sets of information gained through training and experience. Arriving at the correct diagnosis is a disciplined, deductive procedure, in which all possibilities are considered and alternatives supported or refuted based on available data, which may include the history, physical exam, lab tests, and both invasive and noninvasive diagnostic procedures. The following cases illustrate this integrative approach.

CASE HISTORY

Signalment: A female Miniature Poodle, 16 months old presented with a chief complaint of episodic pelvic limb weakness.

History. The onset of the problem began when the dog was 9 months old. When exercised the dog would occasionally become weak in the pelvic limbs, sometimes to the point of collapse. Excessive panting accompanied this weakness. After a few minutes of rest, the dog recovered its strength. Sporadic at first, these episodes slowly progressed in frequency to several per day. The dog had no other significant past medical illness. Other than the weakness, its general physical condition, appetite and excretory functions were normal.

Assessment of History:

FACTS	INTERPRETATION
Pelvic limb weakness to collapse	Disease of the musculoskeletal, nervous, respiratory, cardiovascular or endocrine systems
Episodic event associated with exercise but animal is normal between episodes	Not typical of diseases of the central nervous system
Signs of weakness associated with excessive panting	More likely a respiratory or cardiovascular problem
Increasing frequency of episodes	Suggests an acquired disease, or a congenital problem with secondary complication
No other recent past illness or associated signs	Less likely a systemic infectious disease
Miniature Poodle breed	There is a high incidence of a congenital heart defect called **patent ductus arteriosus** in this breed

Physical Exam: The significant aspects of the physical examination are a normal gait with normal musculoskeletal and neurologic signs. The femoral pulse is normal. Palpation (feeling or examining by hand) reveals that the apex beat of the heart is on the right side. Auscultation (to listen to, as with a stethoscope) of the heart reveals no murmur (a murmur refers to any abnormal heart sound). No abnormal lung sounds (rales) are detected. The dog is exercised and, after a short period, the pelvic limbs become progressively weak until they collapse. The thoracic limbs are normal and the dog remains alert. Increased rate and depth of respiration (hyperpnea) and cyanosis (a blue discoloration of the mucous membranes) are detected.

Assessment of Physical Examination:

FACTS	INTERPRETATION
Normal gait, musculoskeletal and neurological examination	The problem is unlikely to be caused by a disease of these systems
Normal auscultation of lungs	Less likely to be a primary respiratory system disease
No cardiac murmurs	Less likely to be a cardiac disease unless the cardiac lesion (morphologic abnormality) does not restrict blood flow so as to cause an abnormal sound
Palpation of a right apex beat	Normally the apex beat is on the left; enlargement of the right ventricle may cause the apex beat to be felt on the right side
Normal femoral pulse	Less likely the problem is caused by a blockage of blood flow to the pelvic limbs, such as an embolism or thrombosis
Hyperpnea and cyanosis on exercise	Indicates insufficient oxygenation of red blood cells due to a shunt between the venous and arterial blood supplies and an impediment to pulmonary blood flow and oxygenation
Pelvic limb collapse, normal thoracic limbs	Indication that the insufficient oxygenation has mostly affected the blood supply of the pelvic limbs and the shunt is behind the major blood supply to the thoracic limbs and head

Differential Diagnosis: Based on an interpretation of these facts, the most likely clinical diagnosis is a cardiovascular malformation that causes a reduced level of oxygenation in the blood by allowing blood to be shunted from the venous to the arterial systems. The tentative hypothesis is that the animal suffers from a severe **patent ductus arteriosus.**

aortic arch shown in Figure I.1. In the adult the ventral part of each 6th aortic arch forms the pulmonary arteries, carrying blood from the right ventricle to the lungs. However, oxygenation in the embryo occurs in the placenta, not the lungs, and blood entering the right side of the heart via umbilical veins is fully oxygenated. To avoid circulating this blood through pulmonary tissue, the dorsal part of the LEFT 6th aortic remains patent (open) until birth, providing a direct channel for oxygenated blood to enter the systemic circulation. This dorsal part of the left 6th aortic arch is the **ductus arteriosus.** The corresponding segment of the right 6th aortic arch degenerates.

Postnatally, a large patent ductus arteriosus with a pressure in the pulmonary trunk and arteries that exceeds that of the aorta would permit unoxygenated pulmonary blood to flow into the aorta without oxygenation. The ductus arteriosus normally enters the aorta behind the main branches to the head and thoracic limbs so the majority of the unoxygenated blood is flowing to the pelvic limbs. If the patency is large there may be little turbulence in the flow of blood and no murmur will be auscultated.

At this stage in the diagnosis the clinician would obtain lab tests that determine the number and types of cells in the blood and might prepare an electrocardiogram. Other procedures include angiocardiography, in which radiopaque dye injected into the right ventricle via a catheter inserted into the jugular vein is followed radiographically, or echocardiography, in which ultrasound is used to nonsurgically visualize each part of the heart and the major blood vessels.

As will be discussed in detail in Chapters 11 and 12, patent ductus arteriosus is the most common cardiovascular malformation in dogs. However, the signs presented vary considerably, depending upon the age of the animal, the degree of patency in the duct and the level of right ventricular pressure. This is but one of many situations in which an abnormal clinical presentation will be attributable to the persistence of a normal embryonic structure.

CASE HISTORY

Signalment: Stillborn lambs with craniofacial malformations (Fig. I.3).

History: Lambs were delivered from four ewes on two successive days; the rest of the flock was normal. Different rams were used for breeding, and the ewes were unrelated. The flock had occasional access to open pasture.

Physical Exam: Neonates all have severe reduction of facial features, a single fused orbit with double (Fig. I.3*B*) or single (synophthalmia, Fig. I.3*C*) eyes, and a protruding tongue. In addition, they have a prominent proboscis, which is a median, fleshy protrusion above the orbit. The forebrain is reduced in size and has a large single (rather than paired) ventricle.

Diagnosis: Cyclopia and cebocephaly (monkey-face).

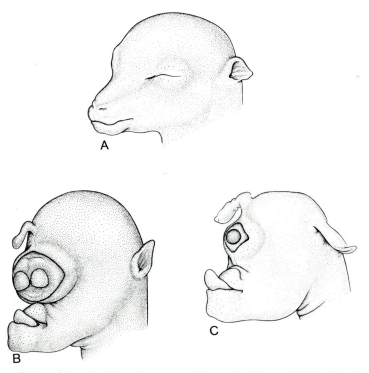

A

B

C

Figure I.3.   The effects of ingested *Veratrum* upon sheep development. *A*, normal ovine fetus at 59 days of gestation. *B*, cebocephalic (monkey-faced) lamb fetus of same age with two eyes in a common orbit, reduced upper jaw, and supraorbital proboscis. *C*, severely effected, cyclopic sheep fetus at 96 days of gestation. (Courtesy of HE Evans.)

Cause: Cyclopia has been reported in most ruminants and, less frequently, in other mammals including man; it is most common in sheep. Experimental studies have proved that ingestion of the wild plant false hellebore (corn lily, *Veratrum*) early in gestation will cause this condition in sheep. While the active alkaloids have been identified, their exact mode of action on the embryo has not been resolved.

From what is known about the development of the vertebrate head, this malformation most likely results from an interference with interactions between the primordium of the eye-forming region of the brain and cell populations located beneath this primordium. Cyclopia can be experimentally produced in fish and amphibian embryos by either applying chemical teratogens or performing surgical lesions at a specific stage of embryogenesis.

By knowing these experimental data it was possible for a team of veterinarians and anatomists to propose that *Veratrum* might be disrupting sheep development at a very precise and short period of time on the 14th day of gestation. Experimental studies confirmed this, and this information has led to a substantial reduction in the incidence of cyclopia in sheep. This situation illustrates how one task of the clinician is to be aware of and able to identify possible teratogenic materials, and to know critical periods of susceptibility during which pregnant animals must be protected from exposure to these agents.

Bibliography

At the end of each chapter are listed selected references that discuss the normal embryology, developmental mechanisms, and common malformations of the system under consideration. The following bibliography provides a list of texts that, while not focusing on domesticated animals, provide general descriptions and analyses of animal development more comprehensive than can be offered in this volume. In addition several recent reviews and tables listing congenital malformations of domesticated animals are included.

GENERAL EMBRYOLOGY TEXTS

Arey LB: *Developmental Anatomy*, ed 7. Philadelphia, Saunders, 1965. (A classic but dated embryology text.)

Balinsky BI: *An Introduction to Embryology*, ed 5. Philadelphia, Saunders, 1981. (Focuses mainly on lower vertebrates; includes mechanisms of development.)

Carlson, BM: *Pattern's Foundations of Embryology*, ed 4. New York, McGraw Hill 1981. (The best of the current comparative embryology texts.)

Evans HE, Sack WO: Prenatal development of domestic and laboratory mammals: growth curves, external features and selected references. *Anat Histol Embryol* 2:11–45, 1973.

Hamilton WJ, Boyd JD, Mossman HW: *Human Embryology*, ed 3. Baltimore, Williams & Wilkins, 1962.

Langman J: *Medical Embryology*, ed 4. Baltimore, Williams & Wilkins, 1981. (Probably the best concise human embryology text available.)

Moore KL: *The Developing Human*, ed 3. Philadelphia, Saunders, 1982. (Many fine schematic illustrations.)

Patten BM: *Early Embryology of the Chick*, ed 5. New York, Blakiston, 1971.

Patten BM: *Embryology of the Pig*, ed 3. New York, Blakiston, 1948.

Phillips JB: *Development of Vertebrate Anatomy*. St. Louis, Mosby, 1975.

Romanoff AL: *The Avian Embryo: Structural and Functional Development*. New York, Macmillan, 1960.

Snell RD: *Clinical Embryology for Medical Students*, ed 2. Boston, Little Brown, 1975.

Torrey TW, Feduccia A: *Morphogenesis of the Vertebrates*, ed 4. New York, Wiley, 1971.

Zietzschmann O, Krolling O: *Entwicklungsgeschichte der Haustiere*. Berlin, Verlag Paul Parey, 1956.

REVIEWS AND COMPILATIONS OF CONGENITAL DEFECTS IN DOMESTIC ANIMALS

Nieberle K, Cohrs P: *Textbook of the Special Pathological Anatomy of Domestic Animals*. London, Pergamon Press, 1967.

Dog and Cat

Earl FL: Abnormalities of intrauterine development in dogs. In Benirschke K, Garner FM, Jones TC, (eds): *Pathology of Laboratory Animals*. Berlin, Springer-Verlag, 1977.

Erickson F, Saperstein G, Leipold HW, McKinley J: Congenital defects of dogs (3 parts). *Canine Practice* 4(4):58–61; 4(5):51–61; 4(6):40–53. (Reprinted by Ralston Purina, St. Louis, MO, 1977: copies available upon request.)

Foley CW, Lasley JF, Osweiler GD: *Abnormalities of Companion Animals*. Ames Iowa, Iowa State University Press, 1979.

Hutt FB: *Genetics for Dog Breeders*. San Francisco, W. H. Freeman & Co., 1979.

Merton DA: Selective breeding in the dog and cat. Part II. Known and suspected genetic diseases. *Compend Contin Educ* 4:332–359, 1982.

Patterson DF: A catalogue of genetic disorders of the dog. In, Kirk R (ed): *Current Veterinary Therapy, VI, Small Animal Practice*. Philadelphia, Saunders, 1977, pp 73–88.

Saperstein G, Harris S, Leipold HW: *Congenital Defects in Domestic Cats*. (Reprinted by Ralston Purina Co., St. Louis, MO, 1978; copies available upon request.)

Horse and Swine

Huston R, Saperstein G, Leipold HW: Congenital defects in foals. *J Equine Med Surg* 1:146–161, 1977.

Huston R, Saperstein G, Schoneweis D, Leipold HW:

Congenital defects in pigs. *Vet Bull* 48:645–675, 1978.

Roberts S: *Veterinary Obstetrics and Genital Disease* (*Theriogenology*), ed 2. Ann Arbor MI, Edward Brothers, 1971.

Cattle and Sheep

Jolly RD, Leipold HW: Inherited disease of cattle. A perspective. *N Z Vet J* 21:147–155, 1973.

Leipold HW, Dennis SM, Huston K: Congenital defects of cattle: nature, cause, and effect. *Adv Vet Sci Comp Med* 16:103–150, 1972.

Saperstein G, Leipold HW, Dennis SM: Congenital defects of sheep. *JAVMA* 167:314–322, 1975.

Laboratory Animals and Miscellanous

deBoom HPA: Anomalous animals. *S Afr J Sci* 61:159–171, 1965.

Gruneberg H: *The Pathology of Development. A Study of Inherited Skeletal Disorders in Animals.* New York, Wiley, 1963.

Kalter H: (1979) Mutant gene effects: mouse. Part I. Congenital malformations. In Altman PL, Katz DD (eds): *Inbred and Genetically Defined Strains of Laboratory Animals. Part I.* Federation for American Societies for Experimental Biology, Bethesda, MD, pp. 55–63, 1979.

Kalter H: A compendium of the genetically induced congenital malformations of the house mouse. *Teratology* 21:397–429, 1980.

Pearson H: Changing attitudes to congenital and inherited diseases. *Vet Rec* 105:318–323, 1979.

Woollam DHM: The long search for the causes of congenital malformations in mammals. *Equine Vet J* 10:43–46, 1978.

CHAPTER 1

Organization of Vertebrate Embryos

HISTORICAL BACKGROUND

The questions of how living organisms develop and what causes malformations to occur have piqued man's curiosity since before recorded history. Since the early Greeks, especially Heraclitus and Aristotle, philosophers, theologians and scientists have wrestled with these problems. Until the last century there were two general schools of thought, the preformationists and epigeneticists. Followers of the **preformation theory** believed that all tissues and the general body form were present in the sperm or egg, and that development proceeded by enlargement of this miniature organism. A 17th century microscopist named Hartsoeker even claimed to have obseved a miniature human (homunculus) in the head of a sperm.

In contrast, the **epigenetic theory** proposed that the tissues and form of an organism arose in a sequential manner from the amorphous contents of the fertilized egg. This theory, which can be traced to Aristotle but was not formalized until the mid 18th century by Wolff, did not gain general acceptance until well into the last century.

It was von Baer (1828) who, based on comparative descriptive studies, first proposed that all vertebrate embryos pass through a stage at which they are anatomically very similar. Only later do class, family, and species-specific structures become evident. This stage is seen in the dog of about 18 days of gestation, the cow at 24 days, and the chick embryo of 48–60 h of incubation.

TERMINOLOGY

After introducing the basic terminology in embryology, this chapter will present the anatomy of this common stage, first in schematic fashion and then as exemplified in the canine embryo.

Germ Layers

Early in development all vertebrate embryos form three layers or sheets of cells, from which all tissues and organs in the emerging fetus will be formed. The outer or uppermost layer is the **ectoderm,** which will form the epidermis, neural tissues, and some of the skeletal and connective tissues of the head. The deepest, innermost layer is the **endoderm**, which will form the lining of the digestive tract, respiratory system and of those organs associated with digestion. Between these two is a more loosely arrayed population of cells called **mesoderm.** This germ layer will form most of the muscles and skeletal tissues, the urogenital system, and the heart and blood vessels of the animal.

It was at one time believed that the anatomy of the embryo was best understood by learning in detail the particular fates of each of these germ layers. However, this theory proved to be unacceptable when it was realized that nearly all organs in the body are derived from more than one germ layer, or from different subsets of the same germ layer. Rather, the importance of the germ layers lies in the fact that all vertebrate embryos form these three layers and use them comparably in constructing the organs and tissues of the animal.

Histological Terms

All cells found in the early embryo, at stages prior to the formation of definitive organs, are either epithelial or mesenchymal in their appearance, as illustrated in Figure 1.1

An **epithelium** lines the surface of an organ structure and is highly specialized to protect, absorb and/or secrete. Epithelial cells are closely apposed to neighboring cells and usually have tight junctions or desmosomes. Also, the basal surface of these cells is underlain by a fibrous meshwork called the basal lamina. Examples of epithelia derived from each germ layer include the surface of the skin (ectoderm), the lining of the digestive tract (endoderm), and the lining of kidney tubules (mesoderm). Two additional terms refer to specialized epithelia. These are **endothelium**, which is the epithelium that lines blood vessels, and **mesothelium**, which is the epithelium that lines the serous (body) cavities and the surface of the organs associated with these cavities.

Mesenchyme is the embryonic precursor

MESENCHYME   EPITHELIA

Midbrain

Pharyngeal endoderm

Surface ectoderm

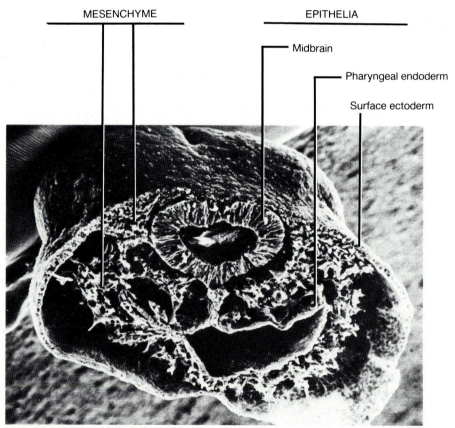

Figure 1.1.   Scanning electron micrograph of a chick embryo at approximately 36 hr of incubation (equivalent to a dog of approximately 17 days gestation). The embryo has been cut transversely at the level of the midbrain (mesencephalon), and this view is looking rostrally at that cut surface with the dorsal side of the embryo towards the top of the micrograph. The midbrain, pharynx and surface ectoderm (presumptive epidermis) are all epithelial tissues, while most of the other internal cells are mesenchymal. (Courtesy of K Tosney.)

of all connective and muscle tissues, and is a component of all organs except the central nervous system. Mesenchymal cells are loosely and usually irregularly arranged with a large volume of **extracellular matrix** between one another. This matrix contains collagen and other macromolecules that affect the behavior and subsequent development of the cells. During early stages of development, mesenchymal cells may aggregate and form an epithelium and, vice versa, epithelial cells may disperse to form mesenchyme.

The term mesenchyme denotes any tissue having this appearance and does not refer to either a specific germ layer of origin or any particular fate. Thus, the terms mesenchyme and mesoderm are not synonymous. As will be discussed later, most embryonic organs and tissues have both epithelial and mesenchymal components, and interactions betweeen them are essential for normal development.

The term **connective tissue** refers to the supporting tissue of the body, which includes loose areolar (subcutaneous) tissue, adipose tissue, dense fibrous connective tissues (ligaments, tendons), cartilage and bone. Throughout most of the body these are mesodermal in origin; in the head they are derived in part from ectoderm. All connective tissues develop from mesenchymal precursors.

COMMON ANATOMICAL FEATURES OF VERTEBRATE EMBRYOS

Vertebrate embryos begin their development with quite disparate appearances. Some, such as the bird, have very large eggs and others, including most domesticated mammals, have eggs that are nearly microscopic. Despite these differences, all vertebrate embryos develop structures that are remarkably similar. This section will describe the anatomy of a "typical" embryo at a stage when the primordia of most organ systems are present but not yet differentiated. The subsequent changes that transform this common anatomical plan into the class and species-unique structures seen in the adult will form the basis for many of the following chapters.

Figures 1.2 and 1.3 show cutaway sagittal and transverse sections of the vertebrate embryo. The body is covered by a layer of ectodermal epithelium, the presumptive epidermis, except at the site where the umbilical stalk (if present) emerges. Beneath this covering in the dorsal midline is the hollow **neural tube,** which has a series of enlarged vesicles located rostrally. These are the primordia of the brain, which is the first part of the nervous system to become specialized. Initially there are three vesicles, the **prosencephalon, mesencephalon,** and **rhombencephalon,** located in a rostrocaudal order. Growing out from the lateral walls of the prosencephalon are a pair of **optic vesicles.** Concomitant with the formation of the lens (Fig. 1.2*A*) the outer wall of each optic vesicle folds inward to form a two-layered optic cup.

Another hollow tube runs the length of the embryo near the ventral midline. This is the future **gut,** which is derived from endoderm. Initially the gut is closed at both ends by layers of endoderm and ectoderm; later in development these areas of apposition open. The rostral end of the gut, the **pharynx,** is quite specialized in the embryo. There are a series of lateral outpocketings of the pharynx that extend out to the surface ectoderm. These are **pharyngeal pouches.** In fishes the areas where pharyngeal pouch endoderm and surface ectoderm are apposed break down, forming channels between the mouth and pharynx and the surrounding water. These channels are gill slits. In higher vertebrates the breakdown, if it occurs (see Chapter 14), is transient. Nonetheless, the embryonic organization of the pharynx in fishes is retained in all vertebrates.

Most of the other tissues in embryos at this stage are mesodermal. Located beside the neural tube is **paraxial mesoderm,** most of which is segmented along the body axis. Each segment is called a **somite,** and these will contribute to the development of all axial skeletal structures and voluntary muscles of the body. Immediately ventral to the

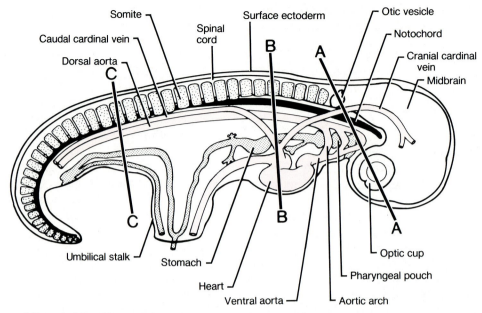

Figures 1.2 and 1.3. *Figure 1.2*, schematic lateral, and *Figure 1.3*, transverse sectional views showing the embryonic anatomical features common to most vertebrate embryos; vascular tissues are shown in red. A few structures, such as the umbilical stalk are found in only some vertebrates, including mammals. Compare these with Figures 1.5 and 1.6, which are a reconstructed lateral view and representative transverse sections of a canine embryo.

neural tube is a longitudinal rod that extends from the level of the midbrain to the tail. This mesodermal condensation is the **noto-chord.** Although it may play a skeletal role in some primitive fishes, the notochord is not fully retained in any of the higher vertebrates (see Chapter 8). However, the development of other axial structures, including the neural tube and paraxial mesoderm, depends upon the notochord, which is one explanation for why it has been retained through the course of evolution.

Located lateral to the paraxial mesoderm are clusters of epithelial ducts and tubules that will form nephrogenic and gonadal structures. The remaining mesoderm, which extends around the gut and beneath the surface ectoderm to the ventral midline, is **lateral plate mesoderm.** It is divided into outer, **somatic** (parietal) and inner, **splanch-nic** (visceral) layers, with a cavity, the **coe-lom,** between them. This organization is found throughout the body of the embryo except in the head and caudal (tail) regions, where no coelomic cavity is present.

The cardiovascular system is also derived

from a simple, common embryonic plan. The **heart,** which is first recognizable as a slightly curved tube, is located midventrally beneath the caudal part of the pharynx. Extending rostrally from it is a single vessel, the **ventral aorta**, from which grow bilateral pairs of blood vessels. These vessels, called **aortic arches,** carry blood dorsally around the pharynx to empty into paired **dorsal aortae.** An aortic arch passes immediately in front of each pharyngeal pouch. The dorsal aortae, which unite to form a single dorsal aorta caudal to the heart, carry blood to the rest of the body.

The venous system is initially more simple. A pair of veins carry blood towards the heart from both the head and the trunk regions. These are the **cranial** and **caudal cardinal veins,** and they empty into the heart via **common cardinal veins.**

Many vertebrate embryos, including all reptiles, birds and mammals and some fishes, have well developed extraembryonic membranes. Branches of the dorsal aorta carry blood out of the embryo either adjacent to the **yolk stalk,** which is attached to

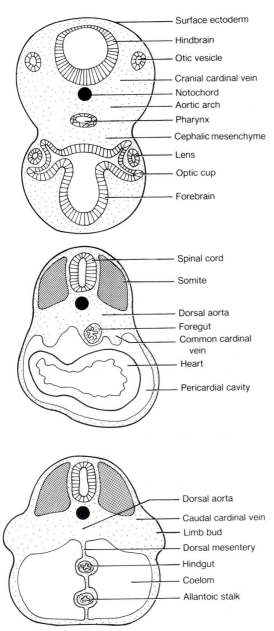

Surface ectoderm
Hindbrain
Otic vesicle
Cranial cardinal vein
Notochord
Aortic arch
Pharynx
Cephalic mesenchyme
Lens
Optic cup
Forebrain

Spinal cord
Somite
Dorsal aorta
Foregut
Common cardinal vein
Heart
Pericardial cavity

Dorsal aorta
Caudal cardinal vein
Limb bud
Dorsal mesentery
Hindgut
Coelom
Allantoic stalk

Figure 1.3.

the midgut, or the **allantoic stalk,** a diverticulum of the hindgut. The former are called **vitelline arteries,** the latter are **allantoic** or **umbilical** arteries.

In summary, all vertebrate embryos share the following common features:

1. A dorsal, hollow neural tube that is enlarged rostrally;
2. A series of somites, which establish the segmental pattern of the embryo;

3. A ventral tube, the gut, that is derived from endoderm, which will form the lining of tissues associated with respiration, digestion, and splanchnic mesoderm. This tube is enlarged cranially as the pharynx;
4. A coelom lined by sheets of lateral mesoderm; and
5. A ventrally located heart and series of bilateral aortic arches that partially surround the pharynx and empty into a pair of dorsal aortae.

ANATOMY OF THE 4-mm (24-SOMITE) CANINE EMBRYO

Embryonic development proceeds in a rostral to caudal sequence. Thus, most of the structures present in an embryo during the initial stages of organogenesis are those associated with the head, neck and thoracic regions.

Figures 1.4 and 1.5 show a 22-somite feline and, schematically, a 24-somite canine embryo, viewed from the right side. By this stage the formerly straight embryo has formed two prominent ventral flexures. That occurring at the level of the first few somites is the **cervical flexure**, that at the level of the mesencephalon is the **cranial flexure.** Most of the tissues that will form the face and jaws are still rudimentary, with the paired primordia of the maxilla and mandible (1st visceral arch) located laterally. The heart, which is located ventral to the level where the otic vesicle (future inner ear) is developing, is in the process of forming a loop. By this stage it has already been contracting for 2–3 days.

Table 1.1 lists the locations in Figure 1.6 of most structures described in the following text. This table can be used as a guide to finding each of these embryonic organs in the serial sections illustrated. By studying these sections and also Figures 1.4 and 1.5 you should acquire an appreciation of both the morphological appearance and spatial relations of each of these primitive organ systems.

Axial Tissues

At this stage, the brain and spinal cord consist of an epithelial cylinder with a large central cavity or lumen. This **neural tube** formed from a flat sheet of ectodermal epi-

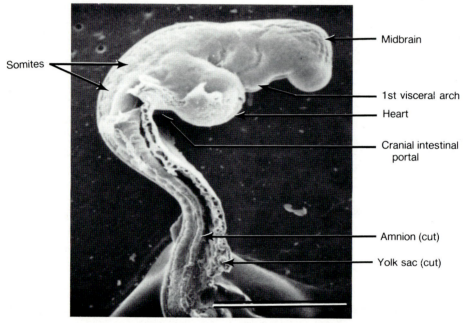

Midbrain

Somites

1st visceral arch

Heart

Cranial intestinal
portal

Amnion (cut)

Yolk sac (cut)

Figure 1.4.　Scanning electron micrograph of the right side of a 22-somite cat embryo, approximately 15–16 days of gestation. The amnion and both the future midgut endoderm and adjacent lateral splanchnic mesoderm were cut off close to the body of the embryo during preparation of this specimen (*bar*, 1 mm).

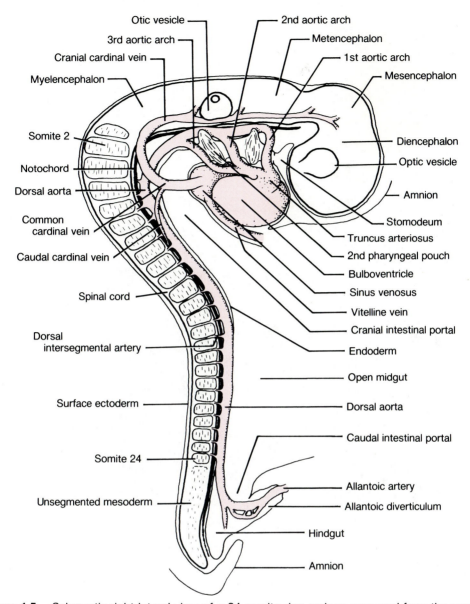

Figure 1.5. Schematic right lateral view of a 24-somite dog embryo prepared from the sections in Figure 1.6. The embryo is bent ventrally at the level of the mesencephalon (cranial flexure) and the first few somites (cervical flexure), and much of the gut is open ventrally. Note that the heart lies ventral to the hindbrain and pharynx at this stage, and that most abdominal and appendicular tissues are rudimentary or not yet present.

thelium that thickened to form the **neural plate.** The lateral margins of the neural plate elevated and fused with one another to form the closed tube (Fig. 6.3).

At this stage, the original three divisions of the brain have formed five recognizable parts. These are, from rostral to caudal, the:

Telencephalon, future cerebrum (forebrain);
Diencephalon, future thalamus, hypothalamus;
Mesencephalon, future midbrain;
Metencephalon, future cerebellum and pons; and
Myelencephalon, future medulla oblongata.

Extending laterally from the ventral part

Table 1.1.
Index of structures present in 24-somite dog embryo sections

Structure	Location in figure 1.6	Structure	Location in figure 1.6
Ectoderm: nervous system and sensory organs		Pleural cavity (continuous with coelom)	E–G
Diencephalon	D–F	Endodermal structures	
Mesencephalon	A–C	Pharynx	E–G
Metencephalon	A–B	Pharyngeal pouch 1	C–D
Myelencephalon	A–F	Pharyngeal pouch 2	C–D
Optic vesicle	E–F	Foregut	H
Otic vesicle	A–B	Cranial intestinal portal	I
Spinal cord	G–N		
Telencephalon	G–H	Open mid- and hindgut	I–K
Paraxial mesoderm		Hindgut (closed)	L–N
Somite 2	C	Allantoic diverticulum	M
Somite 3	D	Cardiovascular system (listed in direction of blood flow)	
Somite 4	F	Arteries	
Somite 5	G	Vitelline vein[a]	J, I
Somite 6	H	Sinus venosus	G, F
Somite 8	I	Atrium	G
Somite 10	J	Bulboventricle	H, I, H, G
Somite 24	K	Truncus arteriosus	F
Unsegmented paraxial mesoderm (presumptive somites)	L, M, N	Ventral aorta	E, D
		Aortic arch 1	E, D, C
		Aortic arch 2	D, C
Dermamyotome (combined dermatome and myotome)	J	Aortic arch 3	D
		Dorsal aorta	C–N
		Dorsal intersegmental arteries	G, H
Sclerotome	J	Allantoic artery	L, M
Notochord	C–N	Veins	
Intermediate mesoderm	I—M	Cranial cardinal vein	A–F
Mesonephric duct	K–L	Caudal cardinal vein	K, J, I, H, G
Mesonephric tubule	K	Common cardinal vein	G
Lateral mesoderm			
Somatic mesoderm	L (E–N)	Sinus venosus	G, F
Splanchnic mesoderm	L (E–N)		
Coelom (intraembryonic)	E–L		
Pericardial cavity (continuous with coelom)	E–H		

[a] Carries blood from yolk sac to embryo; allantoic veins bringing oxygenated blood from the placenta will form later.

of the diencephalon are the **optic stalks** which support the **optic vesicles.** Later, the outer (lateral) part of this vesicle folds medially to form an **optic cup.** The original lateral surface will form the retina, the rest of the vesicle forms the pigmented epithelium.

Lateral to the myelencephalon are the **otic vesicles** that developed from a pair of **otic placodes** located on the surface of the embryo. A **placode** is any focal thickening of the surface ectoderm. Each of these vesicles will form the entire **membranous labyrinth** of the inner ear.

The brain is surrounded by loose mesenchyme that is interrupted only by blood vessels. Beginning at the mesencephalon, the **notochord** lies ventral to the brain and spinal cord, and extends caudally for most of the length of the embryo.

Lateral to the spinal cord and notochord is **paraxial mesoderm,** most of which is segmented into discrete masses called **somites.** Somites form at the rate of approximately 1 per hr beginning during the early stages of neural tube closure and cardiogenesis; somitogenesis occurs in a rostral-caudal sequence. Each somite has three subdivisions: a dorsolateral component, the **dermatome,** which will form the dermis of the skin; a middle component, the **myotome,** which will form axial and appendicular musculature; and a ventromedial component, the **sclerotome,** that will form vertebrae and ribs. The sclerotomal component is closely associated with the notochord.

The mesoderm located just lateral to the somites is called **intermediate mesoderm.** Elements of the excretory system will develop from this mesoderm; therefore, it is also referred to as the **nephrogenic plate.** It is continuous medially with the somites but is not segmented. After the first several somites have formed, short tubules and a longitudinal duct located lateral to the somites develop in this mesoderm. These are most easily seen in the future thoracic level of the animal in the form of the **mesonephric tubules** and **mesonephric duct.** Later, parts of the reproductive system and also the adrenal cortex will be derived from this intermediate mesoderm.

Lateral Mesoderm

Two sheets of mesoderm extend laterally from the intermediate mesoderm. The superficial layer remains adjacent to the ectoderm and is called **somatic** (parietal) **mesoderm** because it will contribute to the formation of the body (soma) wall. The deeper layer remains adjacent to the endoderm and is the **splanchnic** (visceral) **mesoderm** that will form part of the wall of the internal organs (viscera) in the embryo. The space enclosed by these two layers is the **coelom.** A portion of this will be enclosed in the embryo as the body cavity; the remainder is the transient **extraembryonic coelom.**

Endodermal Structures

Prior to the 4-mm stage illustrated here, the region of the initially flat sheet of endoderm located on the cranial end of the embryo is involved in head folding. In this process the endoderm forms a pair of folds ventrally that come together to form a tube. In the head region this tube is called the **pharynx;** more caudally it will be named according to the part of the gut which it will form (esophagus, stomach, etc.). The pharynx becomes flattened dorsoventrally. On each side of the embryo, the pharyngeal endoderm flares laterally and contacts the surface ecotoderm, which has become indented slightly. These outpocketings are the **pharyngeal pouches** (branchial pouches). The surface indentations are **visceral grooves.** A temporary opening often forms at the site of juxtaposition of endoderm and ectoderm; this is a **visceral cleft.** The mesenchyme located lateral to the pharynx between pouches forms a column called a **visceral arch.** The 1st and 2nd visceral arches are recognizable grossly at this stage as lateral bulges located between the brain and heart tissues (Fig. 1.4).

In the 24-somite dog embryo, there are three pairs of pharyngeal pouches and two visceral clefts. Later, 4th and smaller 5th pouches will form. In fishes these pouches and clefts persist to form the gill slits; in higher vertebrates they are transient structures that become highly modified and form such structures as the auditory tube, thymus, and parathyroids.

Immediately caudal to the heart the closed foregut tube opens ventrally, at a site called the **cranial intestinal portal** (window). Caudal to this site, the endoderm is exposed ventrally. Later, the cranial intestinal portal shifts caudally, resulting in the progressive closure of foregut and midgut regions. Concomitantly, a **caudal intestinal portal** shifts cranially to close the hindgut and midgut;

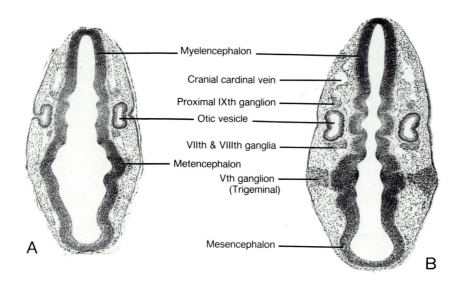

Myelencephalon

Cranial cardinal vein

Proximal IXth ganglion

Otic vesicle

VIIth & VIIIth ganglia

Metencephalon

Vth ganglion
(Trigeminal)

Mesencephalon

A

B

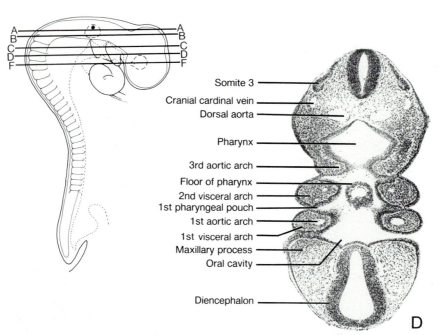

Somite 3

Cranial cardinal vein

Dorsal aorta

Pharynx

3rd aortic arch

Floor of pharynx

2nd visceral arch

1st pharyngeal pouch

1st aortic arch

1st visceral arch

Maxillary process

Oral cavity

Diencephalon

D

Figure 1.6 *A–N.* Representative sections of a 24-somite canine embryo, fixed at approximately 22 days of gestation. The location and plane of each section is indicated on the accompanying sketches and all structures are indexed in Table 1.1. The right side of the embryo is on the left in these photomicrographs. *Arrow* in *I* indicates the site of chorioallantoic fold fusion.

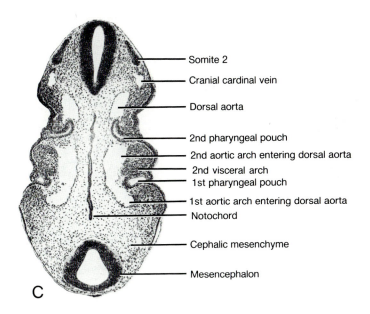

Somite 2

Cranial cardinal vein

Dorsal aorta

2nd pharyngeal pouch

2nd aortic arch entering dorsal aorta

2nd visceral arch

1st pharyngeal pouch

1st aortic arch entering dorsal aorta

Notochord

Cephalic mesenchyme

Mesencephalon

C

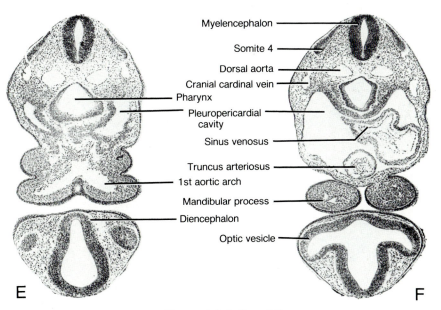

Myelencephalon

Somite 4

Dorsal aorta

Cranial cardinal vein

Pharynx

Pleuropericardial cavity

Sinus venosus

Truncus arteriosus

1st aortic arch

Mandibular process

Diencephalon

Optic vesicle

E

F

Figure 1.6 C, E and F.

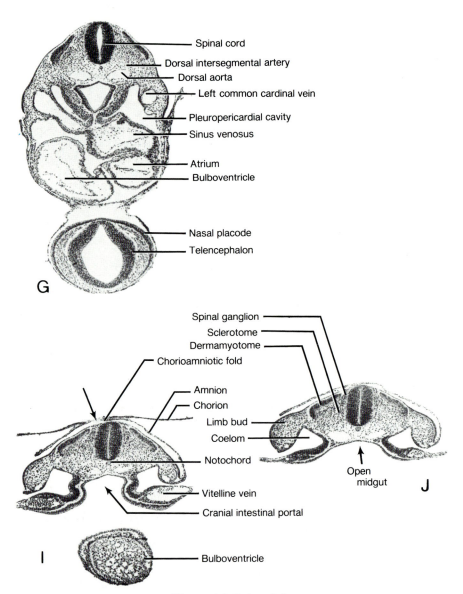

Figure 1.6 G, *I* and *J.*

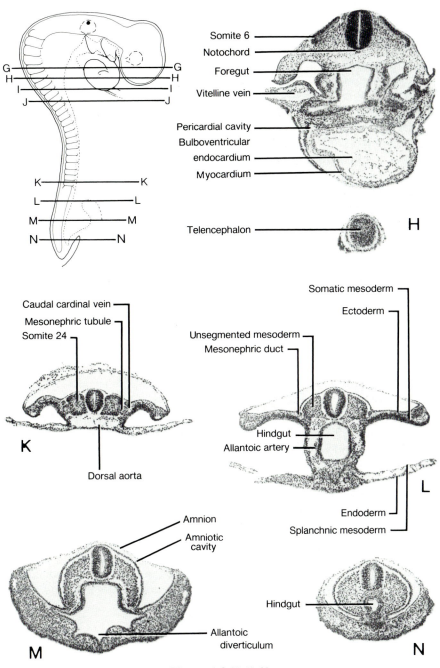

Figure 1.6 *H, K–N.*

the two meet at a transient site, the **vitelline duct** (ileal or Meckel's diverticulum), which is found near the ileojejunal junction.

Cardiovascular System

Prior to and during the early stages of embryo-maternal apposition, embryonic cells absorb necessary metabolites from fluids in the lumen of the uterus. However, the demands of the rapidly growing embryo soon exceed this method, and a vascular system develops to circulate nutrients to the growing cells. As a result, the vascular system is one of the first to be formed and to function in the embryo.

When first formed the heart is a tube *bent slightly to the right* but not subdivided into any chambers. It begins beating within a few hours of its formation. At this time, blood enters the caudal part of the cardiac tube via a pair of large **vitelline (omphalomesenteric) veins,** passes through an enlarged, eccentric **bulboventricle,** and exits rostrally through a **truncus arteriosus.**

By the 24-somite stage, the heart has folded and the beginnings of compartmentalization are occurring. Blood from extraembryonic veins now enters the **sinus venosus,** which is the most caudal part of the heart at this stage and is situated near the midline of the embryo. It then enters a single **atrium** located on the left side of the embryo. From there it flows into the **bulboventricle,** which is a large, U-shaped chamber at this stage. As blood courses through the ventricle, it flows from left to right. Also, it enters the ventricle flowing caudally and leaves it flowing rostrally and dorsally. Finally, the blood exits the heart through the **truncus arteriosus.**

From the truncus, blood enters the **ventral aorta** (aortic sac) from which project a series of paired blood vessels called **aortic arches.** Each of these arches passes through a visceral arch in front of one of the pharyngeal pouches. In the 24-somite dog there are three pairs of aortic arches. Additional arches will form later, but only aortic arches 3, 4, and 6 will be retained as the definitive arteries of the heart, thorax and thoracic limbs.

Blood flows dorsally through the aortic arches into paired **dorsal aortae.** These vessels, which later fuse to form a single dorsal aorta in the trunk, carry blood caudally the length of the embryo. Branching laterally from the dorsal aortae at about the level of the 16th pair of somites are the **vitelline arteries,** which carry blood away from the embryo to a vascular plexus formed in the extraembryonic endoderm and splanchnic mesoderm. The dorsal aorta also gives off intersegmental arteries to the somites and will later supply arterial blood to the viscera and hindlimbs.

At this stage the embryo does not have a closed circulation, which means that there are no capillaries. Blood flows out of arteries into extracellular spaces and channels. It is collected in branches of the large **cranial cardinal veins,** which are located ventrolateral to the mid- and hindbrain. From these paired veins blood flows through a pair of **common cardinal veins** into the **sinus venosus.** Venous drainage of the trunk regions at this stage is slight and is accomplished by the small **caudal cardinal veins.**

The 24-somite embryo is partially enveloped by two extraembryonic membranes, the **amnion** and the **chorion.** Their structure and development will be discussed in Chapter 3.

CHAPTER 2

Early Stages of Development in Birds and Mammals

GAMETOGENESIS

Early in mammalian development, at or prior to the time of neural tube and heart formation, a population of **primordial germ cells** appears outside the body of the embryo in the yolk sac tissue (see Chapter 18). These cells migrate to and enter the embryonic gonad where they proliferate and eventually give rise to the **gametes**.

In the ovary of the female fetus each primordial germ cell forms an **oogonium**. Oogonia and their progeny are mitotically active up to and, in some instances, beyond **parturition** (birth), at which time they enter prophase of meiosis. The female germ cells are now called **primary oocytes** (Fig. 2.1). Homologous chromosomes have become paired (synapsis) and each has replicated to form two chromatids. Thus the primary oocyte contains 4 times the haploid amount of DNA. This is the stage at which exchange of genetic material (crossing over) occurs.

Completion of the first meiotic division does not take place until after the female reaches sexual maturity. The genetic material is then equally divided with one member of each pair of homologous chromosomes being included in the nucleus of each daughter cell. This is called the meiotic reduction division because the number of chromosomes is reduced from diploid to haploid. However, since each chromosome is still composed of two chromatids, the new cells each have twice the haploid amount of DNA.

Cytokinesis (cell division) is unequal during this division. The cell that receives most of the cytoplasm is the **secondary oocyte** and the other, smaller daughter cell is termed the **first polar body**. Each of the cells is theoretically capable of completing the second maturation division upon the stimulus of fertilization. However, this rarely occurs and the first polar body soon degenerates in many species. The products of the second meiotic (maturation) division of the secondary oocyte are an **ovum** and a **second polar body**. Once again, cytokinesis is unequal, and the ovum retains most of the cytoplasm.

Except in the dog and horse, the first meiotic division is not completed until just prior to ovulation. At ovulation a secondary oocyte (Fig. 2.2) and first polar body are released from the follicle. The secondary oocyte must be fertilized by a **spermatozoon** before the second, maturation division is completed. In the dog and horse a primary oocyte resting in prophase is ovulated and **both** meiotic divisions occur after fertilization.

Use of the term ovum is problematic. An ovum is correctly defined as a female gamete containing the haploid number of chromosomes, and the **zygote** is defined as the initial (2N) product of fertilization. As such, a true ovum never exists, since the cell that is

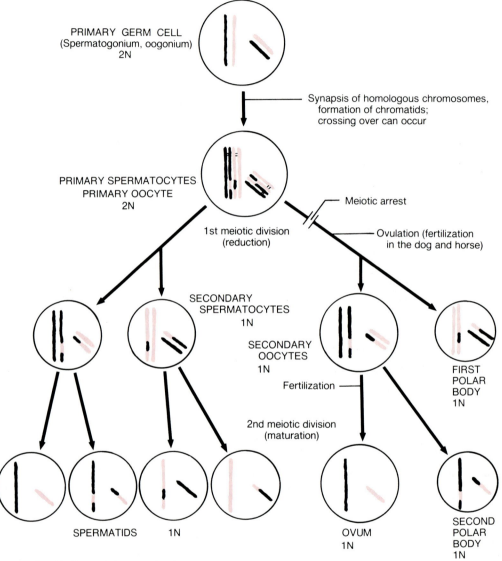

PRIMARY GERM CELL
(Spermatogonium, oogonium)
2N

Synapsis of homologous chromosomes,
formation of chromatids;
crossing over can occur

PRIMARY SPERMATOCYTES
PRIMARY OOCYTE
2N

Meiotic arrest

1st meiotic division
(reduction)

Ovulation (fertilization
in the dog and horse)

SECONDARY
SPERMATOCYTES
1N

SECONDARY
OOCYTES
1N

FIRST
POLAR
BODY
1N

Fertilization

2nd meiotic division
(maturation)

SPERMATIDS   1N

OVUM
1N

SECOND
POLAR
BODY
1N

Figure 2.1. Outline of changes in chromosomal number during meiosis in the formation of male and female germ cells (spermatogenesis, oogenesis). In this example the diploid (2N) chromosome number would be 4, which consists of two pairs of homologous chromosomes.

actually fertilized is a secondary oocyte (primary oocyte in the dog and horse). In common usage the term ovum is used to describe an ovulated female gamete.

The primordial germ cells in the testis of the male form **spermatogonia** that proliferate mitotically throughout most of the life of the animal. Under the appropriate hormonal stimulus a spermatogonium in interphase of its cell cycle replicates its DNA and becomes a **primary spermatocyte**. At the completion of the first meiotic division, two haploid **secondary spermatocytes** are produced which rapidly complete the second division to form four **spermatids**. Further

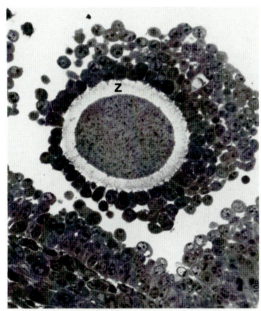

Figure 2.2. Hamster oocyte encased in the zona pellucida (Z) and surrounded by follicular cells comprising the corona radiata. This specimen is from a preovulatory follicle. (From Hafez ESE: *Scanning Electron Microscope Atlas of Mammalian Reproduction.* New York, Springer-Verlag, 1975.)

morphological alterations of cell organelles and the cell membrane of the spermatid result in the formation of the **spermatozoon**.

GAMETES AND FERTILIZATION

Gametes are among the most highly specialized and species-specific cells in living organisms. Their structure and physiology must accommodate three functions: (*a*) to be able to survive in environments quite different from that of the gonad, (*b*) to be able to recognize homologous cells of the other gender and participate in events related to fertilization, and (*c*) to provide sufficient genetic and, depending upon the species, cytoplasmic materials to support development of a new organism.

Ova are classified on the basis of size, which is correlated with both the amount of yolk (lecithin) and its distribution, as summarized in Table 2.1.

In placental mammals the ovum is surrounded with an acellular glycoproteinaceous layer called the **zona pellucia**. Surrounding this are several hundred small follicular cells which are collectively called the **corona radiata** (Fig. 2.2). The ovum itself averages 100–140 μm in diameter.

The male gamete, the spermatozoon, contains three essential components: (*a*) a haploid number of tightly condensed chromosomes; (*b*) an **acrosome**, which is a membrane-enclosed vesicle partly ensheathing the nucleus and containing lytic enzymes important for penetrating the zona pellucida; and (*c*) a set of structures essential for motility, including a tail containing an array of microtubules that extend into a neckpiece in which mitochondria are located.

Following insemination the sperm undergo **capacitation**. This process initiates an enzymatic alteration of surface coat proteins

Table 2.1.
Classification of Vertebrate Eggs

Animal	Size[a]	Yolk distribution
Bird	Macrolecithal	Telolecithal (at one end)
Amphibian	Mesolecithal	Increasing gradient from animal to vegetal pole
Placental mammal	Microlecithal	Isolecithal (equal)

[a] Based on the amount of yolk present.

and a concomitant increase in sperm motility. Sperm are not capable of fertilizing a female gamete, even in vitro, unless capacitation has occurred. Shortly before fertilization the **acrosome reaction** occurs. This partial disintegration of the outer membrane of the acrosome results in the release of acrosomal contents, and is a necessary prerequisite to fertilization. The length of time during which sperm remain active and viable in the female tract differs according to the species, being less than a day in the cow and up to a week in the dog.

Fertilization involves passage of the sperm through the corona radiata and penetration of the zona pellucida (Fig. 2.3). This is followed by the **fertilization reaction**, the first step of which is fusion of the membranes of the two gametes. Beginning at the site of membrane fusion, the resting potential of the zygote cell membrane drops. Also, there is a rapid increase in intracellular calcium, and the contents of many small, subsurface **cortical vesicles** are released between the zygote's membrane and the zona pellucida. This separates the zona pellucida from the surface of the zygote, an event that is often referred to as formation of the "fertilization membrane." Enzymes released by cortical vesicles cause the zona pellucida to become impermeable to other sperm and also to most potentially infectious agents. Changes in the zygote's membrane that prevent additional sperm from fusing are also an effective block to **polyspermy**, which is incorporation of more than one sperm into the female gamete and is usually lethal. Subsequently, the metabolic activity of the cell (respiration, protein synthesis, DNA synthesis), which had been quiescent prior to fertilization, becomes reactivated.

CLEAVAGE STAGES

Development of the embryo continues with the onset of cell division, called **cleavage**. Cleavage, which in mammals occurs while the cells are still surrounded by the zona pellucida (Fig. 2.4), results in the pro-

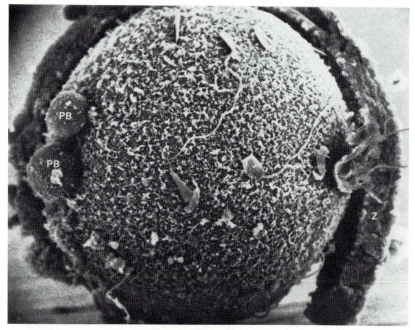

Figure 2.3. Scanning electron micrograph of a rabbit zygote from which much of the zona pellucida (*Z*) has been removed to expose the surface of the zygote, two polar bodies (*PB*), and several sperm that were prevented from penetrating the egg by the fertilization reaction. After Gould, from Hafez ESE: *Scanning Electron Microscope Atlas of Mammalian Reproduction.* New York, Springer-Verlag, 1975.

duction of many smaller cells, the **blasto-meres**. The pattern of cleavage depends upon the amount of yolk present in the zygote. In birds the massive volume of yolk prevents complete division of the zygote; thus, cleavage is **partial** or **meroblastic** (meros, part), as shown later in Figure 2.9. **Total (holoblastic) cleavage** occurs in placental mammals, in which the zygote contains a minimal amount of yolk. This is illustrated in Figure 2.5.

Cleavage in Domestic Animals

In the isolecithal zygote the planes of the second and third cleavages are at right angles to the preceding division plane. Also, after the four-cell stage, cleavage is often asynchronous and it is common to find five-, six-

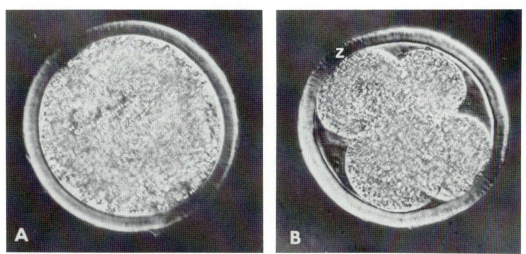

Figure 2.4. Newly fertilized and four-blastomere bovine embryos encased in zona pellucida, photographed with a phase-contrast microscope. Note the reduction in blastomere size during these early cleavage stages. From Seidel GE: *Science* 211:35, 1981, with permission of American Association for the Advancement of Science.

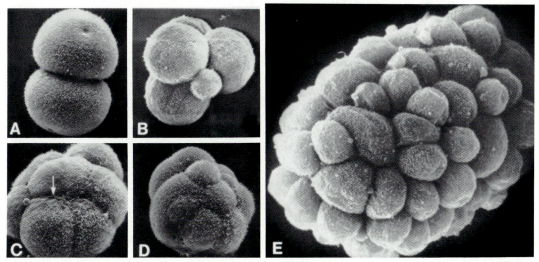

Figure 2.5. Scanning electron microscopic views of early mouse development; the zona pellucida has been removed in each case. *A–D*, early cleavage; *E*, morula at 4 days after fertilization, shown at higher magnification. A polar body is visible in *B*. (From Hafez ESE: *Scanning Electron Microscope Atlas of Mammalian Reproduction.* New York, Springer-Verlag, 1975.

and seven-cell embryos. Cleavage results in the formation of a solid cluster of cells termed a **morula** (Fig. *2.5E*). Prior to this stage the cells of the corona radiata are shed, but the embryo remains surrounded by the zona pellucida. In man the morula consists of 9–16 cells by the 4th day of development; in most domestic animals there are 16–64 cells. The blastomeres of the morula lose their spherical appearance and become tightly apposed to each other; this change is called compaction.

Secretions from the blastomeres collect within the morula causing a fluid-filled cavity, the **blastocoel**, to form. The embryo at this stage, which begins within a week after fertilization (see Table inside front cover), is known as the **blastocyst** or blastula. During the blastocyst stage, the zona pellucida ruptures and the embryo breaks free (hatches), as shown in Figures 2.6 and 2.21. There is a marked increase in the total size and often a change in shape of the organism during this stage, in large part due to enlargement of the blastocoel. For example, the dog blastocyst becomes pear shaped with a diameter

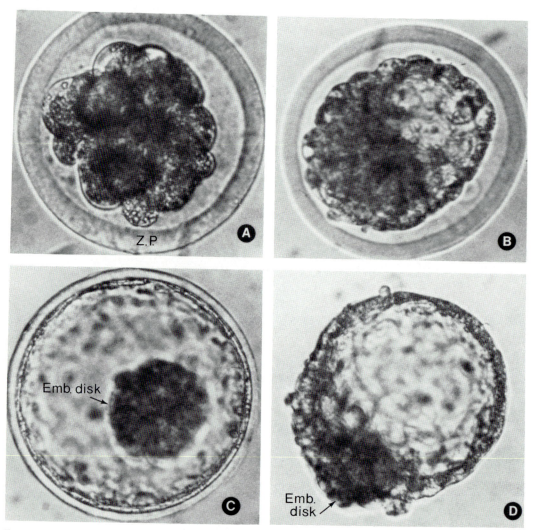

Figure 2.6. Bovine embryos at *A*, morula (5 days postestrus); *B*, early blastocyst (7 days); *C*, expanded blastocyst (8–9 days), and *D*, hatched blastocyst (9 days). The rapid increase in blastocyst size in *C* is due to expansion of the fluid-filled blastocoel. *Z.P.*, zona pellucida. (From GM Lindner and RW Wright: *Theriogenology* 20:407, 1983, ©Geron-X, Inc.)

of 1.5–2.5 mm (Fig. 2.7*A*), which represents a 10- to 20-fold increase in size. Equine blastocysts remain spherical, but pig, cattle and sheep blastocysts undergo a tremendous elongation, expanding at a rate of up to 1 cm per hour and, in the ewe, reaching a length of 1 m by 16 days of gestation.

All the cells of the blastocyst are not identical. Those in one small area become slightly larger than the rest of the cells surrounding the blastocoel. These larger cells constitute the **embryonic disk** (inner cell mass, blastodisk), from which the embryo will develop. The cells on the periphery of the blastocyst are **trophoblast cells**. They facilitate the absorption of nutrients (trophe, nourishment) early in development and later participate in the formation of extraembryonic membranes, which contribute to the formation of the placenta.

In domestic animals the trophoblast cells overlying the embryonic disk degenerate or shift peripherally and the blastodisk becomes exposed on the surface of the blastocyst. In most primates the embryonic disk remains beneath the trophoblastic cover and is referred to as the **inner cell mass**.

Cleavage in Birds

The avian zygote (Fig. 2.8) is the "yolk" that one observes upon breaking open an egg. On the upper side of this large single cell there is a tiny white spot, the **embryonic disk** indicating the location of the nucleus and other cytoplasmic organelles of the zygote. **Meroblastic cleavage** commences at this site, as illustrated in Figure 2.9. Four or five cell divisions occur with complete **karyokinesis** (nuclear division) but incomplete cytokinesis. Cell membranes do not fully surround the new cells and separate them from each other. Thus, the early avian em-

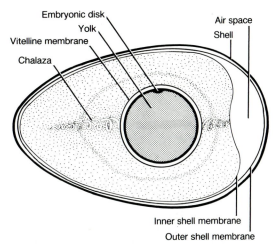

Figure 2.8.   Components of the avian egg. The embryonic disk and yolk are surrounded by an egg membrane; together, these comprise the "ovum" of the bird. All other components are added as the ovum passes down the oviduct.

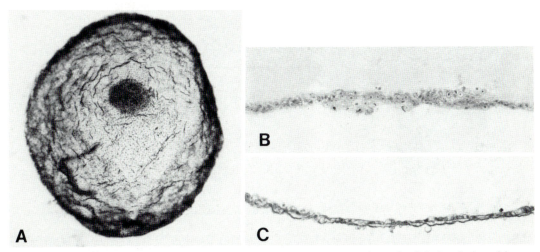

Figure 2.7.   Dog blastocyst. *A*, whole embryo showing dense embryonic disk (center) and large, spherical, less dense trophoblast tissue. *B* and *C* are histological sections through a similar embryo showing *B*, the enlarged cells of the embryonic disk and *C*, the two-layered peripheral region, where the outer (upper) layer is the trophoblast and thin inner layer is the hypoblast.

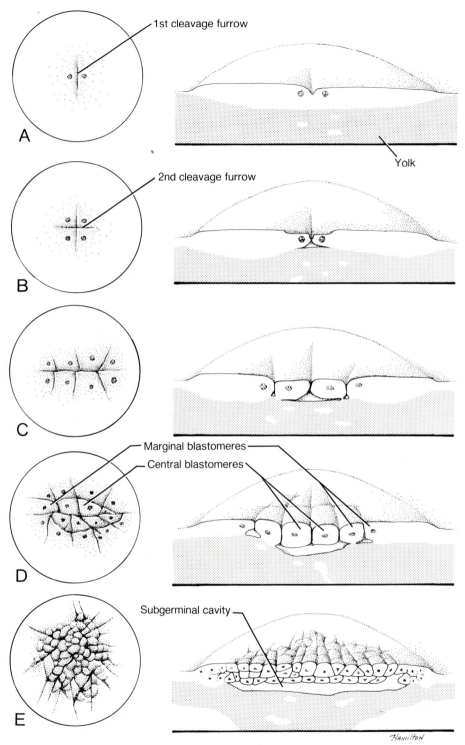

Figure 2.9. Schematic representation of avian cleavage stages shown in dorsal (surface) views on the left, and transverse sections on the right. Until completion of the fourth cleavage the embryonic disk is a syncytium. Then the first cells become fully enclosed by a cell surface membrane; these are the central blastomeres. Marginal blastomeres remain syncytial and continue to spread around the surface of the yolk for several days. *A–D*, first four cleavages; *E*, midcleavage stage.

bryo is a **syncytium**, which is the term describing any multinucleated cell.

Blastomere formation occurs by the growth of membranous furrows between nuclei. These furrows secondarily expand below the nuclei and coalesce with other furrows to form mononucleated cells. Soon this rapidly proliferating mass of blastomeres separates from the underlying yolk. The space thus created is called the **subgerminal cavity**. Cells directly over the subgerminal cavity are the **central blastomeres** and, like the embryonic disk of mammals, these will form the body of the embryo. The more peripherally located cells are called **marginal blastomeres**, and these will form some of the extraembryonic membranes. Marginal blastomeres continue to divide rapidly and the population expands peripherally over the surface of the yolk. Only those located near the outer perimeter remain syncytial.

EMBRYO TRANSFER

The techniques of transferring preimplantation-stage embryos from a donor female to a surrogate recipient can be applied to both laboratory and domesticated animals. Gonadotropin-induced superovulation followed by artificial insemination in cows results in an average of six to seven normal embryos plus an additional two to three that are either abnormal or were not fertilized. The normals may be maintained for a day in an oxygenated, buffered tissue culture medium supplemented with serum or may be frozen in liquid nitrogen ($-196°C$) for long-term storage. Upon thawing these embryos must again be checked since approximately one-third are damaged in this procedure.

The stage of embryo used for transfer is based upon two factors: accessibility and optimal survival. Bovine embryos enter the uterus and become readily obtainable nonsurgically at 4–6 days after estrus (3.5–5 days after ovulation), by which time most are at the 16-cell stage or beyond. Beginning around day 8 postestrus the blastocyst expands (Figs. 2.6 and 2.21), nearly doubling in diameter, and a day later the zona pellu-

cida begins to disintegrate, allowing the embryo to hatch. Following this the embryos are unprotected and thus easily damaged. These events, entry into the uterus and hatching, circumscribe the optimal time for accessibility (after day 5 postestrus) and resistance to physical manipulation (before day 9).

Widespread commercial application of embryo transfer is limited at this time by several factors. First, there is a considerable variation in the number of embryos obtained from superovulated donors, from over 20 to, often, 2 or less. Second, the technology for screening and storing of embryos is highly specialized and costly, much more so than for sperm. While these technical drawbacks may be overcome in the near future, it is unlikely that embryo transfer will equal artificial insemination in practical benefits to the dairy or beef industry. At present the method is most commonly used to expand the number of offspring from cows that have delivered outstanding calves, to quickly introduce new breeds or strains into an area, to increase incidence of twinning, and to test for recessive alleles in daughters of known carriers.

With the advent of quick, nondamaging assays for determining the sex of a blastocyst (cytogenetic analyses are technically possible but not practical), the economic benefits of embryo transfer are increasing. In the future, embryo transfer may be coupled with techniques such as in vitro fertilization, blastomere cloning, nuclear transplantation and gene transfer, which could greatly increase its potential benefits. It is already possible in laboratory animals to transplant specific genes from one organism to another. For example, the growth hormone-producing genes from a rat can be introduced into the zygote of a mouse, and the donor implanted into a pseudopregnant mouse mother. By sexual maturity the genetically modified mouse is nearly twice the size of its normal litter mates. This type of genetic engineering has the potential of affecting not only growth, but resistance to disease, reproductive features, and other parameters of great commercial concern.

GASTRULATION: AVIAN

Gastrulation (gaster, belly) is a critical period in vertebrate development. At this stage cells of the embryonic disk become rearranged to form first two and then three separate, parallel (or concentric) tissues called **germ layers**. When three layers have been formed, the outermost is called **ectoderm**, the innermost is **endoderm**, and that which forms between them is the **mesoderm**. In addition, based on the results of many experiments, it is known that the embryonic genome becomes activated at or shortly before the gastrula stage and the developmental potentials of particular tissues begin to be restricted (see Chapter 4). The intraembryonic features of mammalian and avian gastrulation are morphologically similar. Since most experimental analyses of these many tissue rearrangements have been performed in birds, gastrulation in this class will be presented first.

Gastrulation in the bird occurs in central blastomeres of the embryonic disk overlying the subgerminal cavity. This region is also referred to as the **area pellucida** (clear area), in contrast to the marginal, more opaque area called the **area opaca**, which is adherent to the yolk. During late cleavage stages these central blastomeres become divided into two subpopulations, that are initially intermingled but appear to be of two different sizes (Fig. 2.10A). Subsequently, the larger cells, which contain more yolk, segregate from the smaller cells and form the roof of the subgerminal cavity. In addition, many of these larger cells aggregate at one pole of the embryonic disk (Fig. 2.10 B and C). This site of aggregation marks the future **caudal end** of the animal, and is the first grossly visible asymmetry in the developing embryo.

Some of the larger, more deeply located cells break away from the mass of smaller cells and move into the subgerminal cavity, a process called **delamination**. These are joined by similar cells that have migrated into the subgerminal cavity from the caudal aggregate. As a result of these two processes, a new layer of cells is formed (Fig. 2.10D).

This layer is called **hypoblast**. The cavity below the hypoblast is still the subgerminal cavity, but the newly formed cavity above it is called the **blastocoel**. The more populous layer of smaller cells roofing the blastocoel is now called the **epiblast**.

The accumulation of cells in the caudal part of the embryonic disk is the result of an expansion of the adjacent epiblast. This expansion occurs by a thinning of the multilayered epiblast. Whenever a tissue such as the epiblast expands, either it must occupy a greater area (radial expansion) or else cells must accumulate at one or more sites within the sheet (convergence). Blastulation and, even more so, gastrulation are examples of **convergence**.

Gastrulation begins as soon as the hypoblast layer is established. This process begins caudally, but at its peak involves the entire epiblast. The major stages of gastrulation are as follows:

Oriented Expansion of the Epiblast; Caudal Convergence of Cells

This initial phase, illustrated in Figure 2.11, is a continuation of blastulation. Epiblast populations located at progressively more rostral locations in the embryonic disk begin to undergo expansion. This results in the accumulation of cells in the caudal midline.

Formation of the Primitive Streak

More cells converge towards the midline of the epiblast, causing the caudal condensation to become elongated. This median, thickened area of the epiblast is called the **primitive streak**, and it marks the location of the future longitudinal axis of the embryo. As more of the epiblast undergoes expansion and an increasing number of these cells moves towards the caudal midline, the primitive streak elongates (Fig. 2.11 B and C). In fact, the entire blastodisk is increasing in length as more epiblast cells shift caudally.

The cranial end of the primitive streak is slightly widened, giving the primitive streak a hairpin appearance when viewed from

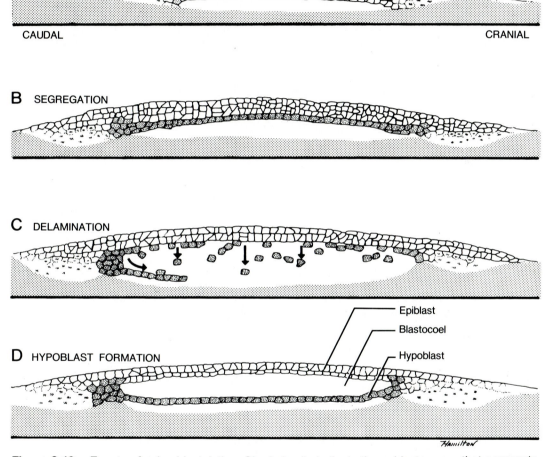

A EARLY BLASTULA

CAUDAL   CRANIAL

B SEGREGATION

C DELAMINATION

Epiblast

Blastocoel

Hypoblast

D HYPOBLAST FORMATION

Figure 2.10. Events of avian blastulation. Shaded cells indicate those blastomeres that segregate then, by delamination, form the hypoblast. A greater number of these cells accumulates at the future caudal margin of the embryo than elsewhere.

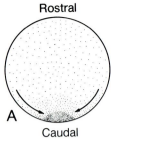

Rostral

A

Caudal

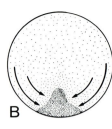

B

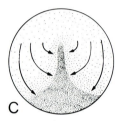

C

Figure 2.11. Dorsal (surface) views showing the movements of epiblast cells caudally and towards the midline during the late blastula and early gastrula stages of avian development. The darkly shaded area indicates the caudal region where epiblast cells accumulate and the primitive streak forms.

above (Figs. 2.12 and 2.13). This enlarged cranial tip is called the **primitive node** (Hensen's node, primitive knot).

Involution of Epiblast Cells: Formation of Endoderm and Mesoderm

In the center of the elongating primitive streak a longitudinal furrow called the **primitive groove** forms, as shown in Figure 2.12. This depression marks the site at which cells are leaving the epiblast. The first cells to break away invade the hypoblast layer, causing the original hypoblast cells to be displaced peripherally. Most of these new, epiblast-derived cells in the deeper layer will form the **intraembryonic endoderm**; the original hypoblast cells become **extraembryonic endoderm**.

However, the majority of the cells that leave the epiblast at the primitive streak form a loose mesenchymal population located between the epiblast and hypoblast (endoderm) layers. This population is called

mesoderm. As gastrulation proceeds, more epiblast-derived cells break away from the primitive streak to join the mesodermal population. This causes the mesenchymal population to expand laterally, as illustrated in Figures 2.12 and 2.15. The entire process, including cells leaving the epiblast, entering the deeper regions of the primitive groove, and then leaving to contribute to endodermal or mesodermal layers, is called **involution**.

Regression of the Primitive Streak: Formation of the Notochord

The cranial third of the epiblast, which was the last area to participate in gastrulation, is the first to cease expanding. Those cells already in the cranial part of the primitive groove migrate away as mesoderm, and no additional cells arrive at the midline to replace them. As a result the streak appears to regress (shorten), with the primitive node shifting position continually closer to the caudal end of the embryo. During this regression phase, cells in or close to the primitive node are deposited beneath the epiblast in the midline; these will form the **notochord** and **paraxial mesoderm**, as illustrated in Figure 2.14.

At its maximum the chick primitive streak is nearly 2 mm long, and extends about two-thirds of the craniocaudal length of the embryonic disk. Avian gastrulation begins approximately 24–30 hr after fertilization, which is usually about 6 hr after the egg is laid by a hen. The primitive streak is maximally elongated at about 18 hr of incubation, and it disappears by 2.5 days of incubation. When the streak has regressed completely and no new mesodermal cells are being generated from the epiblast, gastrulation is completed. The epiblast cells that did not undergo involution and thus remain in the upper surface of the three-layered embryo are now called **ectoderm**.

Mesoderm is formed from the entire length of the primitive streak. As the streak regresses the lateral margins of this mesenchymal population expand laterally and ros-

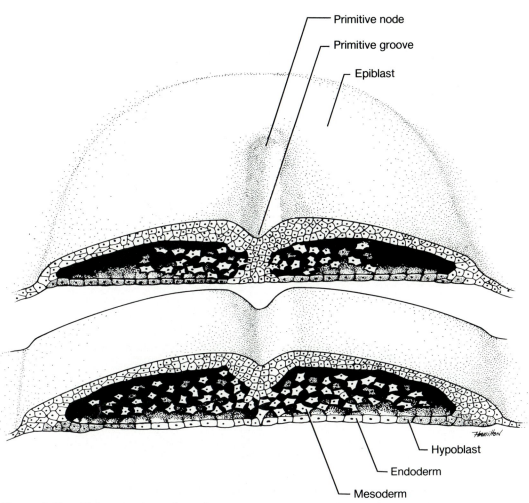

Primitive node

Primitive groove

Epiblast

Hypoblast

Endoderm

Mesoderm

Figure 2.12.   Oblique surface view of an avian midgastrula stage embryo cut transversely at two planes to reveal the locations of internal cells. In the more cranial section, cells derived from the epiblast are displacing hypoblast cells (*shaded*) to form endoderm and are also migrating between the two epithelial layers to form mesoderm, which at this stage is a mesenchymal tissue. The caudal (*lower*) section shows a slightly more advanced stage.

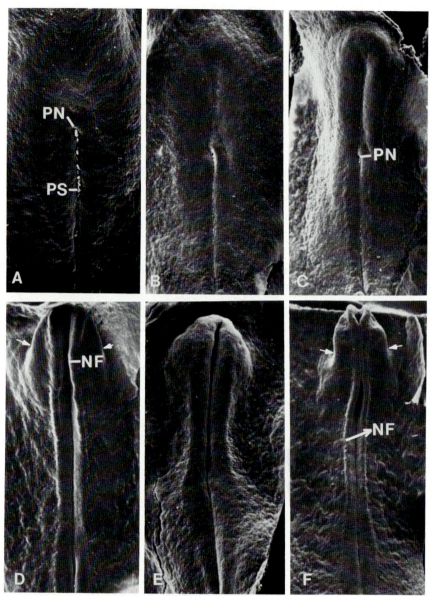

Figure 2.13.   Scanning electron micrographs of six sequential stages in avian gastrulation and neurulation. In *A,* the primitive streak (*PS*) is maximally elongated, with the primitive node (*PN*) at its cranial tip. In *B* and *C* the primitive streak is regressing and, cranial to it, the head process is developing. *D* and *E* show the elevation of cephalic neural folds (*NF*) and in *F,* they meet to form the mesencephalon. At the same time the head process elevates from the surface of the embryonic disk and lateral body folds begin to undercut the cranial part of the embryo (*arrows*). This entire sequence takes only about 10 hr (from 16–25 hr of incubation). (Micrographs courtesy of Dr. Gary Schoenwolf.)

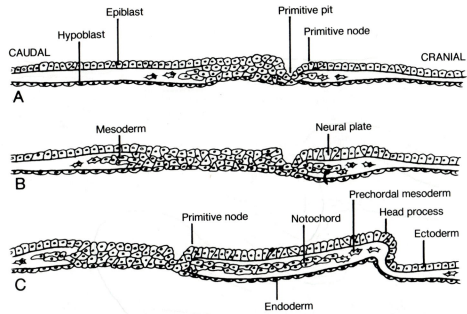

Figure 2.14. Schematic median sections illustrating the avian embryo at early, mid, and late gastrula stages. In *B* the primitive streak is at its maximum length, but by *C* it has regressed caudally, leaving the cranial portion of the notochord and a small population of prechordal mesoderm in the midline. The surface ectoderm overlying and immediately adjacent to the notochord thickens to form the neural plate.

trally, eventually meeting in the midline in front of the embryo, as illustrated in Figure 2.15. The first mesodermal cells to have formed all become extraembryonic and participate in formation of extraembryonic membranes (Chapter 3). The last mesodermal cells formed from the epiblast remain closest to the dorsal midline of the embryo, and form paraxial mesoderm.

GASTRULATION: PRIMATES AND DOMESTIC ANIMALS

Gastrulation occurs during the end of the 2nd week of gestation in most domestic animals, and several days earlier in lab animals. The morphogenetic movements which occur during mammalian gastrulation are similar to those in the chick. The most conspicuous differences are associated with the necessity in mammals of forming extraembryonic tissues very early. As will be discussed in Chapter 3, most mammalian embryos are establishing contacts with the uterine wall concomitant with the onset of gastrulation.

During the blastocyst stage, cells **delaminate** from the inner surface of the embryonic disk and expand beneath the trophoblast. These form a thin, continuous sheet lining the interior of the blastocyst, thus establishing a tube of **hypoblast** inside a tube of trophoblast (Fig. 2.16*B*). Some texts refer to this sparse layer, shown in Figure 2.7*C*, as the exocoelomic membrane. The cavity of the hypoblast tube is called the **archenteron**, or **primitive gut**. Most of this tube will remain outside of the embryo, forming the extraembryonic yolk sac.

Primitive streak formation occurs in the epiblastic cells of the embryonic disk, which occupies a relatively small area of the blastocyst compared with the extraembryonic, trophoblastic portion. Epiblast cells that move inwards at the primitive streak (Figs. 2.16 and 2.17) form the definitive endoderm, the mesoderm of the embryonic axis, including the notochord and presumptive somites, and also the adjacent lateral mesoderm.

In mammals such as the pig, sheep and

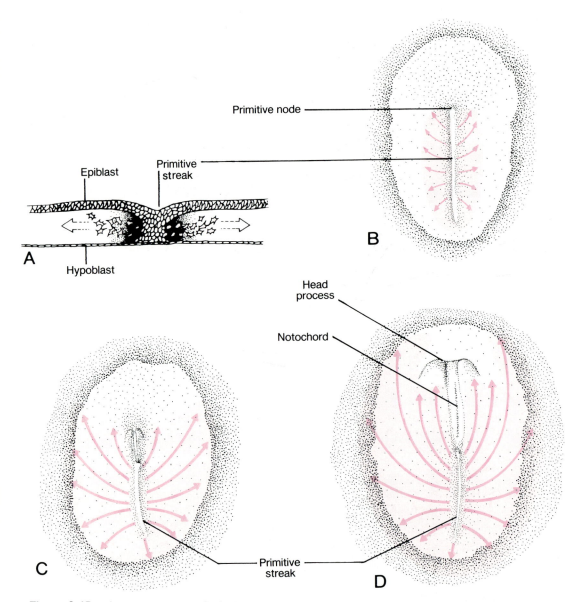

Figure 2.15. *A*, transverse and *B–D*, three dorsal views of the gastrula-stage embryo showing the progressive spread of mesoderm (*red*) away from the primitive streak between surface ectoderm and hypoblast/endoderm. (Redrawn after BM Patten and B Carlson, 1974.)

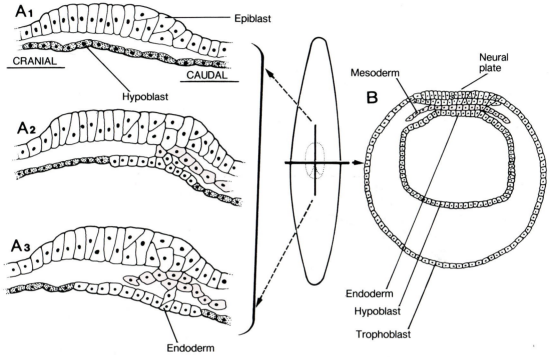

Figure 2.16. Early stages of gastrulation in the pig at 9–10 days of gestation. A_1, A_2, and A_3 are median sections through the embryonic disk at progressively older stages, to illustrate the displacement of hypoblast and formation of mesoderm and endoderm by superficial (epiblast) cells. *B*, tr

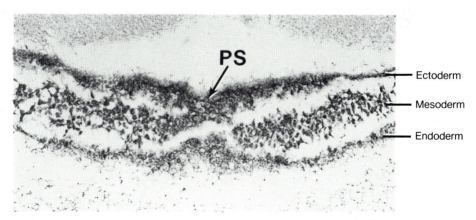

Figure 2.17. Transverse section showing the late primitive streak (*PS*) from a canine embryo of approximately 18 days of gestation.

cow, in which the blastocysts become very elongated, the lateral mesoderm spreads quickly away from the embryonic disk. This population of lateral mesoderm splits into two layers, one associated with each of the epithelial tissues present (Fig. 2.18). The mesoderm immediately beneath the trophoblast and embryonic ectoderm is **somatic mesoderm**, and the two layers combined are referred to as **somatopleure**. Mesoderm surrounding the hypoblast and embryonic endoderm is **splanchnic (visceral) mesoderm**, and the combined layers are called **splanchnopleure**. When the primitive streak becomes inactive and regresses, the cells remaining on the surface of the embryonic disk constitute the ectoderm.

In the primate the inner cell mass usually is retained inside of and attached to the trophoblast (see Fig. 3.12). Early in gastrulation the trophoblast cells separate from the inner cell mass, allowing cells of the epiblast to undergo morphogenetic movements similar to those described above.

NEURULATION

Neurulation marks the formation of the central nervous system, the initial development of the gut and the heart, and the appearance of segmented paraxial mesoderm. At this stage the body of the embryo begins to be delineated within the three germ layers established during gastrulation.

The first feature of neurulation is a thickening of the surface ectoderm along the dorsal midline to form a **neural plate**, which is bounded on both sides by slight elevations called **neural folds**. The plate becomes depressed in the midline, forming a **neural groove**, and the neural folds become more elevated, as shown in Figs. 2.13 *C–F* and 2.19. Subsequently these folds converge towards the dorsal midline, meet and fuse together. This results in the formation of a

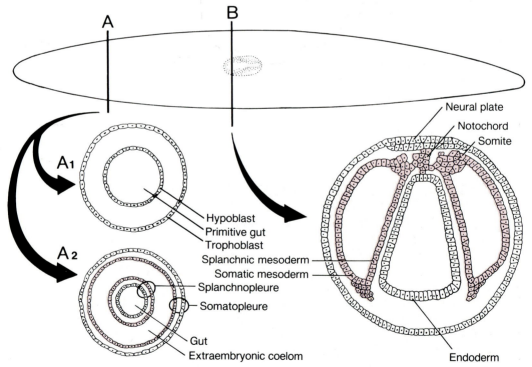

Figure 2.18. Late stages of porcine gastrulation. *A₁* and *A₂* are transverse sections from the peripheral region of the greatly elongated blastocyst at days 12 and 16 of gestation, during which time extraembryonic mesoderm arrives and separates into somatic and splanchnic layers. *B* is a transverse section at the level of the embryonic disk showing the separation of intraembryonic lateral mesoderm into two layers.

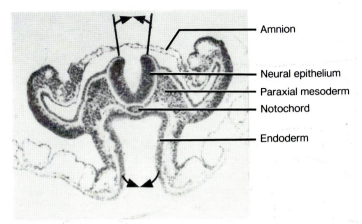

Figure 2.19. Transverse section from the caudal region of a 22-somite cat embryo. Both neural epithelium and endoderm are in the process of closing (*arrows*) to form the thoracolumbar spinal cord and hindgut, respectively.

closed neural tube that is separated from overlying surface ectoderm. This process is discussed in greater detail in Chapter 6.

Concomitant with the formation of a closed neural tube, the cephalic region of the avian embryo begins to grow above the surface of the blastodisk and also to elongate rostrally. This process, which is the first step in forming the body of the embryo, occurs in two stages. First, as the cephalic neural tube elongates rostrally, it overgrows the underlying ectoderm and endoderm. This results in the formation of a transverse furrow called the **subcephalic pocket** located beneath the rostral margin of the forebrain, as shown in Figure 2.20. The elongating cephalic tissues are collectively called the **head process**.

After this initial rostral elevation of the head, the surface ectoderm lateral to the brain begins to fold downward. The furrows that are formed on either side of the head are called **lateral body folds** (Fig. 2.13 *D–F*). These lateral folds are continuous with the subcephalic pocket. They become deeper, eventually undercutting the entire cephalic end of the embryo and separating the head process from underlying extraembryonic tissues. As development proceeds, lateral body folds progressively separate more of the embryo from underlying extraembryonic tissues. Later an identical process will begin at the tail region and proceed progressively cranially. The cranial and caudal sets of lateral

body folds eventually meet at the level of the **umbilicus**, which is the stalk connecting the body of the embryo to its extraembryonic structures.

Formation of the gut tube also begins during neurulation and mirrors the formation of the neural tube. The most rostral tip of the gut tube, the pharynx, is formed when the subcephalic pocket expands beneath the head process (Fig. 2.20). The left and right endodermal folds meet in the ventral midline and fuse, thus forming a closed endodermal tube. This process continues from cranial to caudal and, later, proceeds cranially from the hindgut region. The transient openings from the closed parts of the gut into the subgerminal cavity (in birds) or archenteron (mammals) are called the **cranial** and **caudal intestinal portals** (see Fig. 1.5).

As the gut begins to close beneath the level of the hindbrain, **cardiogenic mesoderm** located beside the paired endodermal folds is brought to the ventral midline. A tube of endothelium on each side will fuse to form a single **cardiac tube**. This will expand to the right, loop 180°, and then become subdivided into a four-chambered heart, as described in Chapter 12.

EMBRYONIC DUPLICATIONS AND TWINNING

Multiple births most frequently result from fertilization of separately ovulated fe-

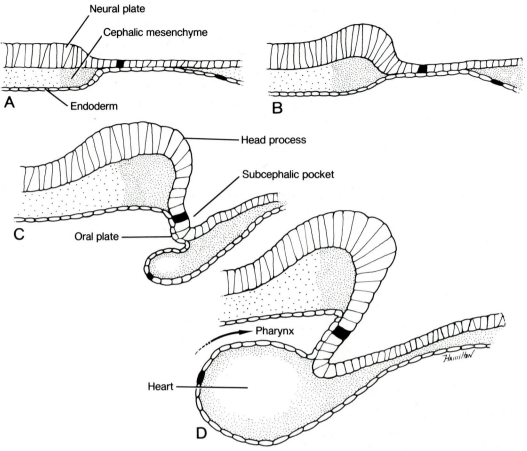

Figure 2.20. Schematic median view of late gastrula and early neurula stages, illustrating in *B*, the elevation of the head process, and in *C* and *D*, initial folding of the surface of the embryonic disk to form the subcephalic pocket and the rostral part of the pharynx. At the same time, the primordium of the heart is folded beneath the embryo (see Chapter 12). Two cells have been blackened to help clarify the translocations occurring at these stages. *Arrow* in *D* passes through the cranial intestinal portal.

male gametes. However, complete or partial separation of cleavage-stage blastomeres and blastocysts, or duplications during gastrulation can also result in the development of multiple organisms. Such embryos are categorized as being **free** (unattached to each other) or **cojoined**, and **symmetrical** or **asymmetrical**.

Free (Separate), Symmetrical, Dizygotic Twins

This category includes most normal twins. Those derived from separate zygotes are called **dizygotic** twins. Each embryo develops independently with its own separate set

of fetal membranes, although in some species the extraembryonic membranes fuse. In the cow this includes fusion of the allantoic blood vessels, which allows blood to be exchanged between the fetuses. If the twins are of different sexes, this exchange results in an abnormal development of the genital system of the female and the production of a **free-martin** (see Chapter 19).

Free, Symmetrical, Monozygotic Twins

These are identical twins derived initially from a single zygote. The separation or duplication can occur at several different stages. The two blastomeres produced by the first cleavage may separate and each form an embryo. More frequently, separation of blastomeres occurs later during cleavage or blastocyst stages. If twinning is initiated during these stages, two separate sets of extraembryonic membranes will usually be formed.

Figure 2.21 illustrates one way in which monozygotic twin bovine embryos can be produced following an abnormally small rupture in the zona pellucida. This permits some but not all of the blastocyst to break free. As long as both hemisected blastocysts

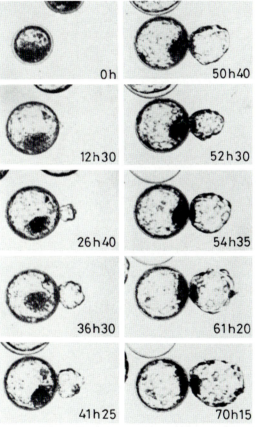

0h

50h40

12h30

52h30

26h40

54h35

36h30

61h20

41h25

70h15

Figure 2.21. Time lapse cinematograph record of atypical hatching by a cow blastocyst developing in culture. Observations began using a fresh 7-day blastocyst (*0 hr*). By *26 hr 40 min*, expansion is complete, and hatching is beginning. Note the subsequent movements of the embryonic disk towards and partially through an opening in the zona pellucida. The two "half embryos" subsequently separated, forming identical (monozygotic) twins (From Massip A, et al. *Veterinary Record* 112:301, 1983, © British Veterinary Association.)

contain part of the embryonic disk, each half may develop normally. Occasionally the embryonic disk will split into two separate parts immediately prior to gastrulation. In these situations there is usually some sharing of extraembryonic membranes between the two fetuses. In the nine-banded armadillo the embryonic disk normally separates into four separate disks, each of which gives rise to an embryo.

Free, Asymmetrical Twins

With asymmetrical free twins one is normal, the other is rudimentary in its development and survives by being attached to the blood supply of the fetal membranes of the normal twin. The origin of these asymmetric twins may be monozygotic or dizygotic.

As a rule, the abnormal twin has no recognizable body form and consists of skin with pigment and hair, connective tissue, bone, teeth, muscle and rudimentary digestive organs. Specific craniofacial structures can sometimes be identified. Although attached to the vascularized fetal membranes of the normal twin, the abnormal twin is usually surrounded by its own amnion.

Various names have been given to the abnormal twin. These include: **amorphous globosus, anidian** (formless) **fetus, acardiac fetus** or holocardius. Originally thought to all be of monozygotic origin, karyotype studies have shown that some are dizygotic twins. It is possible that these represent an abortive attempt at development of a fertilized polar body. Among domestic animals these acardiac twins are most common in the cow.

This abnormal twinning should be distinguished from the condition known as a **mummified fetus** or lithopedion (stone child), in which development of a normal twin is arrested. Rather than become resorbed, the twin becomes dehydrated and shrunken. The presence of a mummified fetus can cause dystocia (abnormal delivery) or, if retained, lead to uterine infection or interfere with a subsequent pregnancy.

Mummified fetuses are most commonly found in cows.

Cojoined or Fused Symmetrical Twins

All cojoined twins are monozygotic in origin and represent incomplete division of one embryo into two components, usually at some time during the primitive streak stage. If the twins are nearly complete, they are generally termed **diplopagus** (2-fold joined), the preferred equivalent of "Siamese" twins. Whenever possible, such twins are identified according to the site of attachment.

Thoracopagus, joined at the sternal region of the thorax, facing each other, often with partially fused or compromised hearts (Fig. 2.22*B*);

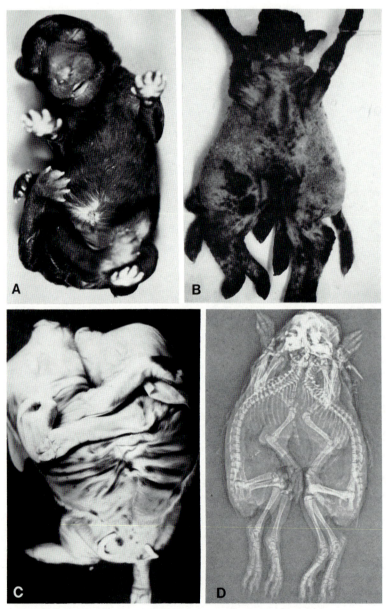

Figure 2.22. Incomplete, symmetrical twinning. *A*, tetrascelus in a puppy; *B*, ovine thoracopagus; *C*, thoracoabdominopagus in pigs; and *D*, radiograph of guinea pigs with cephalopagus.

Abdominopagus, joined at the abdomen, often with partially fused intestines (Figure 2.22*C*);
Pygopagus, joined back to back at the pelvis or sacrum (pygos, buttocks); and
Cephalopagus (craniopagus), joined in the head region (Fig. 2.22*D*).

It is also possible to have duplication of one part of the future axial (and adjacent) structures. These usually arise during primitive streak elongation or regression. This set of anomalies is described by using the prefix di- (or tri-, tetra-, etc.) and the appropriate, region-specific suffix. For example:

Dicephalus, two heads (Fig. 2.23);
Diprosopus, two faces;
Dicaudatus, two tails;
Tetrabrachius, two pairs of thoracic limbs; and
Tetrascelus, two pairs of pelvic limbs (Fig. 2.22*A*).

Cojoined Twins, Asymmetrical

Often the components of the cojoined twins are unequal in size (heteropagus) and consist of one reasonably normal individual, the autosite, with an extra body part, the parasite, attached to it. A frequent manifestation of this is the formation of an extra limb attached along the back of the animal. This is called **notomelus** (noto, back; melus, limb). A normal animal with an extra set of pelvic limbs projecting caudally from its ischial arch is another example of asymmetrical cojoined twinning. This type of duplication usually arises after gastrulation when specific organ-forming regions called fields (limb field, heart field, eye field, etc.) are becoming organized (see Chapter 10).

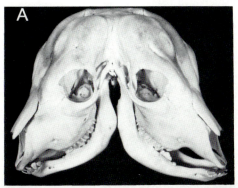

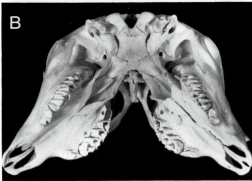

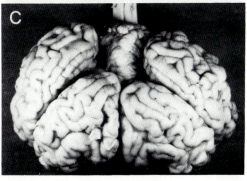

Figure 2.23. Dicephalic cow neonate. *A* and *B*, dorsal and ventral views of the skull; *C*, dorsal view of brain from similar specimen. Most of these animals die due to suffocation resulting from abnormalities of the larynx or glottis.

Bibliography

Note: Early development in avian and primate species is more fully described in most of the general and human embryology texts listed in the Introduction.

EARLY STAGES OF EMBRYONIC DEVELOPMENT IN BIRDS AND MAMMALS

Brackett BG, Oh YK, Evans JF, Donawick WJ: Fertilization and early development of cow ova. *Biol Reprod* 23:189–205, 1980.

Calarco PB, McLaren A: Ultrastructural observations of preimplantation stages of the sheep. *J Embryol Exp Morphol* 36:609–622, 1976.

Eyal-Giladi H, Kochav S: From cleavage to primitive streak formation: a complementary normal table and a new look at the first stages of the development of the chick. I. General morphology. *Develop Biol* 49:321–337, 1976.

Gier HT: Early embryology of the dog. *Anat Rec* 108:561–562, 1950.

Hafez ESE: *Scanning Electron Microscopic Atlas of Mammalian Reproduction.* New York, Springer-Verlag, 1975.

Hill JP, Tribe M: The early development of the cat. (*Felis domestica*). *Q J Microscop Sci* 68:513–602, 1924.

Holst PA, Phemister RD: The prenatal development of the dog: preimplantation events. *Biol Reprod* 5:194–206, 1971.

Hughes PE, Varley MA: Fertilization and conception;

pregnancy. *Reproduction in the Pig*. London, Butterworths, 1980, Chapts 6 and 7.

Linares T, King WA: Morphological study of the bovine blastocyst with phase contrast microscopy. *Theriogenology* 14:212–133, 1980.

Lindner GM, Wright RW: Bovine embryo morphology and evaluation. *Theriogenology* 20:407–416, 1983.

McLaren A: Fertilization, cleavage and implantation. In Hafez ESE (ed): *Reproduction in Farm Animals*, ed 4. Philadelphia, Lea & Febiger, 1980.

Moghissi KS, Hafez ESE: *Biology of Mammalian Fertilization and Implantation*. Springfield, IL, Charles C Thomas, 1972.

Rogers BJ, Bentwood BJ: Capacitation, acrosome reaction, and fertilization. In Zaneveld LJD, Chatterton RT (eds): *Biochemistry of Mammalian Reproduction*. New York, Wiley, 1982, pp 203–230.

Stern CD, Ireland GW: An integrated experimental study of endoderm formation in avian embryos. *Anat Embryol* 163:245–263, 1981.

Tietz WJ, Selinger WG: Temporal relationship in early canine embryogenesis. *Anat Rec* 157:333–334, 1967.

Winterberger-Torres S, Flechon JE: Ultrastructural evolution of the trophoblast cells of the preimplantation sheep blastocyst from day 8 to day 18. *J Anat* 118:143–153, 1974.

BOVINE EMBRYO CULTURE AND TRANSFER

Ayalon N: A review of embryonic mortality in cattle. *J Reprod Fertil* 54:483–493, 1978.

Bowen RA, Howard TH, Pickett BW: Interaction of bluetongue virus with preimplantation embryos from mice and cattle. *Am J Vet Res* 43:1907–1911, 1982.

Hafez ESE, Semm K (eds): *In Vitro Fertilization and Embryo Transfer*. New York, Liss, 1982.

Massip A, Mulnard J, Van der Zwalmen P, Hanzen C, Ectors F: The behaviour of cow blastocyst *in vitro*: cinematographic and morphometric analysis. *J Anat* 134:399–405, 1982.

Massip A, Van der Zwalmen P, Mulnard J, Zwijsen W: Atypical hatching of a cow blastocyst leading to separation of complete twin half blastocysts. *Vet Rec* 112:301, 1983.

Palmiter RD, Brinster RL, Hammer RE, Trumbauer ME, Rosenfeld MG, Birnberg NC, Evans RM: Dramatic growth of mice that develop from eggs microinjected with metallothionein growth hormone-fusion genes. *Nature* 300:611–615, 1982.

Seidel GE, Jr: Superovulation and embryo transfer in cattle. *Science* 211:351–358, 1981.

Seidel SM, Seidel GE: Embryo transfer bibliography X. *Theriogenology* 20:241–256, 1983.

Shea BF: Evaluating the bovine embryo. *Theriogenology* 15:31–42, 1981.

Tervit HR, Cooper MW, Goold PG, Haszard GM: Nonsurgical embryo transfer in cattle. *Theriogenology* 13:63–71, 1980.

Extraembryonic Membranes and Placentation

In order for the early reptilian vertebrates to reproduce outside of an aquatic environment it was necessary to develop structures that would both protect the embryo and allow it to exchange gasses with its environment. This was accomplished by the formation of a shell and, internally, a set of **extraembryonic membranes.** There are four of them: the **amnion** and **chorion**, derived from **somatopleure**, and the **allantois** and **yolk sac** from **splanchnopleure**. Although called membranes, most extraembryonic membranes are in fact initially composed of two layers, somatic or splanchnic mesoderm plus ectoderm or endoderm.

AVIAN

Yolk Sac

In the bird with its megalecithal zygote the yolk serves as a continual source of nutrients via the yolk sac and its vasculature.

Following gastrulation, the extraembryonic germ layers progressively expand over the yolk, which is bound initially by the cell membrane of the zygote and the acellular vitelline membrane. The endoderm and adjacent splanchnic mesoderm that directly cover the yolk comprise the **yolk sac**, shown in Figure 3.1. The outer perimeter of the developing yolk sac is marked by a blood vessel, the **sinus terminalis** or marginal vein, which demarcates the extent of growth of the splanchnic mesoderm over the yolk.

By the 6th day of incubation in the chick, the yolk sac encloses most of the yolk, and is vascularized by vitelline blood vessels in the splanchnic mesoderm. These pass into the embryo along the yolk stalk, which is formed by the completion of body folding and closure of the embryonic gut tube. Yolk does not pass directly into the embryonic digestive tract, but is absorbed through the yolk sac endoderm and endothelial lining of the vitelline vasculature. Thus, nutrients pass into the embryo via the vitelline veins. Beginning on the 19th day of incubation in the chick, which is 2 days before hatching (Table 3.1), the yolk sac is drawn into the abdominal cavity and the remaining undigested yolk is entirely absorbed by about 6 days after hatching.

Amnion and Chorion

The process of body folding, which commences with the previously described head folding, continues caudally along the lateral aspects of the embryo by formation of lateral body folds and, at the caudal end, the tail fold. As a result of this process distinct lateral

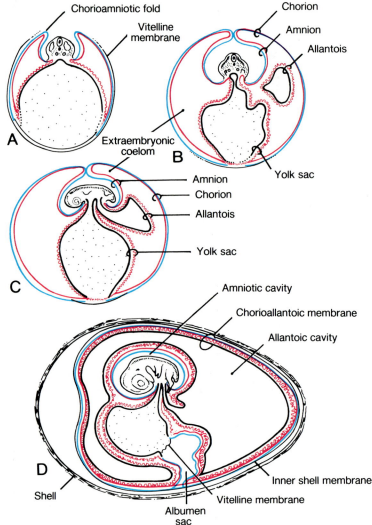

Figure 3.1. Development of avian extraembryonc membranes. *A* and *B* show transverse sections on the 3rd and 5th days of incubation, during which time the large mass of yolk becomes partially encompassed by the yolk sac. *C* and *D* are lateral views of the 5th and 9th days of incubation to illustrate the development of the allantois.

Table 3.1.
Incubation times for domesticated birds

Bird	Days
Quail[a]	16
Budgerigar	18–20
Chicken	21
Pheasant[b]	22–28
Peafowl	28
Duck[c]	28
Turkey	28
Goose	28–32

[a] domesticated Coturnix (Japanese) quail.
[b] Varies according to species.
[c] The Moscovy duck is 35–37 days.

and ventral body walls are formed around the embryo, except at the **yolk stalk**.

Simultaneous with the process of body folding, a pair of folds consisting of extraembryonic somatopleure begins to elevate (Figs. 3.1*A* and 3.2*A*). These **chorioamniotic folds** initially form cranial to the head and elevate at progressively more caudal levels on both sides of the embryo. Later a similar series of events occurs at the caudal end of the embryo, forming a pair of folds that grow progressively cranially.

The chorioamniotic folds expand dorsally

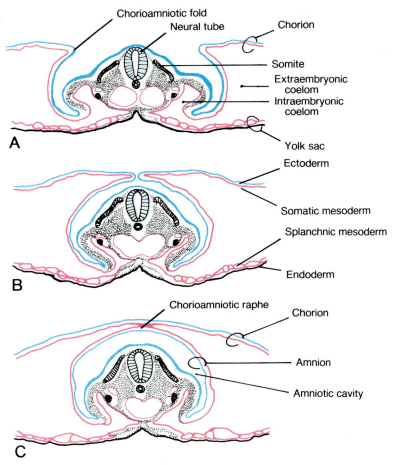

Figure 3.2. The development of the amnion and chorion in the avian embryo. The chorioamniotic folds elevate then fuse dorsal to the embryo. (Redrawn from LG Johnson and EP Volpe, 1973.)

then meet and fuse over the dorsal midline of the embryo. As a result of this growth of folds over the embryo, two layers of somatopleure, separated by the extraembryonic coelom, now extend over the embryo (Fig. 3.2 *B* and *C*). The outer layer of somatopleure is the **chorion**; the inner layer is the **amnion**. The ectoderm of the amnion is continuous with the ectoderm of the embryonic skin at the umbilicus. The site where the left and right chorioamniotic folds meet and fuse is marked by a longitudinal raphe called the **chorioamniotic raphe** or **mesamnion**. In some species of birds (and mammals) it persists; in others it disappears, leaving no connection between the amnion and chorion. In the chick a chorioamniotic raphe persists.

The cavity between the embryo and amnion, the **amniotic cavity**, is filled with **am-niotic fluid.** This is initially a product of secretions from the amniotic ectoderm, but later receives fluids from the fetal kidneys, oral glands and respiratory tract. The amniotic fluid serves to buoy and protect the embryo and provide it with an environment in which the embryo can move its body and limbs.

Initially, there are no blood vessels in the chorion or amnion. However, vessels may later enter these layers of somatopleure from adjacent extraembryonic splanchnic mesoderm. Smooth muscle fibers develop in the somatic mesoderm of the amnion, and their contractions cause agitation of the fluid surrounding the embryo.

The chorion expands quickly (Fig. 3.1) and by 7–8 days of incubation in the chick it becomes closely apposed to the inner shell membrane. Together with the later forming allantois, the chorion mediates gas and water exchange.

Allantois

The **allantois** arises as a diverticulum of the embryonic hindgut. First visible in the extraembryonic coelom of the 3-day embryo as a small vesicle on the right side, by 10 days the allantois fills the cavity between the amnion and the chorion. The allantoic splanchnic mesoderm meets and fuses with the splanchnic mesoderm of the yolk sac and also with the somatic mesoderm of the amnion and chorion.

The allantois is vascularized by **allantoic arteries** that branch off the caudal portions of the two **dorsal aortae**. **Allantoic veins (umbilical)** enter the embryo at the umbilicus and course cranially in the ventral body wall to enter the **sinus venosus** of the heart, along with the vitelline veins. When the allantois fuses with the chorion, its vessels vascularize the somatic mesoderm. This vascular **chorioallantois** is directly apposed to the inner shell membrane, and it is through these allantoic vessels that oxygen from the air around the egg is collected and carbon dioxide is released. The allantoic cavity serves to collect the urinary excretory wastes, most of which precipitate as uric acid in birds.

As the embryo and its extraembryonic membranes develop, the volume of albumen is reduced, mostly by the transfer of its fluid content to the embryo. The space it originally occupied is taken up by the embryo. When the yolk sac and chorion reach the ventral margin of the yolk, a small opening remains where yolk and albumen are continuous. This margin of extraembryonic membrane is the yolk sac umbilicus. Later, when the allantois expands in the extraembryonic coelom and reaches this location, a layer of chorion grows over the surface of the shrinking albumen, creating an albumen sac (Fig. 3.1*D*). Prior to hatching, the albumen sac is enclosed in the abdomen of the embryo, along with the yolk sac.

PLACENTA

The **placenta** of eutherian mammals (all mammals except marsupials and egg-laying monotremes) is a structure that forms by **the apposition of fetal membranes and maternal tissues**. While its primary function is that of selectively mediating physiological exchange between the fetus and mother, it also serves as an important endocrine organ during gestation. The placenta, in particular the fetal components, acts as a barrier to prevent fetal and maternal blood from mixing.

Superficially, the fetal membranes of mammals are very similar to those just described in birds (and reptiles). One major difference is that there is little or no yolk in the mammalian zygote, and as such, the yolk sac is often transient and not as well developed. However, the rudimentary yolk sac does play an essential role in the initial stages of hematopoiesis (blood cell formation) and, in some species, is the source of germ cells. It is the **chorioallantois** that is the principal fetal component of the mammalian placenta.

Prior to apposition with the uterine mucosa (endometrium), the developing mammalian embryo derives essential metabolic substrates from the fluid contents of the uterine cavity. This fluid is called **histotrophe** and is a secretory product of the **uterine mucosal glands**. Histotrophe, which is also called "uterine milk," contains low molecular weight metabolites, fats and glycogen. Following formation of the placenta, histotrophic nutrition is supplemented by **hemotrophic** nutrition, in which essential metabolites are provided by the maternal circulatory system.

Although the placentas of all eutherian mammals share common structural origins and essential functions, in their fully developed state they present contrasting appearances both in the number of tissue layers that remain intact between fetal and maternal circulating blood and in the distribution of contact sites. As outlined in Figure 3.3, there are **three fetal extraembryonic layers** which are present in the chorioallantoic pla-

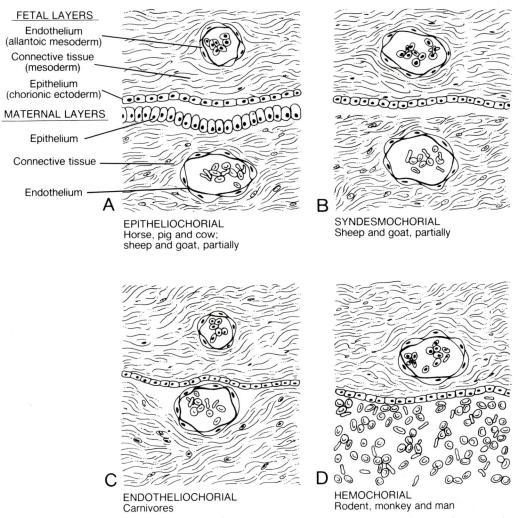

Figure 3.3. Classification of chorioallantoic placentas according to the number of maternal cell layers present. (Redrawn after LB Flexner and A Gellhorn, 1942.)

centa in all mammals. These are the **endothelium**, which lines the allantoic blood vessels, the **chorioallantoic mesodermal connective tissue layers**, and the **chorionic epithelial cell layer**, which is derived from the epithelial layer of the trophoblast.

However, different groups of mammals vary greatly with respect to which, if any, of the **three maternal layers** are retained. The three layers that constitute the **uterine mucosa (endometrium)** are the **vascular endothelium**, the surrounding uterine **connective tissues**, and the **surface epithelium**.

In the domestic animals two types of pla-

centas prevail. An **epitheliochorial placenta** occurs in the horse, pig, and cattle, and in parts of the placenta of sheep and goats. As the name implies, the fetal chorion is in contact with maternal uterine epithelium. There is **no loss** of endometrial tissue during attachment and throughout gestation. Similarly, at birth the maternal endometrium remains intact and is not sloughed off during parturition. Such placentas are called **adeciduate** (a = not; decidius = a falling off). The domestic ruminant is an exception because, although the attachment is epitheliochorial, following parturition a portion of the endometrium that formed the functional placenta is sloughed. Thus, in these species a **partially deciduate** placenta exists.

In carnivores, such as the dog and cat, the functional placenta is **endotheliochorial**. Endometrial epithelium and connective tissue are lost during attachment, leaving uterine vascular endothelium in contact with the fetal chorion. Loss of endometrium occurs during placental development and also at birth. Thus, these animals have **deciduate** placentas. In most rodents and many primates, including the human, the maternal uterine vascular endothelium is also lost, resulting in free maternal blood bathing the chorionic cells. This is a **hemochorial placenta**, which is **deciduate**.

While classification of placentas according to this histological method is the most widely used means of categorization, it is not without difficulties. First, this system describes only chorioallantoic placentas, and in many species the yolk sac forms placental tissues, especially during the early stages of fetal-maternal apposition. Also, in some animals (e.g. sheep and goats) the number of intact maternal layers differs in various parts of the mature placenta.

In addition, it was formerly assumed that the ability of a placenta to function as a restrictive barrier was related solely to the number of maternal layers which persist. This assumption is unwarranted. Factors such as the total area of apposition, species-specific degree of permeability of the various layers, and patterns of fetal and maternal vasculature must also be considered.

Due to these limitations, placentas are further classified according to shape and vascular arrangement. The various shapes, shown schematically in Figure 3.4, refer to arrangement of specialized zones of apposition between fetal and maternal tissues where primary physiological exchanges occur. In some species (e.g. horse and pig) the zone is distributed over most of the chorioallantois; this is called a **diffuse placenta**. In contrast, on the uterine mucosa of ruminants there are discrete areas called **uterine caruncles** to which fetal chorioallantoic tis-

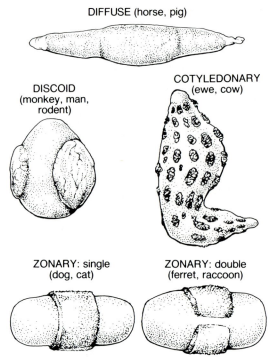

Figure 3.4. Classification of placentas according to the shape and distribution of attachment sites between extraembryonic and maternal tissues. (Redrawn after WJ Hamilton, JD Boyd and HW Mossman, 1962.)

sues adhere (see Fig. 3.8); this is a **cotyledonary** placenta. The other arrangements, **zonary** and **discoid**, will be discussed later.

In most domesticated mammals the chorionic epithelium forms long, branched villi at the sites of apposition with maternal tissues. These villi are epithelial-lined cylinders filled with mesenchyme and allantoic blood vessels, and they establish a **villous placenta**. In some species (carnivores, some rodents and primates) these villi coalesce and the allantoic vessels form irregular, tortuous channels. This vascular arrangement is termed a **labyrinthine placenta**.

APPOSITION AND IMPLANTATION

Embryonic tissues contact the uterine wall shortly after entering the uterus (Table 3.2). In most domesticated mammals the site of permanent contact is **antimesometrial** (opposite to the side of mesenteric attachment) and, in ruminants, the pig, and some ro-

Table 3.2.
Fetal-Maternal Apposition in Domesticated Mammals[a,b]

Animal	Attachment begins[c]	Size of trophoblast at this stage	Attachment complete[c]
Cat	11–12	4 mm	16–17
Cattle	28–32	200+ cm[d]	40–45
Dog	14–17	4 mm	20–21
Horse	35–40	6–7 cm	95–105
Sheep	14–16	10–20 cm	28–35
Swine	12–13	Up to 1 m[d]	24–26

[a] Data adapted from McLaren, 1980; and Evans and Christensen, 1979.
[b] Data refer to definitive, chorioallantoic attachment; in some of these species there are earlier choriovitellinic attachments (see section on the Horse).
[c] Days after ovulation.
[d] Usually equals or exceeds the length of the uterine tube.

dents, this side of the uterus shows an increase in vascularity prior to contact by the blastocyst.

Contractions of the uterine muscle and endometrial ciliary action facilitate the movement of blastocysts, including transuterine movement in many species. However, the mechanisms responsible for spacing of blastocysts in polycotous species, which are those that give birth to more than two offspring per pregnancy, are unknown.

The term **implantation** is commonly used to describe the attachment of the trophoblast to the uterine lining. However, as described earlier, the degree of attachment varies considerably between species. In most of the large domesticated mammals the attachment is noninvasive and fetal tissues can be physically separated from the uterine epithelium. Rodent blastocysts settle into uterine crypts, which are depressions in the uterine lining that subsequently close around the embryo and separate it from the lumen of the uterus. In most carnivores, rodents and primates, including man, attachment is **interstitial**; the trophoblast invades and partially destroys the endometrium. Later, adjacent uterine mucosal tissues may close around the embryo, a process that is called **nidation** (nidus, nest).

PLACENTAS OF DOMESTIC ANIMALS

Pig

(*Sus scrofa*), gestation length: 114–115 days (average).

Close apposition to the uterine wall begins at about 12 days. In pigs the attachment of the chorionic trophoblast is unaccompanied by loss of endometrium or any marked alteration in the morphology of the maternal tissues; thus, the porcine placenta is **epitheliochorial and adeciduate**.

The formation of a tube of hypoblast and the subsequent envelopment of it by splanchnic mesoderm to form the definitive **yolk sac** were described in the preceding chapter (see Figure 2.16). Once underlain by somatic mesoderm the entire trophoblast layer is termed the **chorion**. As in the chick, amniogenesis occurs by a bilateral folding and subsequent fusion of somatopleure tissue (Fig. 3.5). There is a permanent chorioamniotic raphe where the membranes remain attached at the original zone of fusion.

The allantois arises from the hindgut and enters the extraembryonic coelom at about 15 days of gestation (Fig. 3.5*A*). By 25 days it has filled the entire extraembryonic coelom except for the area of the chorioamniotic raphe dorsal to the embryo. Simultaneous with the expansion of the allantois, the yolk sac atrophies. Thus, while the yolk sac and its vitelline vasculature may facilitate histotrophic nourishment of the young embryo, it is quickly replaced by the allantois.

The placenta in the pig is **epitheliochorial**. The trophoblastic epithelium is in direct contact with the maternal uterine epithelium, although some allantoic capillaries may be interposed within the chorionic epithelium to permit more direct exchange across the uterine mucosa. Based on its shape and superficial appearance, the placenta is classified as **diffuse**.

As development proceeds, three zones develop on the chorionic surface, as shown in Figure 3.5*E*. The **placental zone** comprises the central one-half to two-thirds of the chorion. In this region the fetal chorion develops

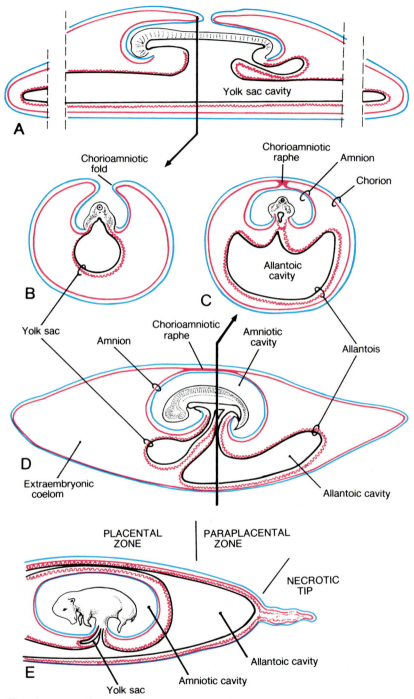

Figure 3.5. Development of extraembryonic membranes in the pig (continued from Figs. 2.16 and 2.17). *A* and *D* are schematic median views at the 10- and 25-somite stages (16 and 20 days of gestation); *B* and *C* are transverse sections at these stages. *E* illustrates the midfetal period. (Redrawn from BM Patten and B Carlson, 1974.)

transverse folds or ridges, which fit into similarly oriented grooves in the endometrium. The development of **microvilli** on the free surface of the chorionic trophoblast cells in the placental zone further expands the surface area of contact. These interdigitate with similarly developed microvilli on the endometrial epithelial cells.

Also prominent in the placental zone are **areolae**. These are shallow, cup-shaped indentations in the chorion that are located opposite the openings of uterine **endometrial glands** and facilitate histotrophic nutrition.

Peripheral to the placental zone are the **paraplacental zones** that consist of a smooth chorion without folds or areolae, giving this region a glistening appearance when examined grossly. The distal extremities of the chorion are markedly reduced in size, often appearing shriveled and dry; they may be colorless or brown. These comprise the **ischemic zones** or **necrotic tips** (Fig. 3.5*E*). Ischemia means lack of blood, and in these zones the allantois atrophies due to the occlusion of peripheral blood vessels.

By the end of the first third of gestation, the pig fetuses and their membranes have grown sufficiently that the ischemic zones of adjacent fetal membranes intertwine and fold into each other. This encroachment of adjacent fetal membranes on each other continues, so that by the end of the second third of gestation the paraplacental zones have adhered to each other. Ultimately, the peripheral borders of the placental zone become apposed, but there is no fusion of fetal vascular tissues between adjacent placentas.

At birth, the placental zone remains attached to the endometrium. Since the amnion is attached to the chorion over the fetus, at the mesamnion, each fetus must rupture its amnion and the fused paraplacental zone immediately before being born. Often a series of pigs will be born before the fetal membranes are shed from the uterus. As a rule, pigs are born without being covered by their amnion because of the persistent mesamnion.

In summary, the pig placenta is classified as a diffuse, epitheliochorial, adeciduate placenta that develops transverse folds in the placental zone.

Horse

(*Equus caballus*), gestation length: 335–345 days.

The equine blastocyst remains spherical as gastrulation occurs. During this stage, it reaches a diameter of 4–5 cm. Within the late blastocyst stage embryo, the yolk sac expands and attaches to the chorion on the side opposite to the embryo. This three-layered zone of apposition (yolk sac endoderm + fused somatic and splanchnic mesoderm + trophoblast) is called a trilaminar omphalopleure (Fig. 3.6). A large blood vessel, the **sinus terminalis**, forms circumferentially around this zone.

The attachment of yolk sac splanchnopleure to chorionic somatopleure establishes a **choriovitellinic placenta**, and this is the primary facilitator of maternal-fetal exchange during the first quarter of gestation in the horse. Histotrophic nutrients transported to the embryo by vitelline veins constitute the primary source of metabolites for the embryo during this period.

A band of elongated trophoblast cells adjacent to the sinus terminalis forms by the 5th week. This is the **chorionic girdle**. Endometrial glands in contact with this band become hypertrophic, forming **endometrial cups**, which contain trophoblast-derived gonadotropin-secreting cells. These large secretory cells atrophy around 150 days of gestation.

Coelom formation occurs around 13–16 days of gestation and is rapidly followed by the elevation and growth of folds of somatopleure over the embryo to form the amnion and chorion. Amniogenesis is completed by about 21 days and **no area of mesodermal fusion persists between the amnion and chorion**. Thus the extraembryonic coelom completely surrounds the amnion.

The allantois appears in the extraembryonic coelom at about this time (21 days). It expands in the extraembryonic coelom over the embryo and on all sides of the yolk sac. By 40 days of gestation, it has com-

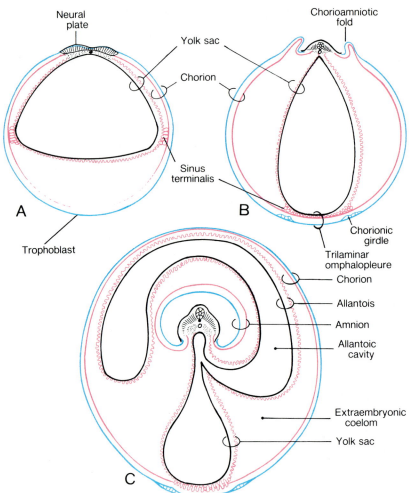

Figure 3.6. Schematic transverse views of the development of the equine extraembryonic membranes at *A*, 15 days; *B*, 18 days; and *C*, 30 days of gestation. Note the persistent attachment of the yolk sac to the abembryonic chorion.

pletely surrounded the yolk sac except for the zone of attachment of the yolk sac to chorion. Allantoic vessels then vascularize the somatic mesoderm of the chorion.

Apposition of the chorion to the endometrial epithelium occurs slowly over the first 7–10 weeks of gestation, and is not complete until about 14 weeks of gestation. There is no loss of maternal tissue; thus, the equine placenta is classified as **epitheliochorial**. Attachment is **diffuse**.

The area of placental contact is expanded by the development of tufts of branched **villi** on the chorion. They are distributed in clusters over the surface of the chorion and project into indentations on the endometrium known as **crypts** (kryptos = hidden). These clusters of fetal tissues are called **microcotyledons**, and are illustrated schematically, later, in Figure 3.8*C*. Microvilli develop both on the surface of the chorionic epithelial cells and on the endometrial epithelial cells; these interdigitate with each other to form the epitheliochorial attachment. This attachment does not compromise the endometrium, and thus the equine placenta is **adeciduate**. Between the microcotyledons are numerous areolae that facilitate absorption of histotrophe.

The mare is monotocous (single offspring

per pregnancy), with twins occurring in less than 1% of pregnancies. The expansion of one twin's placenta is often restricted by growth of the other's, and death of one or both twins in utero is common.

Several additional structures form in the equine fetal membranes and extraembryonic cavities. Starting at about 85 days of gestation, small, soft, usually flat amorphous structures can be found floating in the allantoic fluid. These white or brown masses are **allantoic calculi**, often referred to as **hippomanes**. They vary in size up to about 6 × 14 cm, and consist of a nucleus of cellular debris, probably derived from the endodermal epithelium of the fetal gut, surrounded by concentric deposits of mucoprotein, calcium, and phosphates. These calculi may form as the result of increased amounts of nitrogenous waste products being passed from the fetal kidneys into the allantois via the bladder, which develops in the proximal stalk of the allantois.

Following the 10th week of gestation, the inner surface of the amnion becomes covered with small, white, oval projections. These excrescences of ectodermal epithelium are called **amniotic plaques**, and they contain large amounts of glycogen. Their function is unknown, but they should be recognized as normal structures. Amniotic plaques are particularly prominent on that part of the amnion that covers the umbilical cord, but they are not found on the surface ectoderm of the embryo.

The quantity of both amniotic and allantoic fluids slowly increases throughout gestation. At term a greater volume is present in the allantoic cavity (8–15 liters) than the amniotic cavity (3–5 liters).

The umbilical cord is long in the horse due to the persistent attachment of the yolk sac to the abembryonic wall of the chorion. The proximal three-fifths of the cord is surrounded by amnion, the distal two-fifths by allantois. It varies in length from 50–100 cm and contains the rudimentary yolk sac and allantoic blood vessels. Many practitioners believe it is important for the health of the foal to allow the umbilical cord to remain attached for a few minutes following **parturition** (birth). This allows uterine contraction to force a large quantity of the placental blood present in the chorioallantoic vessels back through the umbilical veins and into the fetus.

Foals may be born covered by the amnion. The reason for this is that the equine amnion completely separates from the chorion. At parturition, after the chorioallantois covering the internal orifice of the uterus ruptures to release the allantoic fluid, the fetus remains attached to the chorion only by the base of the umbilical cord. The amnion does not need to rupture to allow birth of the foal. Even if it ruptures, the collapsed membrane may cover the head of the foal. If not removed by the mare or an attendant, this may result in suffocation of the neonate.

In summary, the equine chorioallantoic placenta is diffuse, epitheliochorial and adeciduate with villi present in tufts called microcotyledons. Amniotic plaques and allantoic calculi are present. The mesamnion does not persist.

Ruminants

Cow (*Bos taurus*), gestation length: 279–282 days.

Sheep (*Ovis aires*), gestation length: 148–150 days.

Goat (*Capra hircus*), gestation length: 150 days.

Except for differences in time and minor structural features, the development of the fetal membranes of domesticated ruminants is similar. After hatching, the blastocyst begins to elongate and, as gastrulation commences, this process occurs so rapidly that the trophoblast extends the entire length of the bovine uterine horn by 19 days. Later the fetal membranes will extend into the opposite uterine horn. In the ovine embryo, elongation of the blastocyst commences on the 12th day and continues through the 14th day at a rate estimated at up to 1 cm per hour.

In ruminants the yolk sac is functional for only a short period of time. Unlike the horse, apposition of the yolk sac splanchnopleure to chorionic somatopleure is transitory because the coelom forms and separates them at an early stage (17 days in sheep). The yolk sac is soon displaced by the developing allantois and degenerates, leaving no visible remnant at term.

Amniogenesis occurs between days 13 and 16 by folding of somatopleure. A mesodermal attachment zone persists between the amnion and chorion at the location where the folds fused dorsal to the embryo.

The allantois first appears in the extraembryonic coelom between days 14 and 21, usually on the right side of the embryo. It extends cranially and caudally along the lateral and ventral aspect of the embryo, and during the 4th week of gestation fills the extraembryonic coelom that now extends between the fetal membranes of each uterine horn. The allantois is shaped like an inverted "T," with the stem located where it passes through the umbilical cord (Fig. 3.7). It cannot pass over the dorsum of the embryo due

to the presence of a broad mesamnion. The allantois fuses with the chorion and much of the amnion.

The umbilical cord is short, consisting only of that portion of the allantoic stalk and blood vessels (two arteries and two veins) that is surrounded by amnion. Beginning at about 3 months of gestation, **amniotic plaques** develop on the amniotic ectoderm, including that covering the umbilical stalk.

Small ischemic zones occur at the poles of the fetal membranes. As in the pig, these regions of atrophied membranes are usually referred to as **necrotic tips**.

Close attachment to the endometrium first occurs during the 5th week of gestation in cattle, and 3rd week in sheep. The areas of fetal membrane attachment and villous development are not diffuse, as in the horse, but rather occur at discrete, specified sites within the uterus. These focal fetal-maternal appositions develop only at preexisting,

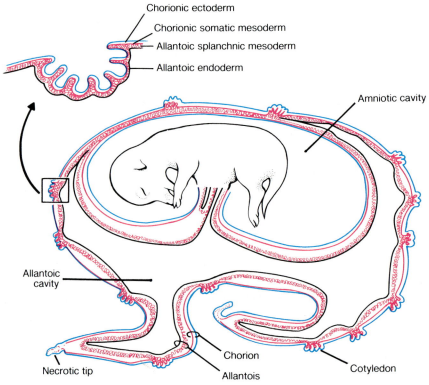

Chorionic ectoderm
Chorionic somatic mesoderm
Allantoic splanchnic mesoderm
Allantoic endoderm

Amniotic cavity

Allantoic cavity

Necrotic tip

Chorion

Allantois

Cotyledon

Figure 3.7.   The extraembryonic membranes of the cow. Cotyledons form at sites of association with maternal uterine caruncles.

oval-to-round elevations of endometrial mucosa, each of which is called a **uterine caruncle** or **endometrial pad**.

Uterine caruncles consist of subepithelial proliferations of connective tissue. They are a normal feature of nonpregnant animals as well. A total of approximately 75–120 caruncles are present in cattle, 80–100 in sheep. They are arranged in two dorsal and two ventral rows throughout the length of the uterine horns. When contacted by fetal membranes, they enlarge and form swellings with a convex surface in cattle, a concave surface in sheep.

Contact with a caruncle causes the fetal chorioallantoic membranes to develop villous processes. This region of specialization in the fetal tissue is termed a **cotyledon**. The villous processes extend into crypts that develop in the proliferating caruncle. A fetal cotyledon and a maternal caruncle together comprise a **placentome**, as illustrated in Figure 3.8.

The fetal chorioallantoic tissues in contact with each uterine caruncle undergo **hyperplasia** (increased cell proliferation) and **hypertrophy** (increased cell or tissue volume) as they form the cotyledon. Some of the cotyledons that develop over the dorsum of the fetus are chorioamniotic but are vascularized by allantoic blood vessels.

These bovine, ovine and caprine placentas are classified grossly as **cotyledonary** or placentomatous. In the region of loose apposition between the placentomes, there is only minimal villous development in the fetal membranes. Uterine **endometrial glands** are found in this intracaruncular area.

Despite considerable debate in the literature, it is now generally accepted that the histological structure of the chorion and maternal epithelium is preserved throughout gestation in the cow; thus, the bovine placenta is classified as **epitheliochorial**. In contrast, parts of the maternal epithelium are lost in sheep and goats; thus, these placentas

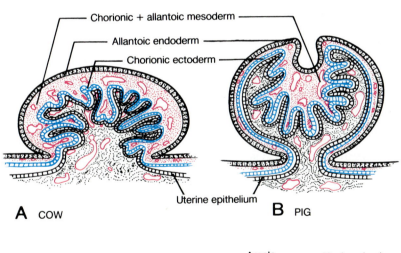

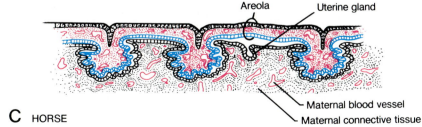

Figure 3.8. Placentomes of the *A*, cow; *B*, ewe; and *C*, horse. The microcotyledons of the horse are indistinct grossly, in contrast to the ruminant cotyledons that become apposed to large uterine caruncles. (Redrawn after SJ Roberts, 1971; and M Silver, et al., 1973.)

are **syndesmochorial**. In the ewe the maternal epithelium in the caruncle usually forms a syncytium as it proliferates.

Between 7 and 10 days following birth, the crypts within each caruncle undergo necrosis due to ischemia, and epithelial cells are sloughed. Thus, the ruminant placenta can be considered as **partially deciduate**. The uterine epithelium later heals over the regressing caruncle. Failure of the fetal cotyledons to separate from the caruncles following birth results in a retained placenta.

Calculi, consisting of protein and calcium oxalate, may be found floating free in either the amniotic or allantoic cavities, more commonly the latter. These are precipitates formed in a manner similar to those in the horse.

The amount and consistency of the extraembryonic fetal fluids varies with the period of gestation. In cattle the volume of allantoic fluid exceeds that of the amniotic fluid during the first third of gestation. This is reversed during the second third, but in the last third the volume of allantoic fluid is again greater, averaging 6–9 liters compared with 3–6 liters of fluid in the amniotic cavity.

During the first half of gestation, the fetal urine that is excreted into the bladder can pass directly into the allantoic cavity via the intraabdominal stalk of the allantois, the **urachus**. This extends from the apex of the developing bladder into the umbilical cord. Alternatively, fetal urine can exit via the cloacal opening into the amniotic fluid.

As a result, fluids in both cavities contain nitrogenous wastes. In the last 2–3 months of gestation, the development of a functional urethral sphincter in the bovine fetus prevents urine from entering the amniotic fluid and all of it passes into the allantoic fluid. Continual swallowing of the amniotic fluid allows nitrogenous wastes to be reabsorbed and then excreted into the allantois.

In contrast, in sheep there are higher levels of nitrogenous wastes in the amniotic fluid. This is due to a loss of patency of the fetal urachus and maintenance of flow through the urethra.

In summary, the bovine placenta is cotyledonary, epitheliochorial, and moderately deciduate, while in sheep and goats it is partially syndesmochorial. The placentome, consisting of a uterine caruncle and fetal cotyledon, is convex in cows and concave in other domestic ruminants.

Carnivores

Dog (*Canis familiaris*), gestation length: 63 days.

Cat (*Felis domestica*), gestation length: 60 days.

Ferret (*Mustela putorius furo*), gestation length: 41 days.

The precise time of initial placenta formation in dogs is controversial, because breeding time is a poor indicator of the actual time of fertilization. Many bitches will mate several days prior to ovulation, and sperm remain viable in the female tract for approximately a week. The presence of only noncornified epithelial cells in a vaginal smear is the best morphological indicator of time of ovulation. In an animal with induced ovulation, such as the cat, or one with a short estrus period, the ferret for example, this is less of a problem.

By the second week of gestation the canine blastocyst has entered the lumen of the uterus. Prior to apposition, which begins at about 14–17 days of gestation in the dog, 11–12 days in the cat and 12–14 days in the ferret, blastocysts move extensively within and between uterine horns. Gastrulation begins shortly before or during the time of initial contact between the oblong trophoblast and the uterine mucosa.

Extraembryonic mesoderm forms quickly, and in the dog the yolk sac splanchnopleure fuses with the chorionic somatopleure in a broad, longitudinal band located along the trophoblast opposite the position of the embryo. Later in gestation this attachment is broken down, except at either extremity, as shown in Figure 3.9. The yolk sac is vascularized by vitelline blood vessels and is functional well after the establishment of a chorioallantoic placenta in these animals. In the dog it persists until term as a clearly visible tubular structure extending throughout the length of the fetal membrane and attached at the poles (Figure 3.10).

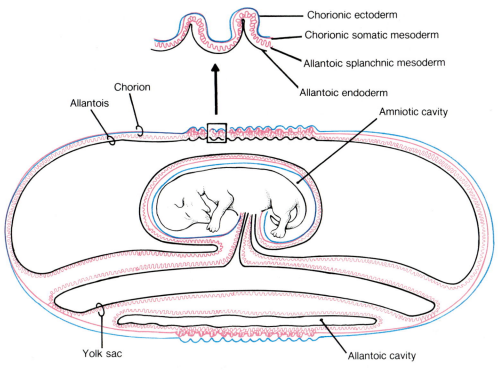

Figure 3.9. Extraembryonic membranes of the dog. The membranes of a cat would appear similar except that the yolk sac is less prominent.

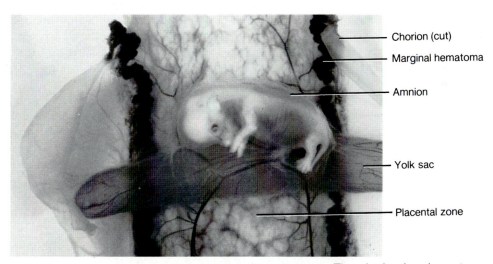

Figure 3.10. Photograph of a midterm canine fetus in utero. The chorion has been torn while opening the uterus.

Amniogenesis occurs by the folding of somatopleure (Fig. 3.11). Fusion of the folds is followed by a complete separation of the amniotic and chorionic mesoderm, so that the amnion-covered fetus floats free in the extraembryonic coelom. The allantois grows into and completely fills the extraembryonic coelom, except for the region of attachment of the yolk sac to the chorion. Calculi and amniotic plaques do not occur in these species.

Shortly before attachment, the tropho-

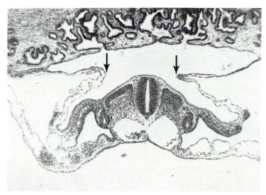

Figure 3.11. Transverse section through a 4-mm feline embryo to illustrate the formation of the amnion and chorion. *Arrows* indicate the chorioamniotic folds.

blast around the central third of the chorion proliferates and forms two distinct types of tissue. The cells adjacent to the chorionic mesoderm remain epithelial and are called **cytotrophoblast**. However, many cells located above the embryonic disk proliferate rapidly and form a syncytium superficial to the cytotrophoblast. This **syncytiotrophoblast** is highly invasive, and wherever it contacts the wall of the uterus the maternal epithelium and underlying connective tissues are destroyed. However, the maternal vascular endothelium remains intact; thus, the carnivore placenta is classified as **endotheliochorial**. Due to loss of maternal tissue during placentation, plus further sloughing at parturition, this placenta is **deciduate**.

The zone of attachment between the chorioallantois and maternal tissues forms a broad band located circumferentially around the central third of the chorion. This topographical arrangement accounts for the carnivore placenta being termed a **zonary placenta**. The zone of specialized attachment is circumferentially complete in dogs and cats, but incomplete in bears and mustelids (ferrets, skunks, weasels, mink).

When the chorioallantoic vasculature develops, it initially forms vascular channels within the cores of syncytio- and cytotrophoblast-covered villi. However, these villi subsequently coalesce to form vascular **labyrinths**. Thus, the mature carnivore placenta is **labyrinthine** rather than villous.

At the peripheral borders of the zonary placenta the maternal endothelium degenerates, which causes bleeding into the spaces surrounded by the labyrinth. These circumferential bands, illustrated in Figure 3.10, are called **marginal hematomas (hemophagous zones)**. Maternal venous drainage of these pools is minimal, but substances secreted by the chorionic epithelium prevent coagulation. This blood is thought to serve as a source of iron to the embryo. It is green in dogs and brown in cats, due to the different nature of the hemoglobin breakdown products. In the ferret and raccoon, the placental hematoma is situated centrally as a hemophagous sac rather than marginally.

The peripheral poles, each comprising about one-third of the fetal membrane surface, remain free of any structural change and are loosely apposed to the maternal epithelium. These **paraplacental areas** are considered to be nonfunctional. Fusion does not usually occur between fetal membranes of adjacent embryos.

Like the foal, the puppy and kitten have a tendency to be born completely surrounded by the amnion. Being unattached to the chorion, the amnion is free to pass out with the fetus during parturition. If it is not removed from around the head, suffocation may ensue.

In summary, the typical carnivore placenta is zonary, endotheliochorial, and deciduate. Neither calculi nor amniotic plaques form, but prominent hematomas are present. The yolk sac, which may be present as an elongated tube, is functional only briefly.

PRIMATE PLACENTAS
Human
(*Homo sapiens*), gestation length: 266 days.

During the 1st week after fertilization, the embryo floats free in the uterine lumen and is nourished by histotrophe. Between 7 and 9 days it attaches to one wall of the lumen and invades the endometrium, and by the 12th day endometrial epithelium adjacent to the site of invasion has surrounded the blastocyst (Fig. 3.12), completing the process of nidation.

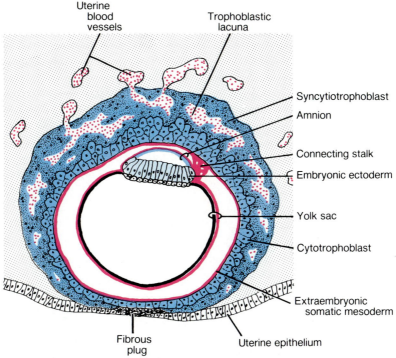

Figure 3.12. Human blastocyst of approximately 12 days of gestation. The process of nidation is nearly complete, and maternal blood vessels have been destroyed by the syncytiotrophoblast. Pools of maternal blood called trophoblastic lacunae are present within the syncytiotrophoblast. Note particularly the precocious formation of extraembryonic mesoderm. The embryo is attached to the chorion by a mesodermal connecting stalk, in which allantoic blood vessels are forming. (Redrawn from J Langman, 1981.)

In the human the inner cell mass remains deep to a layer of trophoblast, and the blastocyst maintains its oval shape. Amniogenesis occurs by **cavitation** within the inner cell mass. As a result a roof of cells, the **amniotic ectoderm**, is formed over the epiblast. During gastrulation, the migration of lateral mesoderm cells above the amniotic ectoderm completes formation of the **amnion**. Body folding further extends the amnion around and ventral to the embryo to the level of the umbilicus. The spread of lateral somatic mesoderm beneath the trophoblast forms the **chorion.**

The **yolk sac** is probably nonfunctional with respect to histotrophic absorption in the primate. It atrophies early and is not usually visible at term in the umbilical cord. The development of the **allantois** as a fluid-filled, epithelial-lined vesicle is similarly rudimentary. It develops only to the extent that allantoic blood vessels grow out from

the splanchnic mesoderm surrounding a hindgut diverticulum and invade the adjacent chorionic mesoderm. Subsequently, the amnion expands, eventually obliterating the extraembryonic coelom, and the amniotic and chorionic somatic mesodermal layers fuse. Although the fetal placental membranes are structurally **chorioamniotic**, they are functionally **chorioallantoic** based on the source of blood vessels.

Cell division is initially similar over the entire surface of the trophoblast. At the time of contact with the uterine wall the trophoblast directly apposed to the mucosal cells proliferates extensively to form a massive labyrinth of **syncytiotrophoblast** and underlying **cytotrophoblast**, all vascularized by allantoic vessels. This region develops into the **chorion frondosum** (leafy), in which chorionic villi become highly branched and then form a labyrinth (Fig. 3.13). The chorion adjacent to the endometrium on the sides

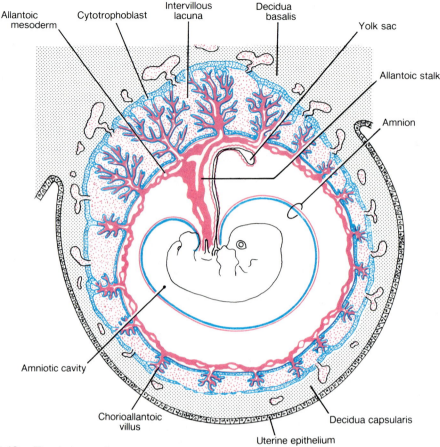

Figure 3.13. The human placenta at approximately 10 weeks of gestation. Large chorionic villi containing allantoic vessels have branched and become surrounded by intervillous lacunae, which are actually channels of maternal blood flow. The cytotrophoblast surrounding the villi degenerates, leaving only a thin layer of syncytiotrophoblast and allantoic vascular endothelium separating fetal from maternal circulatory systems. The umbilical cord is composed of vascular allantoic mesoderm and the vestigial yolk stalk. Later, the amnion expands and also surrounds the umbilical cord.

and abembryonic surfaces proliferates to a lesser extent and is referred to as the **chorion laeve** (smooth). In the zone of contact by the syncytial chorion frondosum there is a massive loss of endometrial tissues, **including the maternal vascular endothelium**. Thus, free blood circulates through and bathes the labyrinth of the chorion. This is structurally and physiologically arranged in such a way that blood is pumped from uterine arteries into the intervillous lacunae lined by chorionic labyrinth and it is drained via uterine veins, insuring a continuous circulation. This is a **hemochorial placenta**.

Cytological changes termed the **decidual reaction** occur in the connective tissues of the endometrium. Three regions of decidual areas are defined. The area apposed to the chorion frondosum is the decidua basalis and that apposed to the chorion laeve is the decidua capsularis. With growth of the embryo and placenta, the lumen of the uterus is soon obliterated and the endometrial decidua capsularis fuses with the endometrial tissue on the opposite side, which is called the decidua parietalis.

The placentome, consisting of the chorion frondosum and the decidua basalis, is oval or disk shaped. This **discoidal placenta** averages 15–20 cm in diameter and 2–3 cm thick. Since loss of the entire endometrium occurs, this is a **deciduate placenta**.

Monkey

(*Macaca mulatta*, rhesus monkey), gestation length: 160 days.

Many species differences exist in extraembryonic membrane formation and placentation among the different groups of primates. Amniogenesis occurs by cavitation if the inner cell mass remains covered by trophoblast, as in man, apes and monkeys. If the embryonic disk is uncovered, as occurs in some lower forms of primates, the amnion is formed by folding.

In the rhesus monkey the yolk sac degenerates early and is probably nonfunctional. Similarly the allantois is vestigial as an endodermal sac, but allantoic blood vessels grow into the somatic mesoderm that attaches the embryo to the adjacent chorionic somatic mesoderm. The amnion expands to obliterate the extraembryonic coelom and fuse with the chorion.

In contrast to the situation in humans, the developing embryo does not undergo nidation, but remains in the lumen of the uterus and attaches to the endometrium at two sites. Usually a pair of **discoid placentomes**, one on each side of the uterine lumen, forms following destruction of the endometrium by syncytiotrophoblast tissues. At the sites of this trophoblastic invasion, there is loss of maternal tissue down through the level of the vascular endothelium, so that free blood circulates throughout the villous development. Thus the **double discoid placenta** is **hemochorial** and **deciduate**.

PLACENTAS OF LABORATORY ANIMALS

Fetal membrane formation and placentation in laboratory animals, including a lagomorph (rabbit), and several rodents, are strikingly different from the other mammalian orders and are similar to one another. Variations between the placentas of these animals are roughly correlated with species differences in the initial rate of development (Table 3.3), which increase progressively from the rabbit to the rat, mouse and guinea pig.

Initial contact between the developing

Table 3.3.
Gestation Period of Laboratory Animals

Animal	Days
Mouse	18–21
Hamster	15
Rat	22–23
Gerbil	24–26
Guinea pig	63–70
Rabbit	30–32

mouse embryo and the uterine mucosa involves the abembryonic trophoblast and the epithelial lining of a **uterine crypt**, which is a deep furrow in the endometrium (Fig. 3.14*A*). Following contact, the surrounding endometrial tissue swells. This decidual reaction causes the lips of the furrow to close partially around the embryo. This is referred to as the **egg cylinder** stage of development.

Concomitantly, the trophoblast overlying the embryonic disc proliferates to form the syncytial **ectoplacental cone** (trager), which has degradative properties similar to the syncytiotrophoblast of carnivores and primates. Thus, the murine embryo undergoes nidation and establishes an **interstitial** attachment. While rabbit embryos also form an interstitial attachment, they remain in the uterine lumen and are not enclosed in the wall of the uterus.

The cavity between the ectoplacental cone and the epiblastic surface of the embryo is the **ectoplacental cavity**. Later, extraembryonic somatopleure will develop folds across this cavity to establish the amnion and chorion (Fig. 3.14*C*). In addition to forming an ectoplacental cone the rodent is unique in that the surface of the epiblast is curved, with the cranial and caudal margins close to one another. This condition, which results from the blastocyst being in a narrow furrow, persists until after the neurula stage, at which time the body axis straightens.

In all of these laboratory animals, the hypoblast (yolk sac endoderm not surrounded by splanchnic mesoderm) expands precociously, and becomes apposed to the trophoblast (Fig. 3.15). Together this pair of epithelial membranes is called a **bilaminar omphalopleure**. Mesoderm does not invade this zone of apposition.

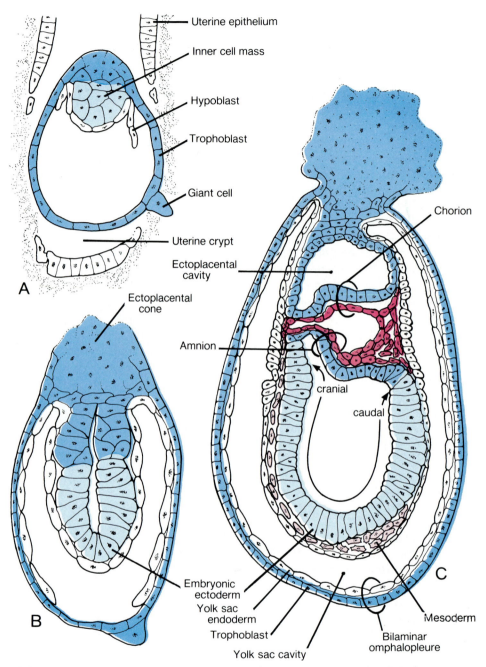

Figure 3.14.   The developing mouse embryo at *A*, 4.5 days; *B*, 5.5 days; and *C*, 7 days of gestation. In *A* the epithelial lining of the uterine crypt has been eroded. *B* and *C* show the egg cylinder stage. Note the formation of the ectoplacental cone and the bilaminar omphalopleure. The embryo is folded so that the cranial and caudal ends of the neural plate are close together. (Redrawn after GD Snell, 1941.)

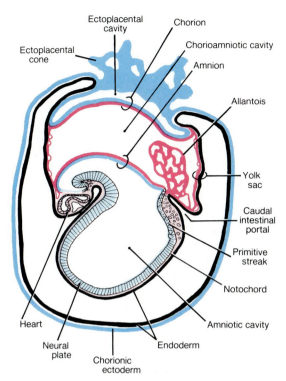

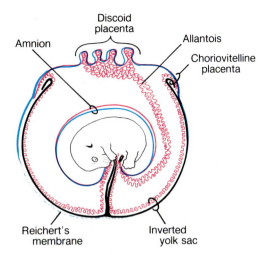

Figure 3.16. The mouse fetus and extraembryonic membranes at midterm. The bilaminar omphalopleure has degenerated except for an acellular remnant, Reichert's membrane. This leaves the inverted yolk sac in contact with maternal tissues. The discoidal chorioallantoic placenta is well developed.

Figure 3.15. The 7½-day mouse embryo, shown in a median view. Neurulation is occurring at this time, and the vascular allantoic mesoderm is expanding. (Redrawn after GD Snell, 1941.)

Continued expansion of the extraembryonic endoderm results in a collapse of the yolk sac, which brings the opposite layer of endoderm onto the bilaminar omphalopleure. In rabbits the latter then degenerates, leaving the single layer of everted endoderm, which is accompanied by splanchnic mesoderm, directly in contact with maternal uterine tissues. This is now called an **inverted yolk sac placenta** (Fig. 3.16).

In most rodents an acellular remnant of the trophoblast called Reichert's membrane persists between uterine blood and the inverted yolk sac. In the guinea pig, the inverted yolk sac forms precociously by an early loss of trophectoderm and replacement by the single layer of original delaminated yolk sac endoderm.

An inverted yolk sac placenta is not the same as a **choriovitelline** placenta, which occurs when the splanchnic mesoderm-covered yolk sac endoderm becomes apposed to the chorion. Such an arrangement is seen around the edge of the yolk sac in these laboratory animals.

The inverted yolk sac placenta is the principal mediator of nutrient transfer during the major stages of organogenesis in rodents and lagomorphs. Many studies have shown that the physiological properties of this placenta are significantly different from those of the chorioallantoic placenta, which forms later in rodents as a result of invasion of allantoic splanchnic mesoderm beneath the chorion. Thus, while rodents are usually the animal of choice as a first test for possible teratogenic effects of a new drug or food additive, they cannot safely be used as the only animal model.

The amnion is free from any attachment to the adjacent chorion in these laboratory animals. The allantoic vesicle is rudimentary. Shortly after contact is made between the lining of the uterine crypt and the bilaminar omphalopleure, large, so-called **giant cells**, derived from trophoblast initiate erosion of the uterine tissues, including the vascular endothelium. Thus, beginning at the inverted yolk sac stage, a **hemochorial** relationship is established.

Later, a tuft of vascularized splanchnic mesoderm grows out of the caudal part of the embryo and attaches to the somatic mesoderm of the chorion overlying the embryo adjacent to the ectoplacental cone. As a result of both the uterine decidual reaction and growth of the embryo, the lumen of the uterus becomes occluded. Following fusion of the two apposed endometrial layers, the ectoplacental tissue and allantoic vessels invade the mesenteric uterine wall, as shown in Figure 3.17. Together they form a **discoid placentome**. Thus, a **hemochorial, chorioallantoic** placenta is also established. This region has a labyrinthine vascular network. Subsequently, endometrial tissues grow beneath the yolk sac placenta, and a new uterine lumen is established.

In summary, lab rodents and rabbits establish two types of hemochorial placentas, an inverted yolk sac and, later, a discoidal, labyrinthine chorioallantoic placenta. During early stages of nidation, lab rodents are arched ventrally (hyperextended), and do not straighten until neurulation is completed.

MALFORMATIONS AND DYSFUNCTIONS

Hydrops

Occasionally, excessive amounts of fluid accumulate in either the amniotic or allantoic cavity. This is termed a **hydrops** condition. Hydrops of the amnion (**hydramnios**) with increased fluid volume of 8–10 times normal is usually associated with some fetal malformation that interferes with its ability to swallow. The condition develops gradually during the last few months of gestation. Hydrops of the allantois, **hydrallantois**, with 10–40 times the normal allantoic fluid volume (up to 50 gallons), is more often associated with some disease of the placenta, causing a vascular disturbance in the endometrium and/or chorioallantois. Hydrallantois may occur anytime during mid or late gestation and may progress rapidly, requiring prompt diagnosis and treatment.

Amniotic Bands

Neonates are occasionally presented either with parts of the amnion attached to

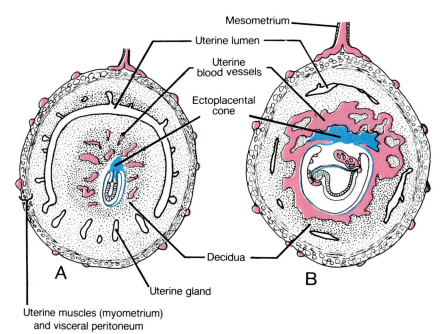

Figure 3.17. Schematic transverse sections through the uterine tube of the mouse to illustrate the extensive dicidual reactions in this tissue and subsequent occlusion of the uterine lumen. At later stages the chorioallantoic placenta will develop on the mesenteric side of the uterine tube, and a lumen will be reformed antimesenterically. (Redrawn after GD Snell, 1941.)

embryonic structures, most commonly the central nervous system or limbs, or with the distal parts of appendages showing evidence of chronic constriction. These result from amniotic folds or fibrous bands of amnion becoming incorporated into or entwined around embryonic structures. Affected limbs may be partially amputated if the fibrous **amniotic bands** form complete constrictions.

Bibliography

Note: All texts on theriogenology or reproduction of domesticated animals discuss the physiology of the placenta and will provide further references.

Hafez ESE: *Reproduction in Farm Animals*, ed 4. Philadelphia, Lea & Febiger, 1980.

Hughes PE, Varley MA: *Reproduction in the Pig*. Boston, Butterworths, 1980.

Kaafman P, King BF: Structural and functional organization of the placenta. *Bibl Anat* 22, 1982.

Liban E, Abramovici A: Fetal membrane adhesions and congenital malformations. In Klingberg MA, Abramovici A, Chemke J (eds): *Drugs and Fetal Development*. New York, Plenum Press, 1972, pp 337–350.

Moor RM, Allen WR, Hamilton DW: Origin and histogenesis of equine endometrial cups. *J Reprod Fertil Suppl* 23:391–396, 1975.

Ramsey EM: *The Placenta: Human and Animal*. New York, Praeger Publ, 1982.

Ramsey EM: *The Placenta of Laboratory Animals and Man*. New York, Holt, Rinehart & Winston, 1975.

Roberts SJ: *Veterinary Obstetrics and Genital Diseases*, ed 2. Ann Arbor, MI, Edwards Brothers, 1971.

Silver M, Steven DH, Comline RS: Placental exchange and morphology in ruminants and mare. In Comline RS, Cross KW, Dawes GS, Nathanielsz PW (eds) *Foetal and Neonatal Physiology*. London, Cambridge University Press, 1973, pp 245–271.

Snell GD: *The Early Embryology of the Mouse*. Philadelphia, Blakiston, 1941.

Concepts and Mechanisms of Development

The preceding chapters have described the formation of a multicellular blastula from a single-celled zygote, and the transformation of this blastula first into a trilaminar gastrula and then into a young embryo that has many recognizable vertebrate characteristics. The experiments presented in this chapter introduce some of the mechanisms by which these complex, integrated events are controlled. With only minor variations these mechanisms operate during the formation and initial differentiation of all organs in the vertebrate embryo.

DEFINITIONS

The following processes operate during early developmental stages.

Growth

Growth is an increase in the size or number of cells in the whole or any part of the organism. During cleavage stages, blastomeres divide rapidly but there is little or no net increase in the volume of the embryo because the size of the blastomeres becomes progressively reduced. With the onset of gas-

trulation and, especially in mammals, the formation of extraembryonic membranes, the size of the organism increases greatly. To a large extent this is brought about by spreading of epithelial sheets (Fig. 4.1*A*) and dispersal of mesenchymal populations. Later in development growth occurs also by the deposition of extracellular materials, such as the matrices surrounding chondrocytes and osteocytes, or by the formation of cell specializations such as neuronal processes and the myelin sheaths surrounding them.

Morphogenesis

Morphogenesis includes any change in the shape or location of a cell or tissue. Examples of **morphogenetic movements** during gastrulation are expansion of the epiblast and involution at the primitive streak, both described in Chapter 2. Neural tube closure, heart tube fusion and bending of the cardiac loop, and formation of the optic vesicle are some of the morphogenetic events associated with the neurula stage. In most situations morphogenesis involves foldings and specializations of epithelial tissues (Fig. 4.1), processes which are usually dependent on adjacent mesenchymal tissues.

Patterning

Patterning is the establishment of programmed subsets of cells in proper relation to each other and to surrounding tissues. Examples of patterning are the positioning of feathers or hair in the skin and of teeth in the oral cavity or the locating and shaping of bones and muscles in a limb. This process usually occurs prior to overt differentiation

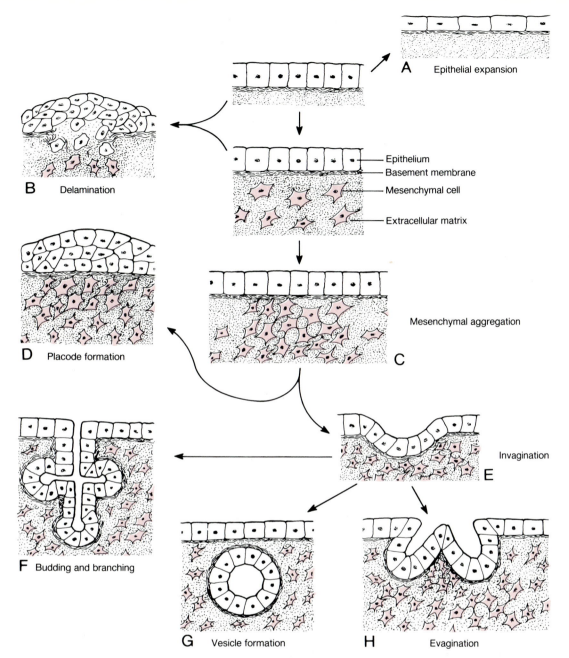

Figure 4.1. Morphogenetic changes exhibited by epithelial and mesenchymal tissues during early embryonic development. *A*, epithelial expansion; example: epiblast expansion during gastrulation. *B*, delamination, in which the basement membrane underlying an epithelium breaks down and cells leave to become mesenchymal; examples: formation of hypoblast and, later, mesoderm from the primitive streak. *C*, mesenchymal aggregation occurs when subpopulations of cells within a mesenchyme become more densely packed together than their neighbors; examples: the initial stages of formation of hair, feathers, teeth, and most skeletal tissues. *D*, placode formation refers to any focal thickening of the surface ectoderm, often in response to an underlying mesenchymal aggregation. *E*, invagination is an infolding of an epithelium, and is often the first stage in a more complex morphogenetic reorganization. *F*, branching is a method of rapidly increasing the surface area of an epithelium, as occurs during the early development of most secretory glands and the lungs. *G*, Vesicle formation occurs when an invaginated tissue separates from the original epithelium; examples: development of the neural tube and lens. *H*, evagination is an outward folding or elevation of an epithelium. The optic vesicles are evaginations from the prosencephalic walls; also, many specialized tissues of the integument, including teeth, will display focal evaginations.

of cells, such as the appearance of keratin or enamel proteins in skin or dental epithelia. The first visible sign of feather or tooth formation is the appearance of discrete condensations in the mesenchyme immediately adjacent to the epithelia, followed shortly by a focal thickening in the epithelium (Fig. 4.1 D and E). The positions at which these mesenchymal aggregations initially form is patterned, not random, and reflects a programming within the mesenchyme. How this programming occurs is not known.

A more complex patterning occurs in the development of musculoskeletal systems, such as the axial system, the face and jaws, and limbs. Shortly after the end of neurulation, the precursors of forelimb and hind limb structures appear as pairs of epithelial-covered mesenchymal swellings called **limb buds**, which are located on the dorsolateral margin of the embryo (see Figs. 1.3 and 1.6J, also Chapter 10). If, as shown in Figure 4.2, mesenchyme from the wing bud of a chick embryo is removed and replaced with leg bud mesenchyme from a duck embryo, a limb having the gross appearance of a duck's

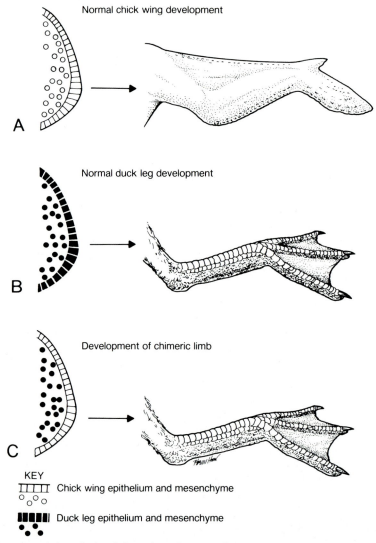

KEY

⊥⊥⊥⊥⊥ Chick wing epithelium and mesenchyme
° ° °

▮▮▮▮▮ Duck leg epithelium and mesenchyme
 • • •

Figure 4.2. Experimental analysis of the roles of mesenchyme and epithelium in patterning of avian limbs. In A and B the two components are separated and then recombined; the resulting limbs are normal. In C, chick wing epithelium has been combined with mesenchyme from the leg bud of a duck; the resulting limb closely resembles a duck's leg.

leg develops in the chick thoracic region. Thus, the information for **patterning** of a complex set of structures was present in the primordium in advance of the formation of any particular tissues.

Cytodifferentiation

Cytodifferentiation is the complex, often tortuous, process by which each cell or cell line attains and expresses a stable phenotype. This process usually occurs over the course of many cell generations, with some of these generations of cells expressing intermediate characteristics.

While the terminal stage of cytodifferentiation is usually easy to define, the starting time is problematical. Some workers define the onset of cytodifferentiation as the time of initial appearance of tissue-specific macromolecules, such as hemoglobin in a hematopoeitic cell line, neurofilaments in a neuron, or amylase in a pancreatic cell line. While this definition is adequate for the expressive phase of a cell's development, it does not encompass earlier stages, during which time a cell may be producing molecules necessary for its embryonic development but different from those of its final phenotype.

Although the actual genetic events marking the onset of cytodifferentiation are not known, it is well established that during early cleavage stages each of the blastomeres has the capability of forming a complete embryo. This was first shown by Hans Driesch near the end of the last century. He placed sea urchin embryos at the two-, four-, and eight-cell stages in flasks containing sea water and shook them until the blastomeres separated from one another. Some blastomeres survived this trauma and, quite unexpectedly, gave rise to small but otherwise normal sea urchin larvae. Thus, at least through the eight-cell stage all blastomeres are identical in their ability to form an entire organism. The same has recently been shown to be true in mammals, and microsurgical separation of blastomeres is being used in conjunction with embryo transplantation to increase the number of progeny from selected breeding stock.

Embryonic cells lose their totipotency during early development. Exactly when this occurs varies depending upon the species and the cell type. In mammals the first visible difference between cell types occurs with the formation of the morula, at which time some blastomeres are located internally and are entirely surrounded by surface blastomeres. However, it has been shown that if the position of any of these blastomeres is experimentally altered, the cell will develop in accordance with its new position. In other words, all the blastomeres are equipotential during early cleavage stages of mammals.

The same is not true by the blastocyst stage. Cells located in the inner cell mass are capable of forming trophoblast if their position is surgically altered, but trophoblast cells have by this stage lost the ability to develop as part of the inner cell mass. By the expanded blastocyst stage, only a few hours later, inner cell mass cells have also become restricted and lost their ability to form certain extraembryonic tissues.

This pattern of gradual, incremental restriction continues as development proceeds. Experimental analyses have shown that once the three germ layers are formed, each has different developmental potentials than the others. Shortly thereafter the first specific cell lines are delineated, including cardiac muscle and blood cells, notochordal cells, somites, and neural cells.

In thinking about these four developmental processes one must appreciate that all are interrelated and, usually, interdependent. It is not the embryo but the embryologist who for convenience separates these four aspects of development. Consider, for example, the development of the mammalian forelimbs. Both are the same length but are mirror images (growth, morphogenesis). The arrangements of cartilages and bone, muscles, nerves and blood vessels, and specializations of the integuments are species-specific but at the same time share major features with members of the same order, family and class (patterning, cytodifferentiation). A genetic or teratogenic insult that disrupts any one of these processes will inevitably cause secondary alterations in all of them.

TISSUE INTERACTIONS

During the gastrula, neurula, and early organogenesis stages, interactions continuously occur between adjacent tissues. These interactions are necessary for the subsequent development of one or all of the tissues involved.

Lens Induction

Shortly after the turn of the century Hans Spemann, a German embryologist who later received the Nobel prize for his research, asked whether the presence of the optic vesicle immediately beneath the surface ectoderm at the future site of lens formation (Fig. 1.6*F*) was in some way necessary for the lens to form. This was, in fact, the first time that the possibility of a **causal relationship** between two events was investigated. He tested his theory by removing the optic vesicle from an amphibian embryo before it contacted the presumptive lens-forming surface ectoderm, as outlined in Figure 4.3. As a result, no lens formed at this site. This was the first demonstration that the action of one tissue, or at least its physical presence, is necessary for the development of another tissue. The mechanism underlying this phenomenon was called **induction**, and the theory of **inductive tissue interactions** has been an essential concept in development ever since.

More recently it has been found that the optic vesicle is not the only tissue to influence the presumptive lens epithelium. During amphibian gastrulation the presumptive lens epithelium is underlain first by endodermal cells that will form the pharynx, and later by presumptive cardiac mesoderm that is shifting towards the ventral midline. To investigate whether these tissues in any way affect the development of the presumptive lens epithelium, each of these tissues was recombined in vitro with this area of surface ectoderm.

The results, outlined in Table 4.1, illustrate two important aspects of tissue inter-

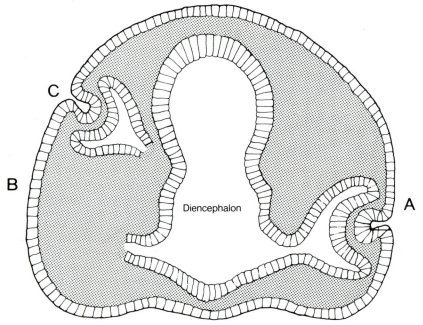

Figure 4.3. Examination of the possible role of the optic vesicle in formation of the lens. *A* shows the normal relationship between these two structures; the lateral wall of the optic vesicle invaginates at the same time as the lens placode invaginates, approximately a day after close contact between the two tissues is established. At *B* the optic vesicle was removed prior to having contacted the surface ectoderm; as a result, no lens forms. If the optic vesicle is placed at an ectopic site, as shown in *C*, an ectopic lens will form. (Redrawn from Wessells NK: *Tissue Interactions and Development.* Menlo Park, CA. Benjamin, 1977.)

Table 4.1.
Tissue Interactions Affecting Lens Development[a]

Tissues in culture	Percentage of cases in which lenses formed
PLE[b] alone	0
PLE + optic vesicle	28
PLE + pharyngeal endoderm	31
PLE + heart mesoderm	14
PLE + endoderm + heart mesoderm	42
PLE + heart mesoderm + optic vesicle	71

[a] After Jacobson A, 1966 and personal communication.
[b] PLE, presumptive lens epithelium.

action. First, inductive interactions are not a singular event, but rather a series of events. Frequently the effects of these interactions are cumulative. Second, inductive interactions may occur long before the final expression of a cell's phenotype. In most cases the molecular effects of each interaction in a sequential series are unknown.

Skin

The integument has been a useful tissue with which to study tissue interactions, because the structures formed by the ectodermal epithelium vary markedly from one region to another. In birds these include different types of feathers, scales on the legs and feet, the beak, the comb and the wattle. The results of recombining embryonic dermal mesenchyme from one region with surface ectoderm of a different site are summarized in Figure 4.4. The structures formed by surface ectoderm are those appropriate to the original location of the underlying mesenchyme. These data reveal that not only is the pattern of epithelial differentiation controlled by the underlying mesenchyme, as discussed under Definitions, but also the types of structures formed.

The range of specialized cell types that surface ectoderm is capable of forming is restricted both by its ontogenetic and phylogenetic histories. It will not, for example, form kidney (mesodermal) or intestinal (endodermal) type cells when grafted adjacent

to the appropriate inducing tissues. These capabilities have been lost during earlier stages. Furthermore, it is not capable of forming tissues not within its genetic repertoire. Avian ectoderm will form rudimentary feathers but not hair when cocultured with mammalian dermis.

A most startling and controversial exception to this is the reported ability of avian oral epithelium to form enamel-producing tooth tissues when grafted adjacent to mouse oral mesenchyme. These data suggest that modern birds have retained the genes coded for enamel proteins for over 100 million years, and that the inductive stimuli emanating from murine oral mesenchyme can elicit this long-quiescent response.

Gut

Many tissue interactions are less consistent than those affecting surface ectoderm. Endoderm forms the lining of most of the gut and associated organs and, beginning at gastrulation, is surrounded by splanchnic mesoderm. If the primordium of the pancreas, which develops from gut endoderm immediately caudal to the stomach, is isolated from mesenchyme it fails to undergo morphogenesis (branching) and cytodifferentiation (appearance of amylase and insulin-secreting cells). When either pancreatic mesenchyme or that from some other gland, such as the lung or salivary gland, is combined with the epithelial rudiment, normal pancreatic development occurs. Both the pattern of branching and the type of cytodifferentiation of the epithelial tissue is characteristically pancreatic, i.e. these properties are programmed within the endodermal tissue.

The development of most internal, glandular organs has been examined using these methods. In a few cases, including the lung, stomach and mammary gland, heterologous mesenchyme can alter the normal course of epithelial differentiation. For example, avian gizzard epithelium combined with proventricular (gastric) mesoderm will develop gastric glands, which indicates that mesoderm can alter the programming of endodermal tissues in certain situations. The importance

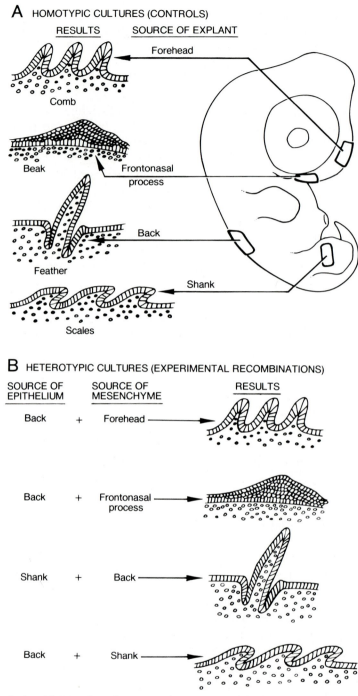

A HOMOTYPIC CULTURES (CONTROLS)

RESULTS   SOURCE OF EXPLANT

Forehead

Comb

Beak

Frontonasal
process

Back

Feather

Shank

Scales

B HETEROTYPIC CULTURES (EXPERIMENTAL RECOMBINATIONS)

SOURCE OF   SOURCE OF   RESULTS
EPITHELIUM   MESENCHYME

Back   +   Forehead

Back   +   Frontonasal
             process

Shank   +   Back

Back   +   Shank

Figure 4.4. Analysis of interactions between dermal mesenchyme and epidermal epithelium in the development of integumentary structures. In series *A*, explants containing both mesenchyme and overlying epithelium were explanted, and they subsequently developed features appropriate to the location from which they were originally taken. In series *B*, mesenchyme from one region was combined with epithelium from another. In all cases the pattern of subsequent development was directed by the mesenchyme.

of these data is 2-fold. First they illustrate the broad range of phenomena encompassed by the term inductive tissue interaction. In some instances the mesenchyme appears to direct or instruct the developing epithelial component; in others it plays a permissive role. In many situations there is a reciprocal exchange between adjacent tissues.

The second important message from these results is that at the stages during which many of these interactions are occurring, one, and possibly both, of the components are already programmed. In the case of the integument, the dermal mesenchyme contains necessary information to pattern itself and the overlying ectoderm. In the case of the pancreas, one specific part of a cytologically homogeneous endodermal tube was specified to form a pancreas, and would develop as such so long as there was an environment that was permissive. In other words, some parts of the gut endodermal tube are inherently patterned, most of the surface ectoderm is not. Clearly, these interactions do not represent the initial step in the development of either the skin or the gut. Rather, they are but one of a series of programming events, a series that must have begun at earlier stages of development.

Primary Induction

Primary induction refers to events occurring during blastula and gastrula stages that lead to the formation of axial tissues (neural plate, paraxial mesoderm, notochord). The term dates back to the early 1920s and an experiment performed by Hilda Mangold, a graduate student working with Spemann. She transplanted pieces of tissue between two species of salamander embryos, one whose cells contained granules of pigment and one without pigment granules. This allowed her to histologically distinguish donor from host tissues in the chimeric embryo. The tissue to be transplanted was excised from the edge of the blastopore, which is a region homologous to the primitive node of a bird or mammal gastrula. As shown in Figures 4.5A and 4.6 it was implanted into

the blastocoel of a host embryo, where it subsequently became apposed to the ventral wall of the abdomen.

The results of this elegant experiment, illustrated in Figure 4.5 B and C, were 2-fold. First, the grafted tissue underwent **self-differentiation**; the transplanted cells formed notochord, somite and spinal cord tissues, the same as they would have done had they not been transplanted to an ectopic (displaced) location. These results indicate that cells originally located adjacent to the blastopore are already programmed to develop along specific pathways of development.

The second and more remarkable result was that the adjacent host tissues, which normally would have formed the ventral wall of the abdomen, developed into an ectopic but complete axial system, including a neural tube, spinal ganglia, somites, intermediate mesoderm, and even a second gut. All these structures develop as a result of placing a fragment of presumptive notochordal and adjacent tissues into the blastocoel.

This experiment, more than any other single discovery in embryology, changed the course of developmental research. Spemann called the implanted piece the "organizer" because it clearly altered the growth, morphogenesis, patterning and cytodifferentiation of all surrounding tissues. It was soon discovered that structures characteristic of different axial levels (forebrain, hindbrain, spinal cord, etc.) could be obtained if cells rimming the blastopore were excised and transplanted at different stages. This is analogous to excising the avian node region at different stages of primitive streak elongation and regression.

There followed an intense pursuit to purify and identify the organizer. One group got positive results implanting proteins into the blastocoel, another claimed to prove that it was a nucleic acid, and others got partial responses by implanting toxic substances into the blastocoel. Another student of Spemann's implanted a piece of boiled blastopore tissue into the blastocoel and got a positive reaction. This led to the very in-

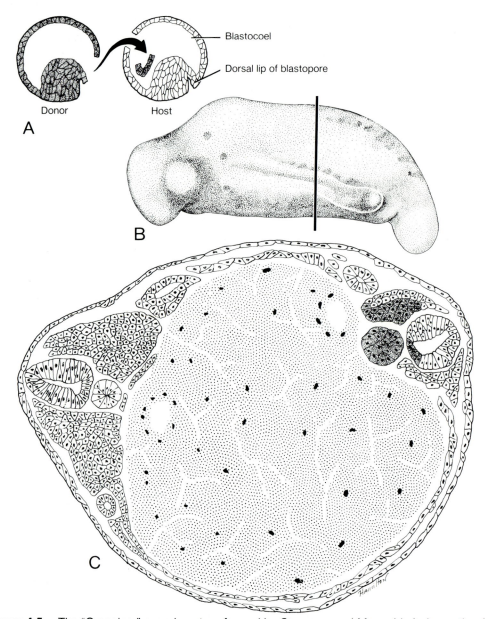

Figure 4.5. The "Organizer" experiment performed by Spemann and Mangold. *A* shows the design of the experiment, in which a piece of the dorsal edge of the blastopore was grafted from a pigment-rich donor to the blastocoel of an unpigmented host. *B* is a lateral view and *C* a transverse section at the region indicated showing the results of this transplant. In *C* the normal host axial structures are on the left. On the right is a complete supernumerary set of axial structures. Some of these are formed by grafted (pigmented) cells; others, however, have developed from host tissues that would normally have formed only superficial ventral abdominal tissues.

sightful but often ignored statement, "A dead organizer is a contradiction in terms." (Spemann, 1938).

Only in the past few years has the importance of this last experiment become recognized. The information to form a neural tube, somites, etc., resides not in the stimulus, but is an inherent component of the **responding** tissues. Belly ectoderm and mesoderm do not form ectopic spinal cord and somite tissues because they are **instructed** to do so, but because they are **permitted** to do

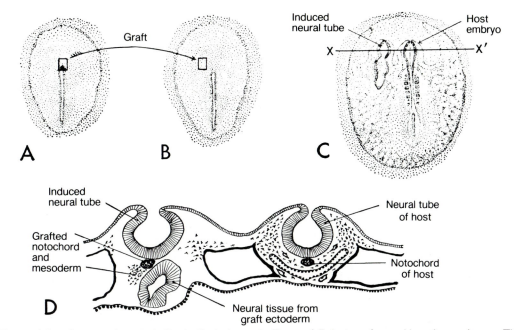

Figure 4.6. An experiment similar to that shown in Figure 4.5, but performed in avian embryos. The results are comparable. (From BM Patten and B Carlson, 1974, based on the work of CH Waddington and GA Schmitt, 1933.)

so, i.e. these ventral tissues have the same programming as do dorsal axial tissues but they normally do not express it. Only the particular regional characteristics of the response depend upon information within the stimulus.

Putting these data into the context of normal embryogenesis, it is clear that during the morphogenetic movements described in Chapter 2 (blastulation, gastrulation) there also occur interactions between developing surface epiblast and underlying mesenchyme, particularly the primordia of the notochord and paraxial mesoderm. As a result of these interactions one part of the surface ectoderm becomes uniquely programmed to form neural tissue, with various craniocaudal regions specified. Paraxial mesoderm becomes committed to form metameric somites, and the mesoderm in the midline condenses to form notochord. The subsequent development of the nervous, muscular and skeletal systems depends largely upon these early interactions. The molecular basis for the programming and expression of these morphogenetic and patterning processes, which are fundamental features in the development of all vertebrates, is unknown.

Bibliography

DEVELOPMENTAL MECHANISMS

Balinsky GI: *An Introduction to Embryology*, ed 3. Philadelphia, Saunders, 1970.

Bodemer CW: *Modern Embryology*. New York, Holt, Rinehart, Winston, 1968.

Browder LW: *Development Biology*. Philadelphia, Saunders, 1980.

Davenport R: *An Outline of Animal Development*. Reading, MA, Addison Wesley, 1979.

Deucher EM: *Cellular Interactions in Animal Development*. New York, Wiley, 1975.

Fleischmajer R, Billingham RE: *Epithelial-Mesenchymal Interactions*. Baltimore, Williams & Wilkins, 1968.

Grant P: *Biology of Developing Systems*. New York, Holt, Rinehart, Winston, 1978.

Hopper AF, Hart NH: *Foundations of Animal Development*. New York, Oxford University Press, 1980.

Karp G, Berrill NJ: *Development*, ed 2. New York, McGraw-Hill, 1981.

Sawyer RH, Fallon JF (eds): *Epithelial-Mesenchymal Interactions in Development*. New York, Praeger Publishers, 1983.

Wessells NK: *Tissue Interactions and Development*. Menlo Park, CA, Benjamin, 1977. (The most readable introduction to developmental mechanisms.)

LENS DEVELOPMENT

Jacobson A: Inductive processes in embryonic development. *Science* 152:25–34, 1966.

Spemann H: The development of the vertebrate eye. In Spemann, H (ed): *Embryonic Development and Induction*. New Haven, CT, Yale University Press, 1938.

SKIN AND GUT DEVELOPMENT

Sengel P: *Morphogenesis of Skin.* Cambridge, England, Cambridge University Press, 1976.

Wolff E: Specific interactions between tissues during organogenesis. In, Moscona AA, Monroy A (eds): *Current Topics in Developmental Biology,* New York, Academic Press, 1968, pp 65–94.

Wolff E: *Tissue Interactions During Organogenesis.* New York, Gordon & Breach, 1970.

PRIMARY INDUCTION

Saxen L, Toivonen S: *Primary Embryonic Induction.* New York, Academic Press, 1962.

Spemann H: *Embryonic Development and Induction.* New Haven, CT, Yale University Press, 1938.

CHAPTER 5

Causes of Congenital Malformations

CONGENITAL MALFORMATIONS

Congenital defects are those abnormalities present at birth that result from errors arising during development. Malformations of neural, muscular and reproductive systems, which are often not manifest until later in life, are also included in this term. Understanding congenital malformations goes beyond identification and, when possible, treatment. It involves knowing the nature of the primary embryonic lesion and attempting to deduce the cause of the defect. This latter is not just a matter of curiosity; breeders of companion animals and valuable, often artificially bred, livestock are anxious to quickly identify any heritable or environmentally (i.e. drug, plant, virus, pesticide) induced malformation. For example, if the owner of a herd of prized purebred cattle has a number of calves born with signs attributable to cerebellar abnormalities, it is crucial to quickly determine if this congenital defect is inherited or the result of an in utero infection. The purpose of this chapter is to introduce the concepts underlying the study of congenital malformations; each of the following chapters will present specific examples.

Precise data regarding the frequency of congenital malformations in domestic animals are not available. In one study (Table 5.1) 1.2–5.9% of the animals studied exhibited a birth defect. These data do not include aborted fetuses, nor is the incidence of unreported malformations known.

HEREDITARY FACTORS

Embryonic development is an interplay between the genome, which needs to be highly conservative to maintain species-specific characteristics, and **epigenetic factors** that create individual differences in many quantitative structural features and metabolic pathways. **Epigenesis** includes all changes in an embryonic cell brought about by interactions with cells and molecules surrounding it. As described in the preceding chapter, some of these interactions may subsequently affect the genetic programming of

Table 5.1.
Incidence of congenital malformations[a]

System	Dog	Cat	Cattle	Horse
Musculo-skeletal	29.0	2.4	2.4	8.0
Urogenital	5.0	1.3	9.6	20.1
Cardiovascular	3.5	0.8	1.2	0.3
Gastro-intestinal	2.2	0.4	1.8	1.5
Sense organs	8.2	1.3	1.2	1.3
Neurologic	1.7	1.7	1.8	1.7
Other defects	9.7	4.3	13.7	10.7
TOTAL	59.3	12.2	31.7	43.6

[a] Data presented as incidence per 1000 births, based on a 5-yr survey of 137,717 patients at ten North American veterinary clinics. (From WA Priester, et al., 1970.)

the cell. Because of the complexity of developmental processes, many aspects of embryogenesis require multiple, sequential gene function. Processes such as limb and facial morphogenesis, brain and spinal cord development, and probably most other examples of organogenesis are under **polygenic** control. Features in which identified single genes exert a known effect include pigment colors and patterns, and the synthesis of major proteins such as hemoglobin, some immunoglobulins, collagen, the components of myelin, and intermediary metabolic enzymes.

Simple dominant and recessive genes can often be identified if pedigree records detailing several generations are available, although test matings are usually necessary to prove the mode of transmission. The expression of deleterious genes, especially those that are recessives, is increased in highly inbred lines.

CASE HISTORY: WEAKNESS IN TIBETAN MASTIFF PUPPIES

Signalment: Several 10- to 12-week-old Tibetan Mastiff puppies presented with a chief complaint of progressive weakness.

History: The onset of weakness began between 7 and 10 weeks and was progressive. These pups were from different litters, each of which contained several normal, healthy animals.

Physical Exam: The affected pups were weak and showed marked hyporeflexia and muscular hypotonia. Most became recumbent within a few days. Some of these recovered, but were chronically weak and displayed a shuffling, plantigrade walk. There was no detectable loss of pain perception.

Ancillary Tests: The nerve conduction velocities of the tibial and ulnar nerves were measured, and found to be reduced by approximately 40% in affected pups. These nerves were examined using the electron microscope and found to show widespread loss of the myelination sheath.

Pedigree: Over a 3-yr period 10 litters containing 15 affected and 47 normal pups had been produced in one kennel. Breeding records indicated that affected pups were produced by breedings involving three sires and five dams, all of which were clinically normal. The ratio of normal-to-affected pups was 3:1.

Conclusion: This neuropathy in Tibetan Mastiffs is inherited as an autosomal recessive trait in which the Schwann cells are unable to form or maintain a stable myelin sheath.

More common and much more difficult to precisely identify are **incomplete dominants.** These typically produce a range of severities, some of which may appear quite different from one another. Often the expression of one gene is modified by other gene products. This process also results in a range of phenotypes, a phenomenon called **variable expressivity.** The frequency with which the phenotypic characters regulated by an incomplete dominant gene are present in each offspring is a measure of the **penetrance** of the gene.

Many genes have several different effects, a situation called **pleiotropy.** Examples of pleiotropic effects include genes whose products act to regulate the transcription of other families of genes, or those that produce part of a hormone receptor complex found on many different types of cell.

CASE HISTORY: CRANIOFACIAL DEFECTS IN BURMESE CATS

Signalment: Two normal-sized kittens (one male and one female) born to a healthy Burmese queen died within a day of birth due to severe head malformations.

History: Three littermates are normal. Both the queen and tom had been bred previously without difficulty, but a sibling of the male had sired a litter that also contained fetuses with a similar malformation.

Physical Exam: Both kittens had severe encephalocele of the forebrain (brain greatly enlarged and protruding through a schisis in the calvaria), no eyes or snout, and four whisker pads (see Fig. 9.29).

Pedigree analysis: Both parents were contemporary-look (Eastern) Burmese cats, which are characterized by a rounded head, heavy eyelids and brows, and a shortened, broader snout. In contrast, the traditional-look Burmese have a more triangular face. The pedigree of these two kittens, organized by phenotype, is shown in Figure 5.1.

Conclusions: The contemporary phenotype results from variable expressivity of an incomplete dominant gene. The mating of two contemporary-look Burmese, regardless of the severity of their expression, is likely to produce litters in which between 25 and 40% of the kittens are malformed. The malformation has never appeared in outcrosses. Thus, the malformation is a severe expression of the same incomplete dominant that causes the contemporary phenotype. All contemporary-look cats are carriers.

The presence in both parents of genetic factors correlated with the changed facial morphology in these cats causes a subtle change in the initial formation and patterning of the rostral neural tube and overlying mesenchyme (discussed in Chapter 9). The basis for this range of phenotypes and also the occasional appearance of litters free of malformed neonates despite both parents having the contemporary phenotype is not known, but such variability is common with incomplete or codominant genetic traits.

This example illustrates the difficulty in making accurate assessments of the cause of a malformation and providing genetic counselling unless extensive pedigree data are available. However, the Burmese story is unique in that introduction of an altered

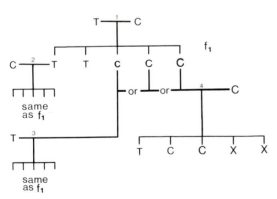

Figure 5.1. Typical breeding record for Burmese cats. Matings of traditional (*T*) with contemporary (*C*) phenotypes produces litters containing a range of facial phenotypes (*small* to *large Cs* represent increasingly rounded heads and shortened snouts). Thus, the contemporary phenotype segregates as an incomplete dominant trait with variable expressivity. Crossing of two contemporary-look cats produces a litter in which there is a high probability that 25–40% of the offspring will have the lethal craniofacial malformation (*X*) described in the text (see Figure 9.29).

genotype into this already highly inbred line happened to produce a phenotype that was viable and made the animals more appealing to owners and prized by judges. These carriers were rapidly introduced across the country before full awareness of the devastating consequences of carrier × carrier matings were known.

There are many instances in which a specific congenital abnormality will occur with higher-than-average incidence in a specific breed of animal, but is not attributable to an identifiable single-gene defect. Examples of these polygenic characters, which are often called a **breed predilection**, include hip dysplasia in some large breeds of dog and patent ductus arteriosus in the poodle. Similarly, many traits will show a familial pattern of inheritance. For example, several reports have described an increased predisposition to develop left displaced abomasum in the descendents of a particular bull. Only through extensive test matings can the mode of inheritance be defined in most of these cases.

PRINCIPLES OF TERATOLOGY

The possibility that extrinsic influences ranging from dietary factors to "evil spirits" might affect embryogenesis has been recognized for centuries. However, it is only in the past few decades that the study of induced birth defects, **teratology** (teras = monster), has been established as a scientific discipline. This was prompted by two discoveries: first, the deleterious effects of hypo- and hypervitaminosis A on pig and rodent embryos. Then, in the early 1960s, it was discovered that severe limb defects in humans resulted from maternal ingestion of the sedative thalidomide during days 20–35 of embryonic development. Since then the list of known and suspected **teratogens** has grown considerably. This section will discuss the general ways in which extrinsic factors may affect development, following which specific examples will be presented.

Maternal-Placental-Fetal Interactions

Some potentially harmful factors are transmitted directly to the embryo; these

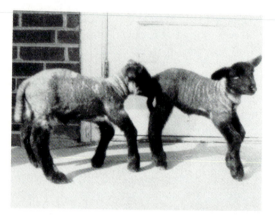

Figure 5.2. Ankylosis (stiffening of joints) of the elbow joint in lambs born to a ewe that was treated with gamma irradiation on day 22 of gestation, at which time the embryos would have been 6- to 7-mm long and the primordia of the forelimbs have just begun to develop. (From BH Erickson and RL Murphree, 1964, courtesy of the American Society of Animal Science.)

include radiation (Fig. 5.2), many viruses, some steroid hormones, and most low molecular weight compounds such as vitamins, metabolic cofactors and their antagonists, ethanol, and heavy metals. However, many agents that enter the mother are modified by her digestive organs or by the placenta. As a result, the actual embryopathic agent may be a catabolic by-product of maternal metabolism. Many suspected mutagens, for example the antineoplasia drug, cyclophosphamide, and some carcinogens, fall into this category. Other compounds activate maternal metabolic enzymes which, at high levels, produce toxic intermediates. This category includes phenobarbitol and related barbiturates, and **dioxin**, a highly teratogenic compound that was a contaminant in the phenoxyacetic acid defoliant called Agent Orange.

Table 5.2 summarizes the results of a study conducted to test the teratogenicity of dioxin (TCDD; 2,3,7,8-tetrochlorodibenzo-p-dioxin) in ferrets. At all doses tested this agent was embryotoxic, often killing an entire litter. At doses above 20 μg/kg, the agent also compromised the health of the mother, producing weight loss and **alopecia** (hair loss). A range of craniofacial defects were

Table 5.2.
Effects of dioxin on ferret development

Condition	Control	10 μg[a]	13.5 μg[a]	20 μg[a]	30 μg[b]
Number of animals	9	1	5	8	9
Average maternal weight change	+29	+29	−89 g	−27 g	−58 g
Number of litters with malformations	0	1	5	5	3
Number of litters with dead fetuses	4	1	5	7	9
Total number of fetuses	86	12	58	101	66
Number of malformed fetuses	0	9 (75%)	6 (10.3%)	18 (17.8%)	6 (9.1%)
Number of dead fetuses	7 (8.1%)	3 (25%)	52 (89.7%)	80 (79.2%)	60 (90.9%)
MALFORMATIONS					
Palatoschisis	0	9	3, 4, 2, 1, 3[c]	4[c]	1, 4, 3[c]
Open eyelids	0	9	4, 1, 6, 1, 3	2	1, 4, 2
Anasarca	0	7	5, 1, 5, 1, 3	1, 5	1, 1, 2
Brachygnatha	0	0	2, 1, 5, 2	5	1, 1, 2
Imperforate anus	0	0	0	0	1, 1

[a] Single injection, day 18
[b] Two injections, days 18 and 20
[c] Each number represents the number of cases in one litter.

seen at all doses used; in addition the fetuses showed severe **anasarca** (edema).

Some heavy metals also cross the placenta. The best defined of these is mercury, which in its organic form (methyl mercury) induces a range of congenital defects in humans, laboratory and domestic animals (Fig. 5.3). In man, neurological deficits and an increased incidence of stillborn result from maternal exposure. Mercury causes **brachygnatha** (shortened jaws), **scoliosis** (lateral deviation or twisting of the vertebral column) and **hypoplasia** (reduced growth) of the kidney, gonad and spleen in ferrets.

Conversely, deficiencies of some maternal metabolites can cause developmental anomalies. The best characterized include vitamins A, E and B$_6$, riboflavin, folic acid, and several cations (copper, magnesium, manganese, selenium, zinc). Both hypo- and hypervitaminosis A induce defects during the closure of the neural tube in several species, resulting in eye, brain and heart defects.

A few agents have been described that

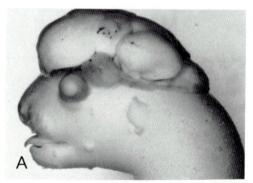

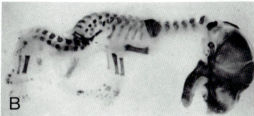

Figure 5.3. This illustrates the effects of methyl mercury on development of the ferret. *A* shows a 35-day fetus with severe exencephaly and secondary facial dysmorphologies. *B* is a neonate that has been cleared and stained to reveal ossified tissue. Note the misalignment of the thoracolumbar vertebrae, a condition called scoliosis.

produce fetal death by attacking the placenta. For example, **brucellosis**, a bacterial (*Brucella abortus*) infection, can have a devastating abortive effect in a herd of cattle. Other organisms, including *Leptospira* and *Campylobacter* also induce abortion in infected cattle. In addition, the toxoplasma protozoan and certain *Aspergillus* fungi compromise the placenta.

Species differences in placental transport function are critically important in attempting to extrapolate the results of drug tests performed on laboratory animals to domestic animals and humans. For example, thalidomide is not teratogenic in rodents, is noxious only at high doses in rabbits and most mammals, but is highly teratogenic at low doses in primates, in which it induces a range of severe limb defects (see Chapter 10). Thalidomide administered to pigs during weeks 2–6 of gestation causes an abnormal coiling of the colon but no skeletal defects. Conversely, acetylsalicylic acid (aspirin) is an extremely potent teratogen in rodents but not in primates. At high doses (400 mg/kg body weight/day) aspirin can induce cleft palate, facial and tail shortening and cardiovascular defects in the dog, but these levels also cause severe gastrointestinal lesions in the mother.

The metabolism and physiology of the embryo differ from those of the mother and are continually changing. This means that some agents readily broken down by the mother can accumulate to toxic levels in the fetus. The rapidly growing embryo is especially sensitive to agents that interfere with DNA synthesis, which explains the teratogenic effect of most alkylating and other antimitotic drugs (Table 5.3).

Critical Periods

The time during which each organ system in the body is being established, when obligatory inductive tissue interactions and morphogenesis are occurring, is called the **critical period** for that system. Generally, it is at this stage that the tissues are most sensitive to disruption by exogenous factors (see Fig. 10.1, limb, and Fig. 12.1, heart critical pe-

Table 5.3.
Teratogenic medications and drugs

Agent	Function	Systems affected
Cyclophosphamide	Antimitotic (alkylating agent)	Embryotoxic: rodents
Folic acid antagonists (aminopterin, pyrimethamine)	Antimitotic (alkylating agent) Antiparasitic	Embryotoxic: dogs, sheep
Hydroxyurea	Antimitotic Antiprotozoan	Embryotoxic: dogs, sheep
Tetracycline	Antibiotic	Teeth, skeleton: all species
Griseofulvin	Antifungal	Head, brain, palate, skeleton: cats, dogs, horses
Parbendazole	Antiparasitic	CNS, kidney, skeleton, limbs: lambs
Metrifonate	Antiparasitic	Cerebellar hypoplasia: pig
Corticosteroids	Steroid hormone	Palate, limbs, edema: several species
Androgen	Steroid hormone	Masculinization: all species
Methallibure	Estrus synchronization	Limb and head defects: pig
Phenytoin (phenylhydantoin)	Anticonvulsant	Cleft palate: cats
Hydroxyzine	Sedative	Embryotoxic: dog
Thalidomide	Sedative	Growth retardation: dog Intestinal defects: pig
Vitamin A	Essential metabolite	Neural tube, heart, limbs

riods). As illustrated in Figure 5.4, critical periods for most structures occur during the first few weeks of development. Agents that disrupt blastula and gastrula stages, or interfere with normal apposition to the uterine mucosa, are usually embryotoxic and induce early abortions. However, beginning at the neurula stage it is more probable that only one or a few systems will be affected.

Often an induced lesion in one system will result in secondary malformations in other structures. This is especially true for defects of the central nervous system and heart. For example, as will be discussed in detail in Chapter 9, the programming of most facial mesenchymal and epithelial tissues is dependent upon interactions between these and the underlying forebrain and eyes, which are themselves programmed during gastrulation as a result of interactions between the neural plate and underlying mesoderm. Chemical disruption of these transient interactions can produce a wide range of facial dysmorphologies, depending on the exact time, dose and target tissue. Possible defects include severe reductions, as exemplified by cyclopia (see Figs. I.3 and 9.28), patterning defects such as described in the Burmese cat earlier in this chapter, and relatively slight deviations from normal devel-

opment, e.g. the **fetal alcohol syndrome** that has been reported in humans and laboratory animals (Fig. 5.5). This last condition is characterized postnatally by reduced head size, narrow forehead, a small nose, short palpebral fissures, a long, thin upper lip and, in humans, mental retardation. Abnormal development in these animals can first be detected during gastrulation in the presumptive rostral neural plate tissues.

The central nervous system is sensitive to teratogenic insult throughout prenatal and, in many species, early postnatal development. As described in Chapter 6, this is due to the relatively late stages at which cortical neurons in the cerebrum and, especially, the cerebellum are formed. In addition, there is increasing evidence that many neuroeffective drugs (tranquilizers, sedatives, anticonvulsants, antidepressants) are **behavioral teratogens.** Some of these bring about irreversible restrictions in cognitive and motor development.

TERATOGENS AFFECTING DOMESTIC ANIMALS
Medications and Drugs

Most medications used in veterinary practice are not harmful to developing embryos.

Critical Periods in Cat Development

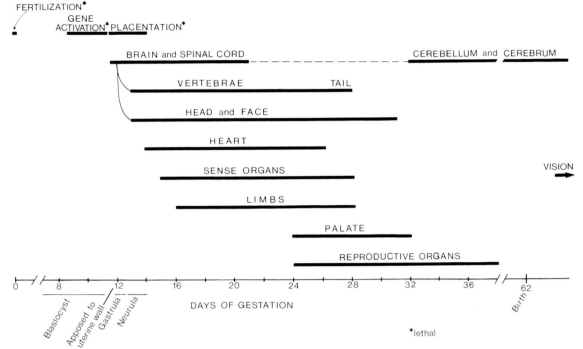

Figure 5.4. The time of maximal susceptibility of the major organ systems in the feline embryo. Embryos of other species would show similar sensitivities at comparable stages and sizes of development (see conversion table inside front cover). *Disturbances at these stages are usually lethal.

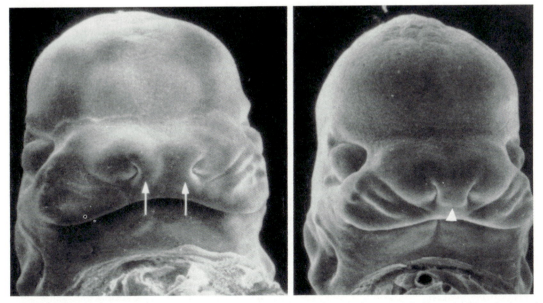

Figure 5.5. Scanning electron micrographs showing the faces of normal (*left*) and ethanol-treated (*right*) 12-day mouse embryos. The experimental group was given injections of ethanol (0.015 ml/g of a 25% solution) at 7 days, and at 7 days, 4 hr, gestation. *Arrows* in the control animal indicate the medial nasal processes that are forming medial to the future external nares. Notice that in the treated embryo these processes (*arrowhead*) have developed as a single median swelling. (From KK Sulik and MC Johnston, 1983, courtesy of AR Liss, Inc.)

Caution should be exercised when prescribing cytotoxic drugs such as the antimitotic and anthelmintic agents listed in Table 5.3. Figure 5.6 illustrates one of the teratogenic

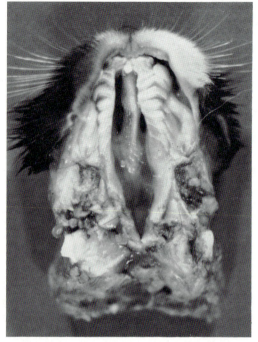

Figure 5.6. Ventral view of the roof of the oral cavity in a neonatal kitten that was born to a queen treated orally with 1000 mg/week of the antifungal agent griseofulvin starting the day after breeding. Note the bilateral cleft palate that exposes the nasal cavity.

lesions frequently produced following treatment of pregnant cats with griseofulvin, a widely used antifungal medication.

The safety of antibiotics is controversial. In most cases extensive retrospective studies of their use in humans have failed to identify significant increases in the number of birth defects, although several of them are teratogenic in laboratory animals. Complicating the issue is the fact that hyperthermia, as frequently occurs during infection, is itself a proven inducer of embryonic malformations and death.

Plants

Herbivorous animals will ingest many plants that contain toxic and teratogenic compounds, usually alkaloids. Some of the more common of these are listed in Table 5.4. Plants that are highly toxic to the mother are frequently embryotoxic as well; these have not been listed. It is not known why appendicular tissues (Fig. 5.7) and vertebrae are the primary targets of these diverse agents: nor, in most cases, has the molecular mode of action of these compounds been identified.

Viruses

Once the blastocyst hatches from its protective zona pellucida, it is vulnerable to attack by viruses. Later, the placenta acts as

Table 5.4.
Common teratogenic plants

Plant	Common name	Affected systems: species
Astragalus lentiginosus	Locoweed, poison vetch	Limbs: cattle
Conium maculatum	Poison hemlock	Limbs: cattle
Datura stramonium	Jimson weed	Limbs: pigs
Lathyrus species	Pea	Limbs: herbivores
Leucaena leucocephala	Mimosine	Multiple: pigs
Lupinus sericeus	Lupine	Limbs, vertebrae[a]: cattle
Nicotiana species	Tobacco	Limbs: pigs
Oxytropus species	Locoweed	Limbs: cattle
Prunus serotina	Wild black cherry	Limbs, caudal structures: pigs
Salsola tuberculata		Prolonged gestation: sheep
Sophora sericea	Silky sophora	Limbs, vertebrae[a]: cattle
Thermopsis montana	False lupine, yellow bean	Limbs, vertebrae[a]: cattle
Veratrum californicum	False hellbore	Craniofacial: sheep, goats
Vicia faba	Common vetch	Limbs, vertebrae[a]: cattle

[a]Crooked-calf syndrome; all these plants contain similar quinolizidine alkaloids.

a protective barrier to some but not all viruses. As indicated in Table 5.5, many viral infections are toxic to the embryo. Some are also stage-specific in their effects. It has been found that treating pregnant sows with attenuated **hog cholera virus** vaccines produces a variety of malformations depending on the time of injection. Application between days 10–16, which is the gastrula-neurula period, is embryotoxic and also induces defects in limbs, kidneys and facial structures. In contrast, injection of the vaccine between 20 and 90 days of gestation produces hypoplasia of the cerebellar hemispheres. A comparable time-response correlation for bluetongue virus is described in Chapter 6, which also discusses the teratogenic effects of the bovine diarrhea, Akabane and feline panleukopenia viruses.

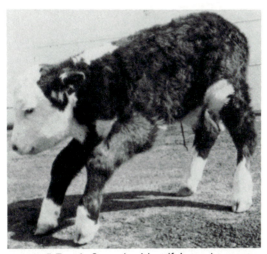

Figure 5.7. A 2-week-old calf born to a cow that had ingested hemlock foliage during days 50–75 of gestation. The forelimbs show ankylosis (immobility of a joint) and arthrogryposis (abnormal limb posture). (From RF Keeler and LD Balls, 1978, courtesy of Marcel Dekker, Inc.)

SUMMARY

The best approach when confronted with a congenital malformation is to be cautious with respect to future breedings or possible environmental contamination, but not to be alarmist. Most cases will not fit an already described inherited pattern for the species concerned or be readily attributable to a known teratogenic agent.

Despite the increasing use of complex medications and household chemicals, the rise of airborn contaminants, and the widespread application of organic herbicides and pesticides, there are very few proven cases of congenital malformations or fetal death in domestic animals attributable to such influences. Similarly, despite the number of suspected inherited malformations in highly inbred strains of domestic animals, only a

Table 5.5.
Common teratogenic viruses

Name	Species affected	Effects
Bovine rhinotracheitis	Cattle	Embryotoxic
Wesselsbron disease virus	Cattle, sheep	Embryotoxic, limb defects
Bluetongue virus	Cattle, sheep	Brain, spinal cord, limb defects
Akabane virus	Cattle, sheep, goats	Brain, limb defects
Bovine viral diarrhea	Cattle, sheep, goat, pig	Forebrain, eye, skeletal defects
Japanese B encephalitis	Pig	Embryotoxic
Hog cholera virus	Pig	Embryotoxic, edema, cerebellar defects
Equine rhinopneumonitis	Horse	Embryotoxic
Equine encephalitis	Horse	Limb defects
Herpesvirus 2	Dog	Eye, brain defects
Feline panleukopenia	Cat, ferret	Cerebellar defects
Rubella	Monkey, rabbit	Heart, eye, brain, skeletal defects

few of these have been carefully studied to determine the mode of inheritance.

Bibliography

REVIEWS

NOTE: Reviews and compendia of inherited congenital malformations in domestic animals are listed in the bibliography of the Introductory Chapter.

Brent RL: Drug testing for teratogenicity: its implications, limitations and application to man. In Klingberg MA, Abramovici A, Chemke J (eds): *Drugs and Fetal Development.* New York, Plenum Press, 1972, pp 31–43.

David LE: Adverse effects of drugs on reproduction in dogs and cats. *Mod Vet Pract* 1:969–974, 1983.

Earl FL, Miller E, Van Loon EJ: Teratogenic research in beagle dogs and miniature swine. In Spiegel A (ed): *The Laboratory Animal in Drug Testing.* Proceedings 5th International Committee on Laboratory Animals, Stuttgart, G Fischer, 1972, pp 233–247.

Fuccillo DA, Sever JL: Viral teratology. *Bacteriol Rev* 37:19–31, 1973.

Harris RE: Viral teratogenesis: a review with experimental and clinical perspectives. *Am J Obstet Gynecol* 119:996–1008, 1974.

Keeler RF: Effect of natural teratogens in poisonous plants on fetal development in domestic animals. In Klingberg M, Abramovici A, Chemke J (eds): *Drugs and Fetal Development,* New York, Plenum Press, 1972, pp 107–125.

Keeler RF, van Kampen KR, James LF: *Effects of Poisonous Plants on Livestock.* New York, Academic Press, 1978.

Juchau MR (ed): *The Biochemical Basis of Chemical Teratogenesis.* Amsterdam, Elsevier Science, 1981.

Langman J: Congenital malformations. In *Medical Embryology,* ed 4. Batlimore, Williams & Wilkins, 1981, pp 102–122.

Michaelis J, Michaelis H, Gluck E, Kollar S: Prospective study of suspected associations between certain drugs administered during early pregnancy and congenital malformations. *Teratology* 27:57–64, 1983.

Moore KL: Causes of congenital malformations. In *The Developing Human,* ed 3. Toronto, Saunders, 1982, pp 140–166.

Palludan B: Swine in teratological studies. In Bustad LK, McClellan RO (eds): *Swine in Biomedical Research.* Seattle, Fryan Printing, 1966, pp 51–75.

Patterson DF: Diseases due to single mutant diseases. *J Am Anim Hosp Assoc* 11:327–341, 1975.

Priester WA, Glass GG, Waggoner NS: Congenital defects in domesticated animals. General considerations. *Am J Vet Res* 31:1871–1879,

Schardein JL: Congenital abnormalities and hormones during pregnancy: a clinical review. *Teratology* 22:251–270, 1980.

Swaab DF, Mirmiran M: Possible mechanisms underlying the teratogenic effects of medicines on the developing brain. In Yanai J (ed): *Neurobehavioral Teratology.* Amsterdam, Elsevier Science, 1984, p 55.

Wilson JG: *Environment and Birth Defects.* New York, Academic Press, 1973.

Wilson JG: Present status of drugs as teratogens in man. *Teratology* 7:3–16, 1974.

TERATOGEN AND GENETIC STUDIES

Akpokodje JU, Barker CAV: Further observations on the teratogenic effect of methallibure in swine. *Can Vet J* 12:125–128, 1971.

Barker CAV: Anti-gestation and teratogenic effects of aimax (methallibure) in gilts. *Can Vet J* 11:39–40, 1970.

Brent RL: Radiation teratogenesis. *Teratology* 21:281–298, 1980.

Brown TT, de Lahunta A, Bistner SI, Scott FW, McEntee K: Pathogenetic studies of infection of the bovine fetus with bovine viral diarrhea virus. *Vet Pathol* 11:486–505, 1974.

Chow TL, Molello JA, Owen NV: Abortion experimentally induced in cattle by infectious bovine rhinotracheitis virus. *JAVMA* 144:1005–1007, 1964.

Clarke ML, Harvey DG, Humphreys DJ: *Veterinary Toxicology,* ed 2. London, Bailliere Tindall, 1981.

Crowe MW, Pike HT: Congenital arthrogryposis associated with ingestion of tobacco stalks by pregnant sows. *JAVMA* 162:453–455.

Cummings JF, Cooper BJ, de Lahunta A, Van Winkle TJ: Canine inherited hypertrophic neuropathy. *Acta Neuropathol* 53:137–143, 1981.

Dolnick EH, Lindahl IL, Terrill CE: Treatment of pregnant ewes with cyclophosphamide. *J Anim Sci* 31:944–945, 1970.

Dyson DA, Wrathall AE: Congenital deformities in pigs possibly associated with exposure to hemlock (*Conium maculatum*). *Vet Rec* 100:241–242, 1977.

Earl FL, Tegeris AS, Whitmore GE, Morison R, Fitzhugh OG: The use of swine in drug toxicity studies. *Ann NY Acad Sci* 111:671–689, 1964.

Edmonds LD, Selby LA, Case AA: Poisoning and congenital malformations associated with consumption of poison hemlock by sows. *JAVMA* 160:1319–1324, 1972.

Emerson JL, Delez AL: Cerebellar hypoplasia, hypomyelinogenesis, and congenital tremors of pigs, associated with prenatal hog cholera vaccination of sows. *JAVMA* 147:47–54, 1965.

Erickson BH, Murphree RL: Limb development in prenatally irradiated cattle, sheep and swine. *J Anim Sci* 23:1066–1071, 1964.

Hall JG, Reed SD: Teratogens associated with congenital contractures in humans and in animals. *Teratology* 25:173–191, 1982.

Hartley WJ, De Saram WG, Della-Porta AJ, Snowdon WA, Shepherd HC: Pathology of congenital bovine epizootic arthrogryposis and hydranencephaly and its relationship to Akabane virus. *Aust Vet J* 53:319–325, 1975.

James LF, Shupe JL, Binns W, Keeler RF: Abortive and teratogenic effects of locoweed on sheep and cattle. *Am J Vet Res* 28:1379–1388, 1967.

James LF: Effect of locoweed on fetal development: preliminary study in sheep. *J Am Vet Res* 33:835–840, 1972.

James LF, Keeler RF: Teratogenic effects of aminopterin in sheep. *Teratology* 1:407–412, 1968.

Johnson RT, Johnson KP, Edmonds CJ: Virus-induced hydrocephalus. Development of aqueductal stenosis in hamsters after mumps infection. *Science* 157:1066–1067, 1967.

Kahrs RF, Scott FW, de Lahunta A: Bovine viral diarrhea-mucosal disease, abortion and congenital cerebellar hypoplasia in a dairy herd. *JAVMA* 156:851–857, 1970.

Kahrs RF, Scott FW, de Lahunta A: Congenital cerebellar hypoplasia and ocular defects in calves following bovine viral diarrhea-mucosal disease infection in pregnant cattle. *JAVMA* 156:1443–1450, 1970.

Keeler RF, Balls LD: Teratogenic effects in cattle of *Conium maculatum* and conium alkaloids and analogs. *Clinical Toxicology* 12:49–64, 1978.

Kilham L, Margolis G: Viral etiology of spontaneous ataxia of cats. *Am J Pathol* 48:991–1011, 1966.

Kilham L, Margolis G: Hydrocephalus in hamsters, ferrets, rats and mice following inoculations with reovirus type I. I Virologic studies. *Lab Invest* 21:183–188, 1969.

Kilham L, Margolis G, Colby ED: Congenital infections of cats and ferrets by feline panleukopenia virus manifested by cerebellar hypoplasia. *Lab Invest* 17:465–480, 1967.

King GJ: Deformities in piglets following administration of methallibure during specific stages of gestation. *J Reprod Fertil* 20:551–553, 1969.

Knox B, Askaa J, Basse A, Bitsch V, Eskildsen M, Mandrup M, Ottosen HE, Overby E, Pedersen KB, Rasmussen F: Congenital ataxia and tremor with cerebellar hypoplasia in piglets borne by sows treated with Neguvon vet. (Metrifonate, trichlorfon) during pregnancy. *Nord Vet Med* 30:538–545, 1978.

LaVecchio FA, Pashayan HM, Singer W: Agent Orange and birth defects. *N Engl J Med* 308:719–720, 1983.

Martin W: Left abomasal displacement: an epidemiological study. *Can Vet J* 13:61–68, 1972.

Robertson RT, Allen HL, Bokelman DL: Aspirin: teratogenic evaluation in the dog. *Teratology* 20:313–320, 1979.

Saunders LZ, Shone DK, Philip JR, Birkhead HA: The effects of methyl-5(6)-butyl-2-benzimidazole carbamate (parbendazole) on reproduction in sheep and other animals. *Cornell Vet* 64:7–40, 1974.

Scott FW, de Lahunta A, Schultz RD, Bistner SI, Riis, RC: Teratogenesis in cats associated with griseofulvin therapy. *Teratology* 11:79–86, 1975.

Selby LA, Menges RW, Houser EC, Flatt RE, Case AA: Outbreak of swine malformations associated with the wild black cherry, *Prunus serotina. Arch Environ Health* 22:496–501, 1971.

Shultz G, DeLay PD: Losses in newborn lambs associated with bluetongue vaccination of pregnant ewes. *JAVMA* 127:224–228, 1955.

Sponenberg DP, de Lahunta A: Hereditary hypertrophic neuropathy in Tibetan Mastiff dogs. *J Heredity* 72:287, 1981.

Stober M, Wegner W, Lunebrink J: Research on the familial occurrence of leftside displacement of the abomasum in cattle. *Bovine Pract* 10:59–61, 1975.

Streissguth AP, Landesman-Dwyer S, Martin JC, Smith DW: Teratogenic effects of alcohol in humans and laboratory animals. *Science* 209:353–361, 1980.

Sulik KK, Johnston MC: Sequence of developmental alterations following acute ethanol exposure in mice: craniofacial features of the fetal alcohol syndrome. *Am J Anat* 166:257–269, 1983.

Suttle NF, Field AC, Barlow RM: Experimental copper deficiency in sheep. *J Comp Pathol* 80:151–161, 1970.

Ward GW, Roberts SJ, McEntee K, Gillespie JH: A study of experimentally induced bovine viral diarrhea-mucosal disease in pregnant cows and their progeny. *Cornell Vet* 59:525–538, 1969.

Webster WS, Edwards MJ: Hyperthermia and the induction of neural tube defects in mice. *Teratology* 29:417–427, 1984.

Wjersig DO, Swenson MJ: Teratogenicity of Vitamin A in the canine. *Fed Proc* 26:486, 1967.

Young GA, Kitchell RL, Luedke AJ, Sautter JH: The effect of viral and other infections of the dam on fetal development in swine. *JAVMA* 126:165–171, 1955.

Central Nervous System and Eye

NEURON

The **neuron** is the parenchymal cell of the nervous system. Although they present many disparate appearances, all neurons have the four basic components shown in Figure 6.1. The **dendritic zone** is the receptor region of the cell where most stimuli are received and converted into impulses. The **axon** conducts impulses from the dendritic zone to the opposite terminal of the neuron called the **telodendron** (telas = end) or axon terminal, where the impulse leaves the neuron. Axons often project in groups or bundles that collectively form **tracts** in the central nervous system or **nerves** in the peripheral nervous system. Impulses are conveyed to other cells at specialized sites called **synapses,** most of which are located on telodendria. The neuronal **cell body** (**soma**; plural = somata) contains the nucleus and cytoplasm that is rich in mitochondria and protein-synthesizing organelles. The soma may be located anywhere along the axon.

In a typical spinal motor neuron the soma and dendritic zone are close together in the ventral region of the spinal cord. The axon leaves the spinal cord in an **efferent** (motor) **nerve** and synapses peripherally on the cell membrane of a muscle cell (see Fig. 7.4). Most primary sensory neurons are located outside of the central nervous system. Their dendritic zones are located at the distal end of an **afferent** (sensory) **axon**, typically in the skin or a neuromuscular spindle. Afferent axons course towards the brain or spinal cord through a peripheral nerve to a **spinal ganglion** (dorsal root ganglion) or **cranial sensory ganglion**. Ganglia are clusters of nerve cell bodies located outside of the neural tube. Afferent axons pass through spinal ganglia without synapsing and enter the dorsal part of the spinal cord, where most have their telodendria synapse on interneurons in the gray matter.

All axons initially arise as outgrowths of the neuronal cell body. At the tip of each developing axonal fiber is an enlarged **growth cone** (Fig. 6.2) from which many long filapodia extend. These processes form and retract quickly, often over the span of a few minutes. Their activity is necessary for both elongation and directed outgrowth of embryonic axons. The growth cone and, later,

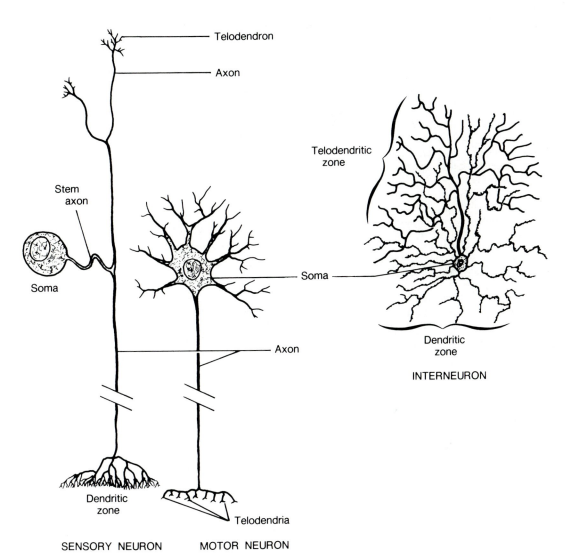

Figure 6.1. Comparative morphology of neurons. A primary sensory neuron, as would be found in a spinal ganglion, has its soma located away from the axon; its dendritic zone is in the skin or an internal receptor, and its telodendria synapse upon interneurons in the dorsal horn of the spinal cord. The interneuron shown is a typical cell from the cerebral cortex. Axons carrying information towards the cell soma are studded with postsynaptic receptor sites; similarly, telodendria are scattered along all branches of axons carrying information away from the soma.

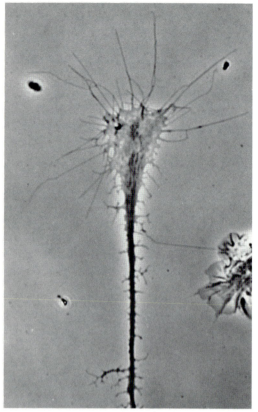

Figure 6.2. The growth cone of an embryonic neuron developing on a plastic substratum in tissue culture medium. Note the elongated filapodia, one of which is contacting a nearby fibroblast. (Courtesy of Dr. RP Nuttall.)

telodendron are the primary sites of axonal membrane synthesis. Membrane precursors along with the enzymes necessary for neurotransmitter synthesis and other regulatory proteins are produced in the soma and delivered to the terminus by **axoplasmic transport.** The movement of metabolites, vesicles and mitochondria through the axon is bidirectional and can be very rapid (several centimeters per hour).

FORMATION OF THE NEURAL TUBE

The development of a dorsal thickening in the cranial surface ectoderm concomitant with primitive streak regression is the first overt sign of neurogenesis. This thickening, the **neural plate,** is bounded laterally by elevations called **neural folds.** A median and

a pair of lateral grooves form in the neural plate (Fig. 6.3), allowing the neural folds to become apposed and subsequently fuse. This process is facilitated by cytoskeletal organelles, including microfilaments and microtubules, located within neural plate cells and also by extrinsic forces generated by underlying paraxial and notochordal tissues.

Neural tube closure begins in the region of the rostral rhombencephalon or mesencephalon, depending upon the species. The tube remains open rostrally for a short period of time at the **rostral neuropore** and caudally for a longer time at the **caudal neuropore.** Neural tube closure occurs similarly throughout the length of the neuraxis except in the lumbosacral region. Here, the spinal cord forms initially as a solid mass of epithelial cells, and a central lumen develops secondarily by **cavitation.**

Initially the **neurepithelial cells** in the wall of the neural tube are organized in a pseudostratified arrangement. Processes of each cell extend to both the inner (apical, luminal) and outer (basal) surfaces of the neural tube. During early embryonic stages all these cells are mitotically active, and the size of the tube increases rapidly as a result of this proliferation. At interphase the nucleus of each cell is located either in the center of the neurepithelium or close to the external surface of the tube; DNA synthesis and chromosomal duplication occur in the latter location (Fig. 6.4). Prior to mitosis, the nucleus shifts towards the luminal surface and contact with the outer surface is broken. The cell becomes spherical and divides, usually parallel to the luminal surface.

The two new daughter cells each reestablish contact with the outer surface of the spinal cord, and the nuclei move away from the lumen. At this time each cell has two alternatives: either to repeat the above proliferative sequence, or to detach from the luminal surface and form either an **immature neuron** or a **spongioblast.** Spongioblasts are the progenitors of two types of **neuroglia** (glia = glue) in the central nervous system, **astrocytes** and **oligodendrocytes.** A third type of glial cell, the **microglia,** is believed to

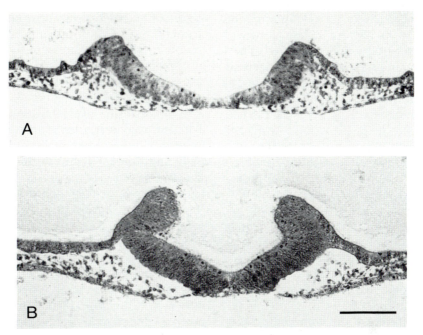

Figure 6.3. Two stages in the closure of the neural plate in a 4-somite dog embryo. *A*, mesencephalic level, and *B*, prosencephalic level. Note that folding occurs in a ventromedian and a pair of lateral sites (*bar*, 0.1 mm).

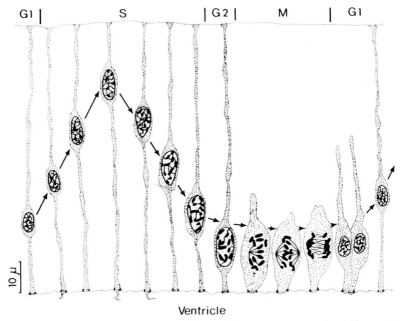

Ventricle

Figure 6.4. Cell division in the neurepithelium. The nucleus moves away from the ventricle, at which time chromosomal replication (S-phase of cell cycle) occurs. Subsequently, the nucleus moves to the ventricular surface, the cell loses connection with the outer margin, and mitotic division (M-phase) occurs. (From M Jacobson (1978) after Sauer (1935), courtesy of Plenum Publishing Corp.)

be of mesodermal origin and presumably enters the central nervous system along with vascular tissues. Generally the period of neuron production procedes that of gliogenesis.

Except for olfactory receptor neurons, all mature neurons are permanently postmitotic. The time at which a prospective neuron undergoes its last division is called its **birthdate.** Generally, neurogenic cells in the ventral part of the spinal cord and hindbrain are the first to stop dividing, with birthdates of dorsal and intermediate neurons following. Cortical neurons in the cerebrum and cerebellum are the last populations to be fully formed, with proliferation not complete until 3–4 months after birth in the dog, and the 3rd yr in humans. In precocial animals such as the foal and calf, most cortical neurons are formed by birth.

The three layers of the embryonic neural tube (Fig. 6.5) are: (*a*) the **ventricular zone,** also called the germinal layer, which is adjacent to the lumen of the neural canal and is the region of active cell division; (*b*) the **mantle layer** or **intermediate zone** which is in the middle and represents the location of cell bodies of proliferating neurepithelial cells, immature neurons and presumptive glial cells; and (*c*) the **marginal layer,** which is on the external surface and contains the axonal processes of developing neurons.

EARLY DEVELOPMENT OF THE SPINAL CORD

The lateral walls of the embryonic spinal cord are thick and packed with proliferating cells. In contrast, the dorsal and ventral margins are thin and are referred to as the **roof plate** and **floor plate,** respectively. A small longitudinal furrow, the **sulcus limitans,** extends along both sides of the neural canal (Fig. 6.6). It is located approximately halfway between the dorsal and ventral margins. This sulcus demarcates the dorsal **alar plate** of the mantle layer and the ventral **basal plate.** Many alar plate neurons have a sensory function, while those of the basal plate have motor functions. Later a shallow **dorsal median sulcus** develops in the dorsal midline of the spinal cord. Also, the basal plate regions on both sides of the spinal cord grow ventrally, creating a deep **ventral median fissure.**

Transformation of this embryonic organization into that of the mature spinal cord occurs as result of massive proliferation, asymmetric movement of immature neurons in the mantle layer, and development

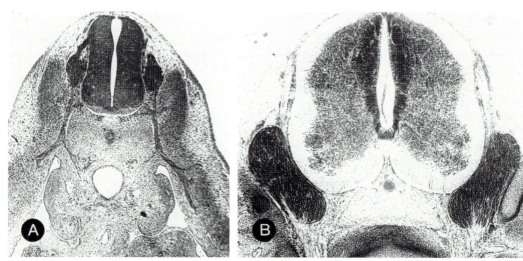

Figure 6.5. Transverse sections of the spinal cord in *A*, 14-mm and *B*, 27-mm calf embryos (32 and 42 days of gestation). The dorsal and ventral roots and mantle layer are well established by the 14-mm stage, but the marginal layer is very small. By the 27-mm stage most of the basal plate neurons are established and the ventricular zone is reduced; the alar plate is less well developed.

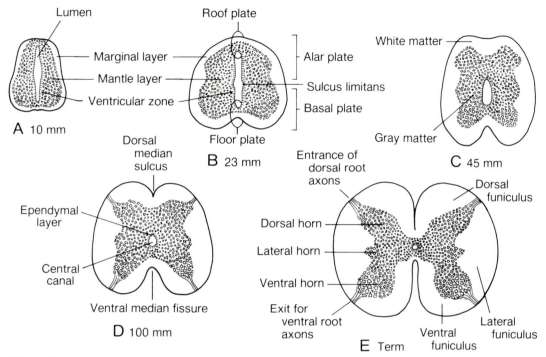

Figure 6.6. Schematic sections illustrating the maturation of the spinal cord. (Redrawn after BM Patten (1954).)

of neuronal processes. The mantle layer becomes the gray matter of the spinal cord, which consists primarily of neuronal cell bodies. Due to differential migrations of immature neurons, the mantle layer becomes shaped like a butterfly (Fig. 6.6E) with prominent **dorsal** and **ventral gray columns (horns).**

Initially the gray columns are uniform along the entire length of the spinal cord (Fig. 6.7). However, as the limbs develop the columns at the corresponding axial levels become significantly enlarged. The presence of a greater number of neuronal cell bodies in these regions is the result of degeneration of immature neurons in nonlimb-innervating regions. Most of these cells die because they fail to form viable contacts with developing muscle tissue. Also, in the thoracic level (T_1 through L_4) immature neurons migrate dorsomedially out of the ventral motor column and form the intermediate gray column. This contains the neuronal cell bodies of the sympathetic neurons. The spinal cord enlargement that occurs from the 6th cervical through the 1st thoracic segments is

called the **cervical intumescence.** The **lumbosacral intumescence,** which provides pelvic limb innervation, is located from the 4th lumbar through the 1st sacral segments.

The marginal layer of the spinal cord is commonly referred to as **white matter,** so named because of the appearance of myelinated axons. This outer layer contains tracts of ascending (projecting cranially) and descending (projecting caudally) axons that are grouped together in bundles called **funiculi.** The **dorsal, lateral** and **ventral funiculi** (Fig. 6.6 E) are separated from one another by the emerging motor and entering sensory roots.

The ventricular zone does not expand proportionately to the other layers. As proliferation of neurons and glia concludes, this epithelium remains as a single layer of ciliated columnar epithelial cells called **ependymal cells** that surround a small **central canal.**

EARLY DEVELOPMENT OF THE BRAIN

As the cephalic neural tube is being formed, three distinct regions of the future

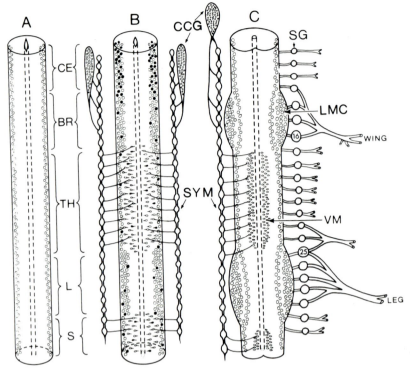

Figure 6.7. Three stages in the development of the avian ventral gray column. As shown in *B*, some immature neurons in the thoracic and sacral levels shift from a ventrolateral to ventromedial (*VM*) position; these form visceral efferent neurons. Other neurons, shown as *solid black cells*, degenerate; this cell death is greatest but not limited to the cervical region, where it is due to an absence of target sites (sympathetic ganglia) for these sympathetic neurons. Much less neuronal degeneration occurs in the limb regions, resulting in the formation of large lateral motor columns (*LMC*) in these regions. *BR*, brachial region; *CCG*; cranial cervical ganglion; *CE*, cervical region; *SG*, spinal ganglion; *L*, lumbar region; *S*, sacral region; *SYM*, sympathetic ganglia; *TH*, thoracic region. (Modified from Levi-Montalcini (1950).)

brain are delineated. An expansion at the most rostral end of the neural tube forms the **prosencephalon.** Growing outward from each side of the prosencephalon is an evagination called the **optic vesicle.** The two enlarged regions of the brain caudal to this become the **mesencephalon** and **rhombencephalon** (Fig. 6.8).

As the optic primordia are developing from the ventrolateral walls of the prosencephalon, the alar region of the rostral end of the neural tube begins to expand bilaterally. This marks the subdivision of the prosencephalon into **telencephalic** and, medially, **diencephalic** regions. The paired telencephalic vesicles will develop into **cerebral hemispheres.** These eventually expand over the diencephalon and mesenceph-

alon, as illustrated in Figure 6.9. The diencephalon remains as the undivided portion of the prosencephalon at the rostral end of the brain stem. It is located in the midline and connected to the laterally expanding optic vesicles. The **thalamus** and **hypothalamus** and the neural component of the pituitary gland **(neurohypophysis)** develop in this part of the brain.

The rhombencephalon becomes subdivided into rostral and caudal components. The rostral division forms the **metencephalon,** which will give rise to the **pons** ventrally and **cerebellum** dorsally. The **myelencephalon,** forms the **medulla oblongata,** which is the caudal part of the brain stem.

Differential growth of these regions gives rise to flexures in the developing brain (Fig.

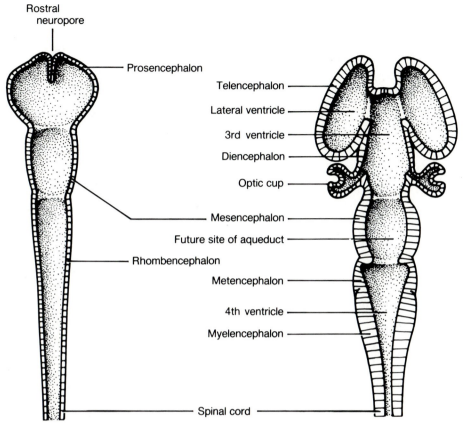

Rostral
neuropore

Prosencephalon

Telencephalon

Lateral ventricle

3rd ventricle

Diencephalon

Optic cup

Mesencephalon

Future site of aqueduct

Rhombencephalon

Metencephalon

4th ventricle

Myelencephalon

Spinal cord

Figure 6.8. Development of the five principal regions of the brain and ventricles, shown in schematic dorsal views.

6.9). As head folding occurs the brain bends ventrally at the level of the mesencephalon to produce the **midbrain flexure.** A second, more gradual ventral bend, called the **cervical flexure** occurs at the junction of the myelencephalon and cervical spinal cord. Later, unequal growth in the rhombencephalon produces a slight dorsal folding, the **pontine flexure.** The final processes in establishing the definitive shape of the mammalian brain are the enlargement of the cerebellar cortex, and the tremendous growth and caudal expansion of the cerebral cortex.

In contrast to the small **central canal** of the spinal cord, the lumen of the brain expands during development (Fig. 6.8). Within each telencephalic vesicle is a **lateral ventricle** (ventricles 1 and 2). The **3rd ventricle** is in the diencephalon. Interventricular foramina connect each lateral ventricle with the

3rd ventricle. The 3rd ventricle is connected caudally via the narrow **mesencephalic aqueduct** to the **4th ventricle.**

As the 4th ventricle expands, the roof plate becomes a thin, dorsal covering consisting of a single layer of ependymal cells closely apposed by meninges. Blood vessels in the pia mater, which is the layer of meninges adjacent to the brain and spinal cord, from a capillary plexus in two longitudinal rows. This plexus with its covering of ependymal cells protrudes into the lumen of the 4th ventricle, forming the **choroid plexus.** The primary function of the plexus is to produce cerebrospinal fluid. A similar choroid plexus develops in the roof of the diencephalon and in the medial wall of each telencephalon.

At the rostral end of the myelencephalon an opening called the **lateral aperture** devel-

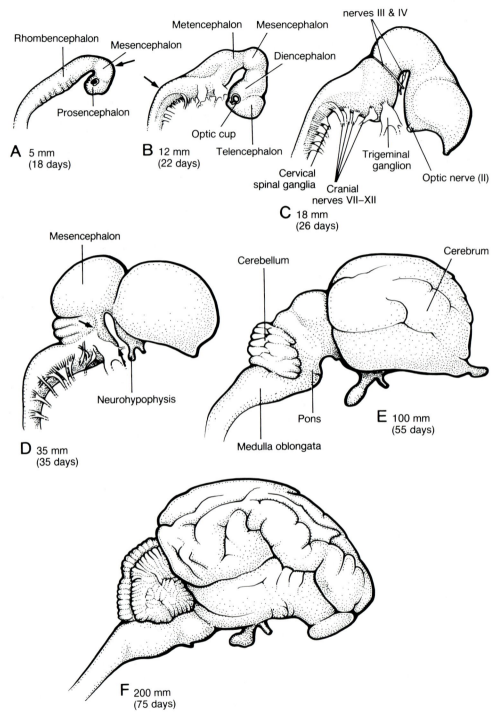

Figure 6.9. Schematic lateral views showing the development of the brain in the pig. *Arrows* in *A*, *B* and *D* indicate the sites of the cranial, cervical and pontine flexures, respectively. (Redrawn after BM Patten (1954.)

ops on both sides of the neural tube. This permits cerebrospinal fluid produced by the choroid plexus to pass out of the lumen of the central nervous system, where it circulates through the meninges and is absorbed by veins.

MATURATION OF BRAIN REGIONS

Myelencephalon

The medulla oblongata extends from the first cervical spinal cord segment to the transverse fibers of the pons. Myelencephalic neurepithelial cells proliferate ventrally in the region of the basal plate and laterally in the alar plate region. These regions are demarcated by a ventrolateral groove in the wall of the neural tube that marks the rostral continuation of the sulcus limitans. The mantle region gives rise to clusters of neurons called **nuclei.** Axons from motor nuclei grow out from basal plate nuclei of the myelencephalon to innervate either striated muscles of the head or peripheral neurons of the autonomic visceral system. These axons comprise the efferent components of cranial nerves VI through XII (see Table 9.1). Axons from neurons in sensory ganglia enter the medulla at the same axial levels as corresponding efferent neurons and synapse

on neurons in nuclei derived from the alar plate region of the mantle layer.

Metencephalon

Development of the basal and alar regions of the metencephalon are very different. The mantle layer of the basal plate gives rise to motor neurons of the 5th cranial nerve, which innervate the muscles of mastication. Some alar plate neurons migrate ventrally to form the **pontine nuclei,** as shown in Figure 6.10. Neurons in the cerebral cortex terminate on pontine neurons that project to the cerebellar cortex. Ventrally, the axons of these pontine neurons form a superficial band of processes known as the transverse fibers of the pons.

The roof of the metencephalon forms the cerebellum. Both the shapes of cerebellar neurons and their spatial arrangement have been highly conserved during vertebrate evolution and thoroughly studied in all classes. Developmental anomalies of this system result in abnormalities of locomotion and posture, which are readily identified and frequently seen in mammals.

The first indication of cerebellar development is a dorsal enlargement of the metencephalic alar plate. This presents a striking

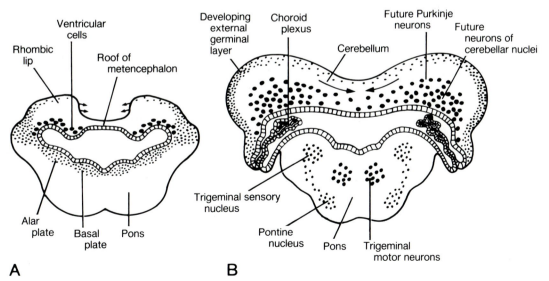

A   **B**

Figure 6.10. Early development of the cerebellum and pons shown schematically in transverse sections through the metencephalon. *Arrows* indicate the direction of movement of cells derived from the rhombic lip.

contrast to the thin roof of the myelencephalon. Bilateral dorsal growths called **rhombic lips** (Fig. 6.10) expand medially through the roof plate of the rostral part of the 4th ventricle, eventually meeting and fusing in the midline to completely cover this part of the ventricle. As the pontine flexure deepens, the enlarged roof of the metencephalon becomes folded against the roof of the medulla, obscuring most of the choroid plexus from dorsal view.

Neurepithelial cells in the rhombic lips develop along several lines. Some occupy a dorsal mantle zone similar to the corresponding lateral region in the spinal cord. From this there develops a population of large, highly specialized cells, the **Purkinje neurons,** which constitute the primary output cells in the cerebellar cortex of all vertebrates. Neurons of cerebellar nuclei located in the floor of the cerebellum and Golgi type II neurons in the cortex also arise from this mantle population.

Purkinje neuron somata become aligned in a single layer near the outer surface of the mantle zone, and each cell develops a large, *uniplanar* superficial dendritic arborization (Fig. 6.11). The plane of this dendritic network is transverse to the longitudinal axis of the folium; when each folium is viewed in longitudinal section the arborization looks very narrow. This layer is well developed in the calf by 100 days of gestation.

Unique to the cerebellum is the formation of a large, superficial population of proliferating neurepithelial cells called the **external germinal layer.** Progenitors of this population arise in the ventricular zone of the rhombic lips, then spread over the entire roof of the cerebellar cortex. These superficial neurepithelial cells continue to divide and subsequently give rise to all remaining cerebellar cortical neurons (granule, stellate and basket neurons). The **granule neurons** are the largest population formed by the external germinal layer. They stop dividing deep within the external germinal layer and become immature bipolar neurons, with their axons running in a plane parallel to the longitudinal axis of the folium. Concomitantly, the soma of each granula neuron moves inward from the external germinal layer (Fig. 6.12), past the layer of Purkinje neuron cell bodies. They form a thick new layer in the cerebellum that is called the **granular layer.**

As the cerebellum grows the cortex forms folds, referred to as folia. The granule layer is thickest over the center of each folium and thinner around the sulci between them. A single axon projects superficially from each granule cell body, then bifurcates at the level of Purkinje dendrites. These granule cell axons are called **parallel fibers** (shown in red in Fig. 6.11), which traverse the cerebellum perpendicular to the plane of Purkinje dendritic trees. Each Purkinje neuron is contacted by several hundred thousand parallel fibers. This superficial zone is called the **molecular layer** of the cerebellar cortex.

The period of greatest development of the external germinal layer varies between species of animals and is closely correlated with the age at which the animal is able to stand and walk in a coordinated manner. In calves, foals and other species that walk within an hour after birth the cerebellum is developed much more than in kittens and puppies who do not walk for about 3 weeks postnatally. In calf fetuses the external germinal layer appears at around 57 days of gestation and reaches maximal thickness at around 183 days. It slowly decreases in size as it produces the neurons of the granule layer of the cerebellar cortex so that at birth the external germinal layer is only a few cells in thickness. Some of the these cells may persist for up to 6–8 months of age and should not be confused with inflammatory cells in the leptomeninges.

In dogs and cats the external germinal layer reaches its greatest development at about 7 days postnatally and begins to decrease in size by 2 weeks of age, concomitant with the formation of the granule neuron layer. Some cells of the external germinal layer will persist for 3 months in these species. In laboratory animals, the peak time of

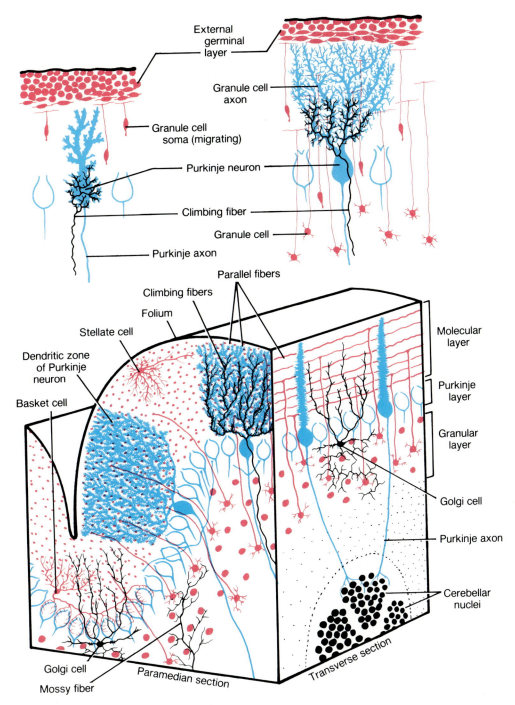

Figure 6.11. Development of the cerebellar cortex. Proliferating cells in the external germinal layer (*red*) stop dividing and begin to develop axons (parallel fibers) while their nuclei migrate inwardly, through the Purkinje cell layer (*blue*). The dendritic area of each Purkinje cell increases as more parallel fibers are formed and synapse upon it. At the same time climbing fibers, which initially establish synapses upon the Purkinje cell bodies, grow into the dendritic arborization of Purkinje neurons and establish new synaptic contacts. Many of the events shown in this figure occur postnatally in altricial mammals (carnivores, primates, laboratory animals) and prenatally in precocial mammals such as the ungulates (horse, cow, sheep, goat).

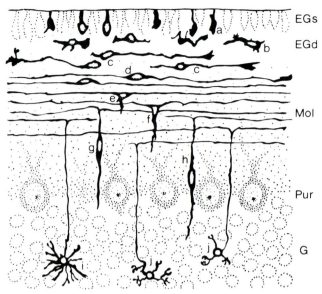

Figure 6.12. This illustrates the sequence of changes (a–j) in the morphology of developing granule cells in the cerebellum during the initial stages of parallel fiber and granular layer formation. *EGd* and *EGs*, deep and superficial strata of the external germinal layer; *G*, granular layer; *Mol*, molecular layer; and *Pur*, Purkinje neuron layer. (From M Jacobson (1978) after Ramon Y Cajal, courtesy of Plenum Publishing Corp.)

proliferation in the external germinal layer is the 2nd postnatal week, but in humans this layer persists until the 3rd yr.

Mesencephalon

The mantle layer of the basal plate gives rise to motor neurons of the 3rd and 4th cranial nerves, which innervate muscles that move the eye. Alar plate neurons form a pair of rostral and caudal bulges called colliculi. Neurons in each **caudal colliculus** are involved with auditory function; those in the **rostral colliculi** are concerned with visual function. In most vertebrates the rostral colliculus (optic tectum) acts as a primary integrator of visual inputs; in mammals this function is assumed by the visual cortex (telencephalon).

Alar and basal plate mantle layers contribute neurons to the region of the mesencephalon ventral to the aqueduct known as the **tegmentum.** These will be part of the core of the brain stem known as the **reticular formation** that extends from the myelencephalon to the diencephalon. This has components that ascend into the diencephalon and are concerned with the state of consciousness of the animal.

Diencephalon

The sulcus limitans does not extend cranially beyond the mesencephalon, and the walls of the neural tube rostral to the midbrain are considered analogous to components of the alar plate. The mantle layer of the diencephalon gives rise to the neurons that comprise the many nuclei of the **thalamus** and **hypothalamus.** These connect with each other, with other brain stem nuclei, and a large component project to the cerebral cortex.

Initially the neural canal of the diencephalon expands vertically in the median plane. The central region of this ventricle becomes obliterated by the **interthalamic adhesion,** which is formed by medial enlargements of the developing thalamic primordia. Ventral to the adhesion the 3rd ventricle forms a vertical slit located between the walls of the developing hypothalamus and extending ventrally into the stalk of neurohypophysis.

Dorsal to the interthalamic adhesion the 3rd ventricle is covered by a narrow strip of roof plate which consists of a single layer of ependymal cells. A choroid plexus similar to that of the 4th ventricle develops the full length of this roof plate on both sides of the midline.

Telencephalon

Each telencephalic vesicle will give rise to a **cerebral hemisphere.** The mantle layer of the neural tube of the telencephalon gives rise to neurons whose cell bodies migrate to the surface of the neural tube to form the cerebral cortex. Many of the axons of these neurons then grow inward to project to other areas in the same or opposite hemisphere or to the brain stem. As a result of this process the cerebral cortex consists of superficially located neuronal cell bodies that comprise the gray matter, and underlying axons that form the white matter. This is the opposite of the gray and white matter relationship in the spinal cord.

As these immature neurons migrate from their origin on the surface of the mantle layer to the external surface of the telencephalon they establish layers of neurons that comprise the **cerebral cortex.** The first neurons to organize on the surface will be found in the deepest layer of the mature formed cerebral cortex. As more cells stop dividing and leave the ventricular zone, they must migrate through layers of neurons already present. The last neurons to form are found in the most superficial layer of the cerebral cortex. In addition to populating the cerebral cortex, neurons derived from the mantle layer of the telencephalon form collections of cell bodies deep to the surface known as **basal nuclei.**

The processes of neurons in each cerebrum comprise three groups based on their termination. The association neurons have processes that course between adjacent gyri (short association neurons) or distant gyri (long association neurons) of the same cerebral hemisphere. These axons always terminate on another neuron within the same hemisphere. Neurons whose axons cross to the opposite cerebrum, in a pathway referred to as a commissure, are called commissural neurons. The largest commissure is the **corpus callosum.** The primordium for this pathway is first established by primitive glial cells that migrate medially and form a bridge-like structure between the adjacent surfaces of each telencephalon just rostral to the lamina terminalis, which is the most rostral surface of the diencephalon. The axons of commissural neurons grow through this pathway to establish the primitive corpus callosum. As the telencephalic vesicle expands dorsally and caudally over each side of the brain stem this commissural pathway expands so that the corpus callosum ultimately extends over the entire diencephalon.

In each telencephalon there is a narrow zone of neural tube that does not develop into parenchyma but remains as a single layer of ependymal cells similar to the roof plates of the 3rd and 4th ventricles. The pial blood vessels proliferate along this layer of ependymal cells to form the choroid plexus of each lateral ventricle. It projects into the lateral ventricle and is continuous rostrally at the interventricular foramen with the choroid plexus of the third ventricle.

EYE, LENS AND CORNEA

The area of the neural plate destined to form the eyes is initially a single median region, the **optic field,** located near the rostral margin of the future prosencephalon. Interaction of this area of neuroectoderm and the underlying head mesoderm and, in amphibians, the foregut endoderm, causes the single optic field to separate into two lateral eye-forming regions. Failure of separation to occur completely is the basis for the cyclopian malformation, in which a single eye develops in the center of the head (see Fig. 9.28, and Fig. I.3 of the Introduction).

After closure of the cephalic neural tube, lateral expansion of the prosencephalon forms the **optic vesicles** (Fig. 6.13), which remain attached to the prosencephalon by the **optic stalks.** Each optic vesicle grows laterally until it contacts the adjacent surface ectoderm. As a result of this contact (see Chapter 4), the ectoderm thickens to form the **lens placode.** This subsequently invaginates and forms a **lens vesicle,** which breaks away from the surface ectoderm; the latter becomes the anterior (superficial) layer of the **cornea.** The deeper layers of the cornea are derived from neural crest mesenchymal cells. Concomitantly, the lateral surface of the optic vesicle invaginates to form a nearly complete, bilayered **optic cup,** (Fig. 6.14). The inner surface layer of the optic cup will give rise to the **neural retina** with its layers of neurons that function in visual reception. The outer layer of the optic cup becomes the **pigmented epithelium** of the retina. The **optic stalk** persists, connecting the optic cup with the diencephalon and serving to guide axons of neurons in the retinal ganglion layer back to the developing brain. Table 6.1 outlines the stages at which these events occur in the dog and cow.

The ciliary body and the posterior surface

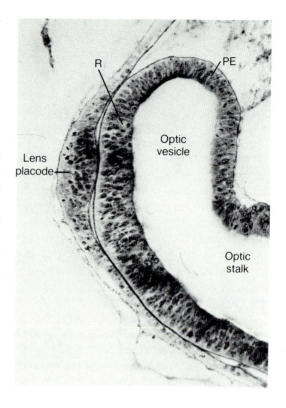

Figure 6.13. Transverse section showing the close contact between the evaginating optic vesicle and the overlying surface ectoderm in an avian embryo. Interactions between these tissues result in the formation of the lens placode, which will subsequently invaginate and form the lens. *R* and *PE* indicate the future retinal and pigmented epithelial layers of the eye.

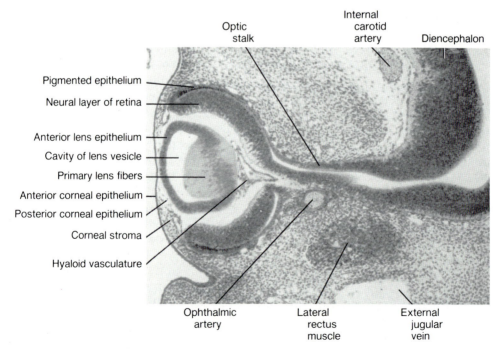

Figure 6.14. Transverse section through the optic cup of a 10-mm cat embryo. At this stage the posterior cells of the lens vesicle are elongating to form lens fibers, and the primordia of the cornea are beginning to migrate over the anterior surface of the lens.

Table 6.1.
Timetable of embryonic eye development (days)

Structures formed	Dog	Ox (mm)
Optic vesicle	17	25–30(6)
Optic cup	19	30(10)
Lens vesicle	25	30(10)
Retinal ganglion cell layer	33	30(10)
Eyelids fused	33	50(40)
Inner plexiform layer	Birth	
Inner and outer retinal nuclear layers	+7–13[a]	40–50(14–33)
Eyelids open	+14[a]	Birth
Rods and cones	+16–35[a]	150–180(410)

[a] Days after birth.

of the iris are formed by cells of the pigmented epithelium that extend towards the lens from the anterior lip of the optic cup. Connective tissues in the choroid, sclera and iris are derived from the neural crest, with minor contributions from mesoderm. Periocular blood vessels in the choroid, ciliary body and iris are derived from mesodermal angiogenic cords originally associated with the first aortic arch.

The muscles of the eye are derived from three different precursors. The extrinsic ocular muscles, which move the eye in the orbit, are derived from cephalic paraxial mesoderm (see Chapter 9). There are two sets of intrinsic ocular muscles. Those in the iris are formed from pigmented epithelial cells originally located at the edge of the optic cup. Ciliary muscles, in contrast, are derived from neural crest mesenchymal cells.

The retina develops circumferentially, with new cells being added peripherally during embryonic development. In fishes this process continues throughout the life of the animal. Since the brain is fully formed in juvenile stages, new retinal axons entering the fish's mesencephalon displace preexisting nearby visual projections, which then compete for synaptic terminals with adja-

cent optic nerve axons. All this occurs in a spatially ordered manner, with no compromise of visual acuity. In mammals, retinal ganglion cell neurons that fail to establish synapses on brain neurons degenerate.

ONTOGENY OF VISUAL NERVE PATHWAYS

The basic wiring of the visual system, especially the connections from the retina to the lateral geniculate nucleus and from there to the visual cortex, develops prenatally as a result of genetically-based mechanisms. However, in some altricial mammals, particularly the cat and monkey, it has been proven that functional inputs play a significant role in the establishment and maintenance of precise synaptic terminals. The critical period for this process is the 1st 3–4 months after birth in cats and 1st yr in monkeys, although these animals are especially sensitive during weeks 2–4 (cat) and 2–12 (monkey).

Visual input from both eyes is especially important in the development of binocular vision. Information about a specific point or object in front of the animal converges on each neuron in one layer of the visual cortex. While some of these neurons are stimulated equally by both eyes, most are driven preferentially by one or the other (Fig. 6.15*A*). Typically, groups of central neurons driven by projections from the contralateral eye alternate across the visual cortex with groups driven by the ipsilateral eye.

Many studies using kittens and monkeys have shown that if visual input in one eye is temporarily reduced, as a result of inherited cataracts or short-term surgical closure of the eyelids, normal binocular vision never develops (Fig. 6.15*B*). Moreover, in these animals the projections carrying information from the normal eye form functional synapses upon cortical neurons normally contacted by the deprived eye. Thus, cortical neurons that would normally have received and maintained inputs from the deprived eye have shed these inputs and acquired and maintained inputs from the normal (stimu-

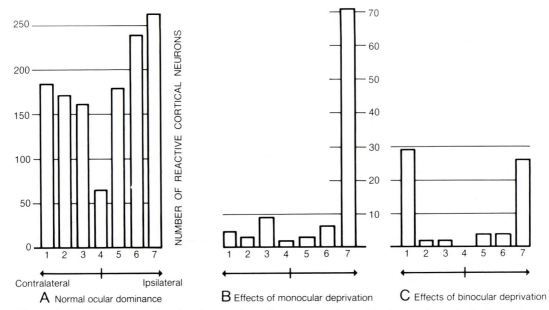

Figure 6.15. Histograms showing the number of neurons activated by inputs from the ipsilateral eye (*column 7*), the contralateral eye (*column 1*), or both eyes (*columns 3–5*), based on electrophysiological analysis of visual cortical neurons in the rhesus monkey. *A*, normal pattern; *B*, after monocular deprivation for 1.5 yr after birth; and *C*, following binocular deprivation for 1 month. In *B*, the deprived eye generated no cortical response. Data on cats is very similar. (Redrawn after DH Hubel (1982).)

lated) eye. These results were obtained only when deprivation occurred during the critical, early postnatal period, and the animals never recovered. In contrast, animals will recover if the period of deprivation is much shorter (several days) or occurs after the most sensitive stage of the critical period.

Interestingly, the effects of temporarily depriving *both* eyes of normal input are less severe. After restoring normal input to the retinas, the electrical activity of visual cortical neurons remains depressed, but the pattern of left- and right- dominant cells is intact (Fig. 6.15*C*). This proves that the development of normal binocular vision depends upon synchronous, balanced, spatially-aligned inputs from both eyes.

MALFORMATIONS OF THE SPINAL CORD

Myelodysplasia

The general term for a malformation of the spinal cord is **myelodysplasia.** This can include one or more of the following:

Hypoplasia, (aplasia): reduced (absence of) development of one or more segments of the spinal cord;

Hydromyelia: dilation of the central canal due to excess accumulation of cerebrospinal fluid;

Syringomyelia: abnormal cavitation of the spinal cord;

Diplomyelia: two spinal cords developed beside each other usually in one set of meninges and in one vertebral canal; and

Diastematomyelia: two spinal cords developed with a partition between them. These are usually in separate vertebral canals and have separate meninges (Fig. 6.16).

The origin of most of these abnormalities can be traced back to events occurring during neurulation, beginning with interactions between the notochord and paraxial mesoderm and the dorsal surface ectoderm (future neural plate). Abnormalities associated with the central canal in the lumbosacral region may be related to errors in cavitation. Also, as documented in the experiments illustrated in Figure 6.17, defects in the spatial arrangements of somites or the notochord can result in gross asymmetries in the neural tube. Because of this close relationship between the developing neural tube, notochord and paraxial mesoderm, a primary abnor-

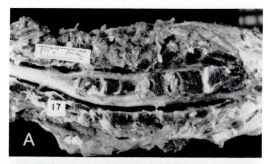

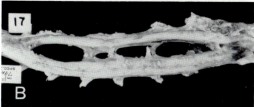

Figure 6.16. Diastematomyelia in the lumbosacral region of a newborn Holstein calf. *A*, dorsal view of specimen following laminectomy. *B*, same perspective with spinal cord isolated. Note in *A* that vertebral processes project between the two spinal cords, indicating that two separate embryonic axial systems must have formed at this region.

mality in one may compromise the development of the others (see also Fig. 8.6).

Myelodysplasias occur commonly in cattle and are often accompanied by vertebral malformations. These are usually sporadic occurrences on farms and are of unknown cause. The majority of these involve the thoracic, lumbar or sacral segments. Animals with these malformations are often unable to generate normal coordinated movements of the pelvic limbs, and attempts to walk often result in simultaneous hopping motions of the pelvic limbs. The signs are evident at birth and usually do not change.

A dominantly inherited myelodysplasia described in Weimaraner dogs has been called **spinal dysraphism**, a terminology used for the same condition in children. This term infers a failure of the neural folds to appose and close to form the neural tube. In this sense it is incorrectly used, because in this disease the neural folds close correctly. Subsequently, the spinal cord develops a number of abnormalities including hydromyelia, syringomyelia, absence or duplication of the central canal, absence or divided

ventral median fissure, and aberrant migration of neuronal cell bodies.

The neurologic signs resulting from this malformation are usually apparent by 6 weeks of age. As these puppies begin to walk, they move their pelvic limbs simultaneously, producing a "bunny hopping" type of gait. They may also stand in a crouched posture on these limbs, with both limbs partially abducted or with one limb overextended. Other abnormalities that have been observed in these dogs include scoliosis, abnormal hair patterns on the dorsal midline of the neck, and koilosternia, which is a gutter-like depression on the midline of the sternum. This spinal cord abnormality has also been reported sporadically in other breeds of dogs.

Myeloschisis, Meningocele

Spina bifida includes all abnormalities in which the vertebral arches fail to close dorsal to the spinal cord to form the vertebral canal (see Fig. 8.11). As such it is a vertebral anomaly, not one of the spinal cord. However, in the majority of these cases there is some compromise of adjacent neural and/ or meningeal tissues. In some instances the cord is normal but the meninges protrude through the opening in the vertebral arches and form a cyst beneath the skin; this is spina bifida with **meningocele** (Fig. 6.18*F*). More often the spinal cord also has a dorsal cyst, in which case the condition is called spina bifida with **meningomyelocele** (Fig. 6.19). The spinal cord segments adjacent to the meningomyelocele frequently show additional signs of myelodysplasia.

If any part of the neural tube fails to close during neurulation a permanent cleft (schisis) will result. This is called **myeloschisis** (Fig. 16.18*D*). When the neural tube remains open it is impossible for vertebral arches to form and fuse normally. Generally this condition will involve several vertebral segments.

The severity of peripheral functional loss in these vertebral-spinal cord schises depends on the amount of neural tissue lost or damaged. If large portions of the luminal surface of the lumbosacral spinal cord are

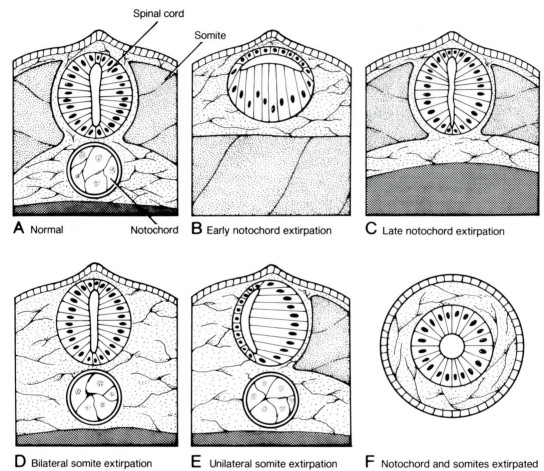

Figure 6.17. Tissue interactions affecting the early development of bilateral symmetry in the spinal cord. *A*, normal; *B*, effects of early removal of the notochord (somites have fused together beneath the spinal cord); *C*, effects of later removal of the notochord; *D*, *E*, effects of bilateral and unilateral somite extirpation; and *F*, effects of removing all adjacent tissues except the surface ectoderm. These experiments were performed on amphibian embryos. (Redrawn after J Holtfreter and V Hamburger (1955).)

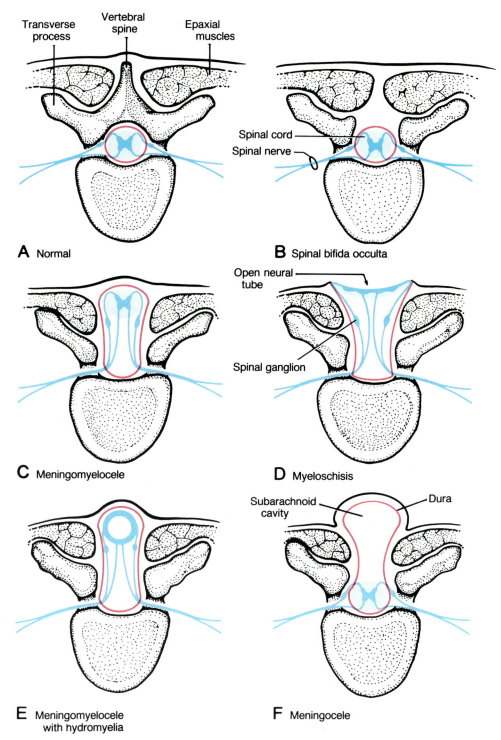

Figure 6.18. The principal types of vertebral-spinal cord-meningeal malformations, shown in schematic transverse section. The dura is shown in *red*, neural tissue in *blue*.

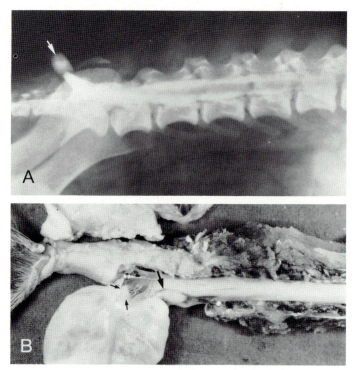

Figure 6.19. Meningomyelocele in a 4-month old Bulldog. The animal was presented because of lack of voluntary control over urinary and fecal excretions. There was a dimple in the skin overlying the sacrum. *A*, myelogram showing that dye injected subdurally leaves the vertebral canal and enters a sac (*white arrow*) located above the first two sacral vertebrae. *B*, dorsal view of the lumbosacral cord and vertebral region following laminectomy. This shows the presence of a large miningocele. The dura has been torn open (*small arrows*), revealing the presence of neural tissue entering the enlarged dural sac; this is a meningomyelocele. The *large arrow* indicates an abnormal cleft in the spinal cord which, upon histological examination, was a syringomyelia.

exposed early in development the neurepithelium usually degenerates, which would lead to neurogenic atrophy of pelvic limb and flank musculature by the time of parturition. A localized area of myeloschisis in the thoracic or cranial lumbar spinal cord segments might interrupt the spinal cord tracts to and from the pelvic limbs, perineum and tail. Paralysis of motor function and loss of all conscious sensation from these regions would result, but the local reflexes would persist.

In humans it is usually possible to diagnose neural tube defects during fetal stages. Detection is based in part on elevated amounts of α-**fetoprotein** in amniotic fluid. This protein is normally present in several fetal tissues including cerebrospinal fluid, which leaks into amniotic fluid when a myeloschisis is present. Ultrasonic scanning can also be used to examine the vertebral column and skull of a fetus, especially when elevated extra-embryonic levels of α-fetoprotein are found.

A malformation of the sacrocaudal vertebrae and associated spinal cord and nerves is observed most commonly in Manx cats and English Bulldogs. In Manx cats it is the result of selective breeding for **anury**, which is absence of the tail, or **brachyury**, a shortening of the tail (see Fig. 8.13). In the process of selectively breeding for this skeletal abnormality, an associated spinal cord abnormality commonly occurs. Many of these kittens are culled at birth or shortly after because they are unable to use their pelvic limbs. Others may walk normally but have no voluntary control of urination and defecation due to abnormalities in the sacral spinal cord or related peripheral nerves. These kittens can never be house trained.

The abnormalities that accompany the caudal vertebral aplasia or hypoplasia in Manx cats include sacral or lumbar spina bifida and meningocele or, more commonly, meningomyelocele. Myelodysplasia is common in the associated lumbar and sacral spinal cord segments. This exemplifies how inbreeding for one characteristic may cause another that is incapacitating to the animal.

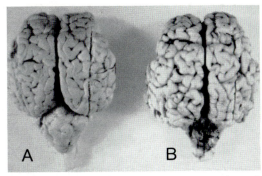

Figure 6.20. Dorsal view of brains taken from *A* a normal newborn calf and *B* one infected in utero with bovine virus diarrhea virus. Note the absence of the cerebellar cortex in the affected calf.

MALFORMATIONS OF THE BRAIN

Cerebellar Hypoplasia and Atrophy

The developing cerebellum is susceptible to a number of in utero or perinatal (at birth) viral infections, two of which have been studied extensively in domestic animals. In the cat the **feline panleukopenia virus** infects the rapidly dividing cells of the external germinal layer. Destruction of these cells causes a hypoplasia of the granular layer of the cerebellar cortex. Infection and subsequent cell destruction can occur in utero or in the immediate postnatal period. In severe infections the Purkinje neurons will also be affected and destroyed.

The **bovine virus diarrhea** (BVD) **virus** has a predilection for the developing cerebellum in calves. Infection of the fetus between 100 and 200 days of gestation regularly produces varying degrees of destruction of the cerebellum. An acute inflammation occurs 17–21 days postinfection with hemorrhage, necrosis, edema and inflammation. This results in a malformed cerebellum observed at birth that is hypoplastic and atrophic (Fig. 6.20). The clinical signs will be present when the newborn first walks; they will not progress but will remain static for the life of the animal.

CASE HISTORY

Signalment: A 1-day-old Holstein calf, delivered normally without assistance, presented with a chief complaint of inability to get up and stiff limbs.

History: When this calf was at 134 days of gestation, the dairy herd had an illness in many of its cattle with diarrhea, anorexia and fever as the clinical signs. Erosions of mucous membranes were observed in half the animals. Serological tests supported a diagnosis of infection with the bovine virus diarrhea (BVD) agent. Of 29 cows pregnant at that time, 19 delivered normal calves, 8 aborted and 2 had calves that were unable to rise at birth.

Physical Examination: The calf was alert and responsive; all cardiovascular, pulmonary, digestive and excretory functions appeared normal. It sucked vigorously and swallowed normally when fed milk. All cranial nerves were normal.

The calf laid in lateral recumbency with its head and neck hyperextended (opisthotonos). The limbs were rigidly extended. When it attempted to get up, it struggled vigorously with its limbs and rolled from side-to-side and had wide excursions of the head and neck. If the animal was held up, its limbs extended rigidly and they occasionally made stiff, hypermetric movements. However, the ataxia and stiffness (spasticity) were too severe to allow the calf to walk, and it was unable to balance without assistance. The limbs were hypertonic and all spinal nerve reflexes were normal.

Assessment

FACTS	INTERPRETATION
Unable to stand and use limbs at birth	Suggests a congenital neural or musculo-skeletal problem

Alert, responsive, cranial nerves functional; strong voluntary movements and normal spinal reflexes

Ataxic, unable to balance, all limbs affected

Herd infected with bovine virus diarrhea during midgestation

Unlikely to be a cerebral, brainstem or spinal cord problem

Suggests a congenital cerebellar abnormality

BVD is a known teratogen in cattle that primarily affects the developing cerebellum

Cerebellar Abiotrophy

A postnatal or occasionally prenatal Purkinje neuronal death has been observed in many of the domestic animals and numerous strains of laboratory animals. In affected individuals some abnormality intrinsic in the development of the Purkinje neuron does not permit it to survive and it dies prematurely (Table 6.2). This premature degeneration is referred to as cerebellar abiotrophy (a = lack of; bios = vital substance; trophy = nutrition). The primary defect in the Purkinje neuron is unknown and may reside in its metabolic apparatus or in the chemical environment to which it is exposed, including synaptic relations with other neurons. In those breeds of animals where adequate study has occurred, a genetic basis for this abiotrophy has been found; it is usually inherited as an autosomal recessive gene. Whereas in domestic animals most inherited abiotrophies affect Purkinje neurons, in laboratory mice there are examples that primarily affect granule neurons.

Hydrocephalus

Hydrocephalus is the accumulation of an excessive amount of cerebrospinal fluid in the cranial cavity. If an acquired lesion or developmental abnormality interferes with the circulation of cerebrospinal fluid from the ventricular system to the external surface

Table 6.2.
Purkinje neuron abiotrophy

Breed	Onset of clinical signs
Kerry Blue Terrier	3–4 months
Rough Coated Collie	1–3 months
Gordon Setter	6–24 months
Arabian horse	Birth–4 months
Gotland Pony	3–9 months
Holstein cattle	3–9 months
Yorkshire pigs	3–5 weeks

of the brain for absorption into the venous system, fluid will accumulate between the site of production from the choroid plexus and the obstruction. Ventricles exposed to this elevation of fluid pressure will enlarge, thereby compressing and usually destroying cortical neurons. This is called **obstructive hydrocephalus.**

A common site for such obstruction is the mesencephalic aqueduct. Developmental abnormality of the aqueduct results in expansion of the 3rd and especially the lateral ventricles, causing secondary atrophy of the cerebral cortex and, usually, enlargement of the cranial cavity covered by the calvaria. In utero inflammation of the lining of the mesencephalic aqueduct produces the same result. This is a rare manifestation of the feline panleukopenia virus in kittens.

If brain tissue fails to develop or is lost due to a destructive process, such as injury or inflammation, cerebrospinal fluid takes the place of the lost parenchyma. This condition is called **compensatory hydrocephalus.**

Hydranencephaly

When a destructive process destroys either the neurepithelial cells that give rise to the telencephalon or the fetal telencephalon itself, this leaves only a thin layer of glial and meningeal connective tissue where the neural parenchyma should be located. The resulting cavity, which is a greatly enlarged lateral ventricle, fills with cerebrospinal fluid. In domestic animals this most commonly results from in utero viral infection or, more rarely, an interruption of blood supply to the telencephalon.

Hydranencephaly has in some cases been shown to result from in utero viral infection. In Australia hydranencephaly and arthrogryposis (crooked limbs, see Chapter 10) have been found separately or together in newborn dairy calves of all breeds. These calves are blind, dull ("dummy calves"), ataxic, and unable to suckle. At necropsy the telencephalic tissue is necrotic; both already differentiated neural cells and actively mitotic germinal cells are affected. In those animals with arthrogryposis, somatic efferent neurons in the ventral gray column of nearby limb-innervating parts of the spinal cord are absent or degenerative. The cause of these defects has been identified as the **Akabane virus.**

Mature sheep infected with **bluetongue virus** exhibit fever, lameness, and erosions and ulcerations of the oral and nasal mucosae. The live-virus vaccine produced to establish immunity in sheep was found to cause brain malformations including hydranencephaly in lambs born from ewes immunized during gestation. Experimental studies of direct innoculation of this vaccine virus into fetal sheep have demonstrated that innoculation between 50–58 days of gestation consistently produces a severe necrotizing encephalitis which is manifest at term as hydranencephaly. Innoculation between 75–78 days of gestation produces multifocal encephalitis, which presents at term as **porencephaly**, congenital cystic cavities in the cerebrum that may communicate with the lateral ventricle. Innoculation after 100 days of gestation causes mild focal encephalitis with no significant malformation.

Unilateral hydranencephaly was found in an 8-month-old miniature poodle with a visual deficit. No data was available to establish an in utero infection as the cause but the lesion was predominantly in the area of the neopallium supplied by the middle cerebral artery. In humans, considerable emphasis on the pathogenesis of this malformation has been placed on prenatal occlusion or agenesis of the carotid artery and this has been experimentally produced in puppies.

Prosencephalic Hypoplasia

A malformation appears in calves in which there is a small opening on the surface of the calvaria, which is abnormally flattened. This hole communicates with a malformed diencephalon, and cerebrospinal fluid may be draining from it. There are no cerebral hemispheres and the space where they are normally located is filled with bone from the reduced calvaria. The rest of the brain stem and cerebellum are present although their shape is altered. The development of the face, nasal openings and oral cavity is normal. This malformation, called **prosencephalic hypoplasia,** may represent a failure of the neural tube to separate from the surface ectoderm at its most rostral extent (rostral neuropore), which would prevent the normal development of the telencephalic vesicles.

CONGENITAL OCULAR AND VISUAL MALFORMATIONS

Numerous malformations of the eye have been described in domestic animals, most commonly in dogs and cattle. One study found that 17% of the congenital malformations reported in cattle involved the eye. Many of these were anomalies in the pigmentation of the iris and did not seriously compromise the animal's vision. In the following discussion only the more common, vision-impairing malformations will be presented.

A large percentage of Collie dogs have an hereditary malformation called the **Collie eye syndrome.** This results from a defect in the growth of the optic cup, and is usually seen in the retina and choroid as a focal dysplasia. A defective area in the sclera (ectasia) may be present. Also, a schisis of the optic nerve and a pigment-free zone in the retina and iris may be present; these are called a **coloboma** and are usually the result of abnormal closure of the ventral margin of the optic cup. Many ophthalmologists believe that the incidence and severity of Collie eye syndrome are correlated with an increased length-to-width ratio in the face of these dogs, a morphology for which some breeders have selected.

Retinal dysplasia is an abnormal development of the inner layer of the optic cup. This is inherited in the English Springer

Spaniel, American Cocker Spaniel, Bedlington Terrier, Sealyham Terrier and Labrador Retriever. Retinal dysplasias can also result from an in utero inflammation as occurs in kittens infected with the feline panleukopenia virus.

Anophthalmia and **microphthalmia** result from the failure of formation of an optic vesicle or, more commonly, from severe interference with normal growth of the optic cup. Often rudiments of the pigmented retina are found in the orbits of these animals. Along with other facial malformations, microphthalmia has been observed in kittens exposed to griseofulvin during gestation and as a part of an inherited craniofacial malformation in Burmese kittens (see Chapter 9). Hereditary microphthalmia has been reported in all species and breeds, but most frequently in Akitas, Collies, Schnauzers, Australian Shepherds, Great Danes and White Short-Horn cattle. In Guernsey cattle it is sometimes associated with a cardiac malformation and a twisted or missing tail. In pigs, dogs and cattle, microphthalmia often results if the diet of the mother is deficient in vitamin A.

Optic nerve hypoplasia has been observed in dogs, cats, and horses. In these animals the optic disk is small, as are the optic nerves, chiasm and optic tracts. The only evidence of optic nerves may be the meningeal coverings that extend from the eye to the optic chiasm. This condition is observed most commonly in Miniature Poodles.

Progressive retinal atrophy is a common disease in many breeds of dogs and is usually inherited. The onset can begin from prior to birth to after several years. It is a progressive disease that may include an abiotrophy of various components of the nervous coat of the retina. In some animals the initial sign is reduced night vision; in others a loss of object detection is the first function compromised. Electroretinographic examination often reveals reduced responsiveness to light in dogs under 3 months of age, well in advance of overt behavioral signs. This permits affected dogs to be removed from breeding stock, thereby reducing the incidence of this form of inherited blindness.

The term **cataract** defines any loss of clarity in the lens or lens capsule, regardless of the exact cause or time of onset. While the precise mode of transmission is unresolved in most breeds, it is clear that in several strains of dogs there is a heritable predisposition for cataracts. Cocker Spaniels are most commonly affected, with one study identifying lens opacities in 88% of the dogs examined. Beagles, Boston Terriers, Staffordshire Terriers, Old English Sheepdogs, Miniature Schnauzers, Poodles (all sizes), Fox Terriers and Afghans also show increased incidence of congenital primary cataracts. Congenital cataracts appear occasionally in cattle, and rarely in horses and cats.

Most Siamese cats have a medial deviation of the eyeballs, **medial strabismus**, and a few have a fine rapid involuntary oscillation called a **pendular nystagmus**. For normal vision there is a very precise anatomical relationship between the afferent visual pathway from the retina into the central nervous system and the efferent neurons that innervate the muscles that move the eye. Interneuronal connections from the visual cerebral cortex to the motoneurons in brain stem nuclei of cranial nerves III, IV, and VI cause the eyes to move conjugately together so that the appropriate portion of the retina of each eye will receive the light stimulus from the object being viewed. This will be the medial retina of the eye on the same side as the object and the lateral retina of the opposite eye.

In the normal cat about 65% of the axons in each optic nerve cross in the optic chiasm and project to the contralateral lateral geniculate nucleus. These come from neurons in the medial portion of each retina. Axons projecting from the lateral part of the retina do not cross in the optic chiasm. Rather, they terminate in the ipsilateral lateral geniculate nucleus. Thus, objects observed in the left area of the visual field stimulate neurons in the medial retina of the left eye and lateral retina of the right eye. These impulses will be conducted centrally to the right lateral geniculate nucleus and ultimately stimulate cortical neurons in the right cerebrum where binocular integration and visual perception occur. Visual inputs from the right visual field are transmitted to the left cerebrum.

Many Siamese cats have a developmental abnormality in this precise anatomical system; too many axons from each lateral retina cross in the optic chiasm. Developmentally this causes changes in the anatomical organization of neurons in the lateral geniculate nuclei and the visual cortices. As a result, different points in space project to the same site in the visual cortex. In order to unscramble this abnormal input, the inappropriate cortical projections are functionally suppressed in many Siamese cats. While this permits normal vision, with reduced binocularity, the link to ocular efferents remains abnormal and results in the strabismus and, occasionally, nystagmus.

This condition is due to incomplete expression of the gene for albinism. Most true albinos, white tigers, the pearl mink and Siamese cats show this anomaly. The light coat color of the Siamese is a temperature-sensitive variant for the albinism gene.

Bibliography

EMBRYOLOGY OF THE BRAIN AND SPINAL CORD

Angevine JB, Sidman RL: Autoradiographic study of cell migration during histogenesis of cerebral cortex in the mouse. *Nature* 192:766–768, 1961.

Berry F: Untersuchungen uber die Entwichlung der Motilitat und die histologische Differenzierung des kleinhirns bei der katze in den ersten Lebenswochen. In Aug Diss, Zurich, University of Bern, 1963.

Fujita S, Shimada M, Nakamura T: H³-Thymidine autoradiographic studies on the cell proliferation and differentiation in the external and the internal granular layers of the mouse cerebellum. *J Comp Neurol* 128:191–208, 1966.

Holfreter J, Hamburger V: Amphibians. In Willier BH, Weiss PA, Hamburger V, (eds): *Analysis of Development*. Philadelphia, Saunders, 1955.

Houston ML: The early brain development of the dog. *J Comp Neurol* 134:371–384, 1968.

Jacobson M: *Developmental Neurobiology*, ed 2. New York, Plenum, 1978.

Kaufmann J: Untersuchungen uber die Fruhentwicklung des kleinhirns bein Rind. In Aug Diss, Zurich, University of Bern, 1959.

Levi-Montalcini R: The origin and development of the visceral system in the spinal cord of the chick embryo. *J Morphol* 86:253–284, 1950.

Patten BM: *Embryology of the Pig*, ed 4. Philadelphia, Blakiston, 1954.

Phemister RD, Young S: The postnatal development of the canine cerebellar cortex. *J Comp Neurol* 134:243–254, 1968.

Purpura DP, et al: Comparative ontogenesis of structure-function relations in cerebral and cerebellar cortex. *Prog Brain Res* 4:187–221, 1964.

Rakic P: Extrinsic cytological determinants of basket and stellate cell dendritic pattern in the cerebellar molecular layer. *J Comp Neurol* 146:335–354, 1974.

Sidman RL: Cell-cell recognition in the developing central nervous system. In Schmitt FO, Worden FG (eds): *The Neurosciences: Third Study Program.* Cambridge, MA, MIT Press, 1974, pp 743–757.

Smith DE, Downs I: Postnatal development of the granule cell in the kitten cerebellum. *Am J Anat* 151–527, 1978.

Woodward JS. Origin of the external granule layer of the cerebellar cortex. *J Comp Neurol* 115:65–73, 1960.

Yamada KM, Spooner BS, Wessels NK: Ultrastructure and function of growth cones and axons of cultured nerve cells. *J Cell Biol* 49:614–635, 1971.

VISUAL SYSTEM DEVELOPMENT AND MALFORMATIONS

Acland GM: Developmental anomalies. In Blogg JR (ed): *The Eye in Veterinary Practice*, Philadelphia, Saunders, 1980, pp 106–166.

Aguirre GD, Rubin LF, Bistner SI: Development of the canine eye. *Am J Vet Res* 33:2399–2413, 1972.

Bistner SI, Rubin LF, Aguirre GD: Development of the bovine eye. *Am J Vet Res* 34:7–12, 1973.

Blasdel GG, Pettigrew JD: Effect of prior visual experience on cortical recovery from the effects of unilateral eyelid suture in cats. *J Physiol* 274:601–619, 1978.

Gelatt KN, Leipold HW, Coffman JR: Bilateral optic nerve hypoplasia in a colt. *JAVMA* 155:627–631, 1969.

Greiner JV, Weidman TA: Histogenesis of the cat retina. *Exp Eye Res* 30:439–453, 1980.

Greiner JV, Weidman TA: Histogenesis of the rabbit retina. *Exp Eye Res* 34:749–765, 1983.

Guillery RW: Visual Pathways in Albinos. *Sci Am* 230:44–54, 1974.

Guillery RW, Casagrande VA, Oberdorfer MD: Congenitally abnormal vision in Siamese cats. *Nature* 252:195–199, 1974.

Guillery RW, Kaas JH: Genetic abnormality of the visual pathways in a "white" tiger. *Science* 180:1287–1288, 1973.

Hubel DH: Exploration of the primary visual cortex. *Nature* 299–515–524, 1982.

Hubel DH, Wisel TN: Binocular interaction in striate cortex of kittens reared with artificial squint. *J Neurophysiol* 28:1041–1059, 1965.

Hubel DH, Wiesel, TN: The period of susceptibility to physiological effects of unilateral eye closure in kittens. *J Physiol* 206:419–436, 1970.

Hubel DH, Wiesel T: Aberrant visual projections in the Siamese cat. *J Physiol* 218:33–62, 1971.

Hughes WF, McLoon SC: Ganglion cell death during normal retinal development in the chick: comparisons with cell death induced by early target field destruction. *Exp Neurol* 66:587–601, 1979.

Johns PR, Rusoff AC, Dubin MW: Postnatal neurogenesis in the kitten retina. *J Comp Neurol* 187:545–556, 1979.

Kern TJ, Riis RC: Optic nerve hypoplasia in three miniature poodles. *JAVMA* 178:49–54, 1980.

Noden DM: Periocular mesenchyme: neural crest and

mesodermal interactions. In: Jakobiec FA (ed): *Ocular Anatomy, Embryology and Teratology.* Philadelphia, Harper & Row, 1982, pp 97–119.

Ozanics V, Jakobiec FA: Prenatal development of the eye and its adnexa. In Jakobiec FA (ed): *Ocular Anatomy, Embryology and Teratology.* Philadelphia, Harper & Row, 1982, pp 11–96.

Peiffer RL: Inherited ocular diseases of the dog and cat. *Compend Cont Ed* 4:152–166, 1982.

Pettigrew JD: The effect of visual experience on the development of stimulus specificity by kitten cortical neurons. *J Physiol* 237:49–74, 1974.

Rakic P: Prenatal development of the visual system in rhesus monkey. *Philos Trans R Soc Lond* 278:245–260, 1977.

Rubin LF, Lipton DE: Retinal degeneration in kittens. *JAVMA* 162:467–469, 1973.

Saunders LZ: Congenital optic nerve hypoplasia in collie dogs. *Cornell Vet* 42:67–80, 1952.

Shatz C: A comparison of visual pathways in Boston and midwestern Siamese cats. *J Comp Neurol* 171:205–228, 1976.

Shively JN, Epling GP, Jensen R: Fine structure of the postnatal development of the canine retina. *Am J Vet Res* 32:383–392, 1971.

Spaeth GL, Nelson LB, Beaudoin AR: Ocular teratology. In Jakobiec FA (ed): *Ocular Anatomy, Embryology and Teratology.* Philadelphia, Harper & Row, 1982, pp 955–1080.

West-Hyde L, Buykmihci N: Photoreceptor degeneration in a family of cats. *JAVMA* 181:143–247, 1982.

Wiesel TN: Postnatal development of the visual cortex and the influence of the environment. *Nature* 299:583–591, 1982.

Yakely WL, Wyman M, Donovan EF, Fechheimer NS: Genetic transmission of an ocular fundus anomaly in collies. *JAVMA* 152:457–461, 1968.

MALFORMATIONS OF THE SPINAL CORD

Bailey CS: An Embryological approach to the clinical significance of congenital vertebral and spinal cord abnormalities. *J Am Anim Hosp Assoc* 11:426–434, 1975.

Bone DL, Wilson RB: Primary syringomyelia in a kitten. *JAVMA* 181:928–929, 1982.

DeForest ME, Basrur PK: Malformations and the Manx syndrome in cats. *Can Vet J* 20:304–314, 1979.

Engel HN, Draper DD: Comparative prenatal development of the spinal cord in normal and dysraphic dogs: Embryonic stage. *Am J Vet Res* 43:1729–1734, 1982.

Engel HN, Draper DD: Comparative prenatal development of the spinal cord in normal and dysraphic dogs: Fetal stage. *Am J Vet Res* 43:1735–1743, 1982.

Leipold HW, Huston K, Blauch B, Guffy MM: Congenital defects of the caudal vertebral column and spinal cord in Manx cats. *JAVMA* 164:520–523, 1974.

McGrath JT: Spinal dysraphism in the dog. *Pathol Vet* 2:1–36, 1965.

Michael-James CC, Lassman LP, Tomlinson BE: Congenital anomalies of the lower spine and spinal cord in Manx cats. *J Pathol* 97:269–276, 1969.

Patten BM: Embryological stages in the establishing of myeloschisis with spina bifida. *Am J Anat* 93:365–395, 1953.

MALFORMATIONS OF THE BRAIN

Altman JW, Anderson WJ: Experimental reorganization of the cerebellar cortex. I. Morphological effects of elimination of all microneurons with prolonged X-irradiation started at birth. *J Comp Neurol* 146:355–406, 1972.

Altman JW: Experimental reorganization of the cerebellar cortex following X-irradiation. *J Comp Neurol* 165:31–65, 1976.

Brown TT, de Lahunta A, Bistner SI, Scott FW, McEntee K: Pathogenetic studies of infection of the bovine fetus with bovine viral diarrhea virus. I. Cerebellar atrophy. *Vet Pathol* 11:486–505, 1974.

Brown TT, de Lahunta A, Scott FW, Kahrs RF, McEntee K, Gillespie, JH: Virus-induced congenital anomalies of the bovine fetus. II. Histopathology of cerebellar degeneration (hypoplasia) induced by the virus of bovine viral diarrhea-mucosal disease. *Cornell Vet* 63:562–578, 1973.

Cho DY, Leipold HW: Congenital defects of the bovine central nervous system. *Vet Bulletin* 47:489–504, 1977.

Cho DY, Leipold HW: Anencephaly in calves. *Cornell Vet* 68:60–69, 1978.

Cork LC, Troncosco JC, Price DL: Canine inherited ataxia. *Ann Neurol* 9:492–499, 1981.

Csiza CK, de Lahunta A, Scott FW, Gillespie JH: Spontaneous feline ataxia. *Cornell Vet* 62:300–322, 1972.

Csiza CK, Scott FW, de Lahunta A, Gillespie JH: Pathogenesis of feline panleukopenia virus in susceptible newborn kittens. II. Pathology and immunofluorescence. *Infect Immun* 3:838–846, 1971.

de Lahunta A: *Veterinary Neuroanatomy and Clinical Neurology,* ed 2. Philadelphia, Saunders, 1983.

de Lahunta A, Averill DR, Jr: Hereditary cerebellar cortical and extrapyramidal nuclear abiotrophy in Kerry Blue Terriers. *JAVMA* 168:1119–1124, 1976.

de Lahunta A, Fenner WR, Indrieri RJ, Mellick PW, Gardner S, Bell JS: Hereditary cerebellar cortical abiotrophy in the Gordon Setter. *JAVMA* 177:538–541, 1980.

Dennis SM, Leipold HW: Anencephaly in sheep. *Cornell Vet* 62:273–281, 1972.

Halsey JH, Jr, et al: The morphogenesis of hydranencephaly. *J Neurol Sci* 12:187–217, 1971.

Hartley WJ, De Saram WG, Della-Porta AJ, Snowdon WA, Shepherd, NC: Pathology of congenital bovine epizootic arthrogryposis and hydranencephaly and its relationship to Akabane virus. *Aust Vet J* 53:319–325, 1977.

Hartley WJ, Barker JSF, Wanner RA, Farrow BRH: Inherited cerebellar degeneration in the rough coated Collie. *Aust Vet Pract* 8:1–7, 1978.

Herndon RM, Margolis G, Kilham L: The synaptic organization of the malformed cerebellum induced by perinatal infection with the feline panleukopenia virus. *J Neuropathol* 30:196–205, 557–570, 1971.

Johnson RH, Margolis G, Kilham L: Identity of feline ataxia virus with the feline panleukopenia virus. *Nature* 214:175–177, 1967.

Johnson, RT: Effects of viral infection on the developing nervous system. *N Engl J Med* 287:599–604, 1972.

Kahrs RF, Scott FW, de Lahunta A: Congenital cerebellar hypoplasia and ocular defects in calves following bovine viral diarrhea-mucosal disease infection in pregnant cattle. *JAVMA* 156:1443–1450, 1970.

Kilham L, Margolis G: Viral etiology of spontaneous ataxia of cats. *Am J Pathol* 48:991–1011, 1966.

Kilham L, Margolis G, Colby E: Congenital infections of cats and ferrets by feline panleukopenia virus manifested by cerebellar hypoplasia. *Lab Invest* 17:465–480.

Llinas R, Hillman DE, Precht W: Neuronal circuit reorganization in mammalian agranular cerebellar cortex following panleukopenia virus infection. *J Neurobiol* 4:69–94, 1973.

MacLachlan NJ, Osburn BI: Bluetongue virus-induced hydranencephaly in cattle. *Vet Pathol* 20:563–573, 1983.

Margolis G, Kilham L: Virus-induced cerebellar hypoplasia. In Zimmerman, HM (ed): *Infections of the Nervous System*, Baltimore, Williams & Wilkins, 1968, pp 113–146.

Osburn BI, et al: Experimental viral-induced congenital encephalopathies. I. Pathology of hydranencephaly and porencephaly caused by bluetongue vaccine virus. II. The pathogenesis of bluetongue vaccine virus infection in fetal lambs. *Lab Invest* 25:197–205, 206–218, 1971.

Richards WAC, Crenshaw GL, Bushnell RB: Hydraencephaly of calves associated with natural bluetongue virus infection. *Cornell Vet* 61:336–348, 1971.

Scott FW, Kahrs RF, de Lahunta A, Brown TT, McEntee K, Gillespie JH: Virus induced congenital anomalies of the bovine fetus. I. Cerebellar degeneration (hypoplasia), ocular lesions and fetal mummification following experimental infection with bovine viral diarrhea-mucosal disease virus. *Cornell Vet* 63:536–560, 1973.

Trautwein G, Meyer H: Experimentelle Untersuchungen uber erbliche Meningocele cerebralis beim Schwein. II. Pathomorphologie der Gehirnmissbildungen. *Pathol Vet* 3:543–555, 1966.

CHAPTER 7

Peripheral Nervous System and Ear

Formation of the Peripheral Nervous System

Shortly after the fusion of the neural folds and separation of the neural tube from overlying surface ectoderm, a population of cells derived from the neurepithelium condenses dorsal to the tube. This population, which is called the **neural crest** (Fig. 7.1), forms most of the cells, including neurons and Schwann cells, located in the peripheral nervous system (PNS).

Subsequently all neural crest cells migrate away from the dorsal midline. In the trunk region they disperse along several pathways. Most of them move ventrally, passing either between the spinal cord and somites, as shown in Figure 7.2, or in intersomitic spaces.

Upon emerging from beneath the somites, some of these crest cells aggregate segmentally dorsolateral to the aorta, where they will subsequently form **sympathetic trunk ganglia.** Any aggregation of neuronal cell bodies located outside of the CNS is called a ganglion. As shown in Figure 7.3, other crest cells continue migrating ventrally to form the **abdominal sympathetic ganglia** and secretory cells of the **adrenal medulla.**

Some neural crest cells stop their ventral migration as soon as they contact the somites. These will form the metameric (segmental) **spinal ganglia,** which contain sensory neurons. In addition to forming neurons, crest cells form all of the accessory and glial cells within ganglia and all the Schwann cells that ensheath peripheral nerves.

A second, smaller group of neural crest cells migrates laterally from the dorsal midline beneath the presumptive epidermis. This group will form the **melanocytes** (pigment cells) of the integument. Pigment cells associated with visceral organs and mesenteries are also of neural crest origin.

There are two exceptions to this basic pattern of neural crest development. First, some crest cells emigrating from the sacral level of the spinal cord and the caudal part of the brain (occipital level) invade the wall of the gut and other internal organs and blood vessels. Those that populate the length of the gut form ganglia of the **enteric plexus.** Other crest cells from these regions develop into the **parasympathetic ganglia**, which are located in tissues throughout the body (see Autonomic Nervous System, Parasympathetic Components).

The second exception is that some of the neural crest cells arising from the cephalic neural folds have a much broader range of derivatives. In addition to forming most of the peripheral neurons in the head, these crest cells contribute to the development of facial skeletal and connective tissues, as will be discussed in Chapter 9.

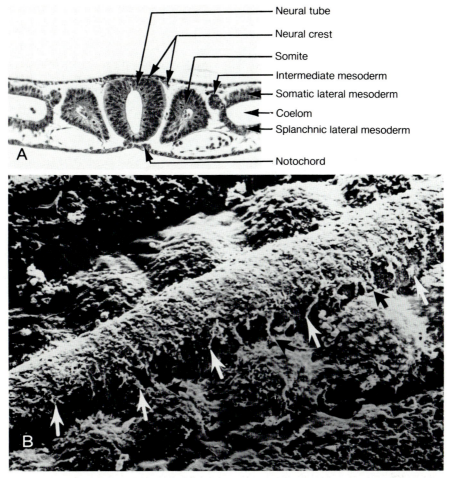

Figure 7.1. Early migration of neural crest cells. *A* is a transverse section at the level of the 8th somite from a 14-somite feline embryo. Crest cells are beginning to emigrate from the roof of the neural tube. *B* is a dorsal view of a chick embryo from which the dorsal surface ectoderm has been removed to reveal the spinal cord and somites. *White arrows* illustrate the leading edge of the migrating neural crest population, some of which (*black arrows*) are contacting somites. The cranial end of this embryo is to the right. (*B* courtesy of K Tosney.)

CLASSIFICATION OF PERIPHERAL NERVES

The PNS consists of motor or **efferent** components that conduct impulses away from the CNS, and sensory or **afferent** components that conduct impulses towards the CNS. Most nerves contain both kinds of fibers, and it is not possible to functionally identify individual axons unless neuroanatomic mapping or electrophysiological methods are used.

Virtually every tissue in the body except the CNS is innervated by efferent and afferent neurons, although the relative numbers of each type varies greatly. Muscle, for example, has a large number of efferent terminals, with fewer afferent endings present. Conversely, the integument primarily receives afferent innervation, although efferent neurons to peripheral blood vessels, skin glands, and feather or hair muscles are present.

Separation of the PNS into afferent and efferent components distinguishes two subdivisions that are both functionally and, as

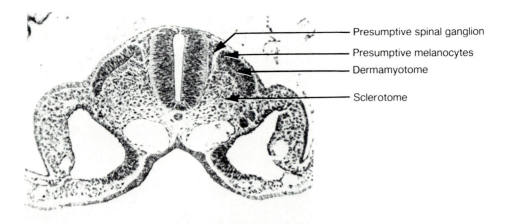

Figure 7.2. Transverse section at the 8th somite of a 24-somite cat embryo. Some crest cells are moving ventrally between the dispersing sclerotome and wall of the neural tube. Others, the prospective melanocytes, are moving laterally between the surface ectoderm and somites. The primordia of the spinal ganglia have ceased their ventral migrations.

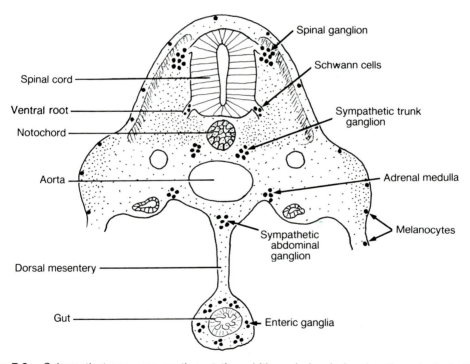

Figure 7.3. Schematic transverse section at the midthoracic level showing the principal sites of neural crest cell distribution. All except those in the gut wall are derived from the thoracic spinal cord; the enteric population migrated caudally along the gut from the occipital level of the brain.

shown in Figure 7.4, anatomically very different. Motor neuron dendritic zones and cell bodies are located in the CNS or in peripheral ganglia and their axons extend to target tissues. In contrast, the dendritic zones of sensory neurons are located in peripheral tissues and the axons project centrally. The cell bodies of most afferent neurons are located in spinal and cranial sensory ganglia. The exceptions are those associated with vision and olfaction, which are found in the retina and olfactory epithelium. These are not derived from the neural crest.

All neurons of the PNS are categorized as

being **visceral** or **somatic**. Originally this subdivision was based on whether their peripheral terminals (efferent telodendria or afferent dendritic zones) were located in tissues derived from splanchnopleure, i.e. visceral tissues, or somatopleure, i.e. body wall tissues.

However, the term visceral includes innervation of all **involuntary muscles,** including those of peripheral blood vessels and the integument, parts of which are derived from somatic mesoderm or, in the head, from the neural crest. In these cases the categorization of visceral versus somatic innervation is usually assigned based on analogous tissues in the trunk. As a general rule, **somatic afferent** and **somatic efferent** neurons innervate voluntary muscles and related connective tissues plus structures in which ectodermally-derived epithelia are present (skin, mouth, most sense organs). **Visceral efferent** neurons are involved with control of involuntary muscle movement in the digestive tract, glands and the cardiovascular system. **Visceral afferent** fibers project to these same tissues.

SOMATIC EFFERENT AND SOMATIC AFFERENT SYSTEMS

Voluntary muscles in the vertebrate body are derived from paraxial mesoderm, which includes the somites in the trunk region and similar but less well developed condensations of paraxial mesoderm in the head. These muscles are striated and are innervated by somatic efferent neurons. The somata and dendritic processes of these neurons are located in the **ventral gray column** of the spinal cord or within discrete motor nuclei in the brain stem, and their axons project directly to target muscles.

Somatic efferent neurons are among the earliest neural cells to develop in the embryo. The first of these axons begin to emerge from the ventrolateral margin of the neural tube shortly after neurulation. The pattern of axon emergence is always segmen-

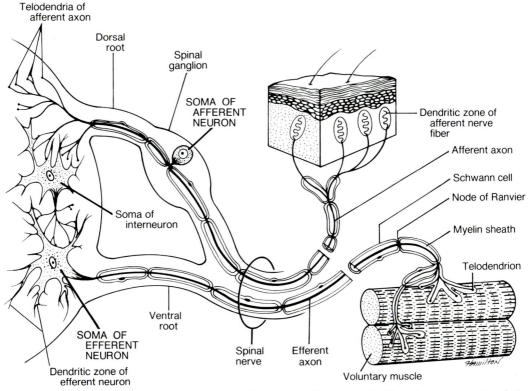

Figure 7.4. The anatomical organization of somatic efferent and afferent components of the peripheral nervous system. (Redrawn after Mader, 1976.)

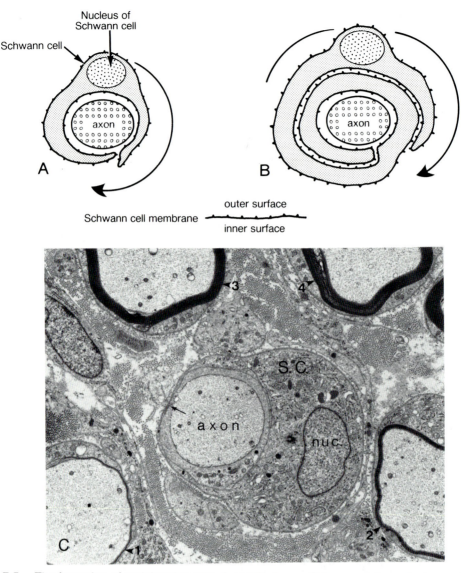

Figure 7.5.   The formation of peripheral myelin. *A* and *B* show a Schwann cell enveloping and then wrapping around an axon. Subsequently, the original outer surfaces of the Schwann cell membrane will fuse and most of the cytoplasm will be removed from all but the outmost layer of the cell. *C* is an electron micrograph of the ventral root from a neonatal puppy. The Schwann cell (*S.C.*) in the center is enveloping an *axon. Numbered arrows* indicate progressive stages of myelin deposition in adjacent efferent axons of this root. *Nuc.*, nucleus of Schwann cell. (Courtesy of John F. Cummings.)

tal, even though the somata are usually distributed continuously along the ventral gray column of several segments. The growth cones of these axons often establish contacts with immature myogenic mesenchyme cells before the latter have moved to their definitive location.

   As soon as they emerge from the neural tube, bundles of somatic efferent axons are enveloped with **Schwann cells.** Later the bundles become separated into individual axons, a process called **fasciculation.** Schwann cells ensheathing each axon begin to wrap around the axon and deposit myelin, as shown in Figure 7.5.

   Somatic afferent neurons transmit information about any physical or chemical stimulus impinging upon the animal. These are called **exteroceptive** functions, and involve receptors in the skin. In the head there are somatic afferents projecting to specialized mechanoreceptors associated with the vestibular and auditory systems as well as photoreceptors in the eye and, in lower vertebrates, the pineal.

Somatic afferent neurons projecting to voluntary muscles and associated connective tissues (fasciae, tendons), or to ligaments and joint capsule tissues mediate **proprioceptive** functions. These provide information necessary for control of posture and movement intensity.

In the trunk the somata of these afferent neurons are located in spinal ganglia associated with the segmental spinal nerves. **Cranial ganglia** with sensory function are less regular in their location than the segmental spinal ganglia. Some of their neurons are derived from thickenings of the lateral surface ectoderm called **neurogenic placodes** (Fig. 7.6 and 7.7) rather than from the neural crest. For example, the vestibular and cochlear (spiral) ganglia are formed entirely from cells that break away from the medioventral wall of the otic placode. The functional significance of this dual origin of cranial afferent neurons is not known.

Neurons in sensory ganglia are initially bipolar, with peripheral and central projections emerging from opposite sides of the soma. As the cells mature these two outgrowths join together, and remain attached to the soma only by a single convoluted stem axon. Thus, sensory impulses traveling centrally from the skin can enter the CNS directly, without involvement of the neuronal cell body. The central projections from spinal ganglia course through dorsal roots and enter the spinal cord segmentally. Most of these axons have their synapses upon neurons in the dorsal grey column.

AUTONOMIC NERVOUS SYSTEM

While the axons of the somatic efferent system project from cell bodies located within the CNS directly to their target mus-

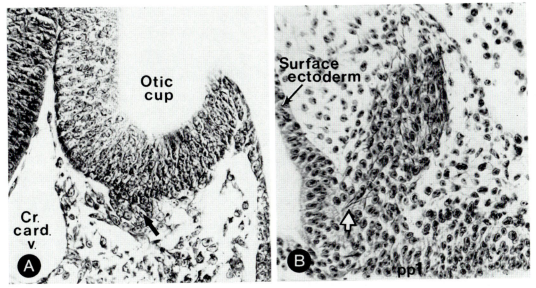

Figure 7.6. Neurogenic placodes. *A* shows neuroblasts (*arrows*) breaking away from the epithelium of the *otic cup* in a 2-day quail embryo. These neuroblasts will subsequently form neurons in the vestibular and cochlear ganglia. The wall of the myelencephalon is to the left. *Cr. card. v.*, cranial cardinal vein. *B* illustrates the development of neurons forming the geniculate (VIIth cranial nerve) ganglion. These arise from surface ectoderm located close to site of contact by the first pharyngeal pouch (ppl) in a 3-day chick embryo. *Arrow* indicates afferent axons. (From D'Amico-Martel and Noden, 1983.)

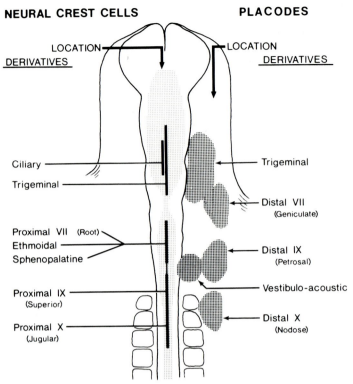

Figure 7.7. Schematic drawing showing the locations of neural crest and placodal primordia of cranial ganglia in a neurula-stage avian embryo. The ciliary, ethmoidal and sphenopalatine contain parasympathetic second neurons; all the rest are sensory ganglia. The avian acoustic (cochlear) ganglion is homologous to the mammalian spiral ganglion. (From D'Amico-Martel and Noden, 1983.)

cles, the visceral efferent network always involves *at least two neurons,* as shown in Figure 7.8. One cell body is in the CNS, the other is in a peripheral ganglion. Collectively the visceral efferent neurons are part of the autonomic (involuntary) nervous system. Visceral afferent neurons and interneurons in the spinal cord and brain, especially the hypothalamus, are also included in the autonomic nervous system.

The peripheral component of the autonomic system has three principal subdivisions, the **sympathetic, parasympathetic** and **enteric** systems. All share several common properties. Each has both a **first** or **preganglionic neuron** and one or more **second neurons.** The soma of a preganglionic neuron is located in the **intermediate gray column** of the spinal cord or equivalent nucleus of the brain, and its axon projects onto the cell body of the second neuron, which is located

in a peripheral ganglion. The axon of the second neuron is the **postganglionic axon**; it usually projects to the target tissue. All second neurons are derived from the neural crest.

Sympathetic Components

The **sympathetic** cells of the visceral efferent system are generally concerned with the response of the body to stress. Sympathetic preganglionic neurons are all located in the intermediate gray column of the spinal cord between the 1st thoracic and 4th lumbar segments. For this reason the sympathetic system is often referred to as the **thoracolumbar** component of the autonomic nervous system.

Sympathetic preganglionic axons course through the ventral gray column and white matter (marginal zone) then enter the ventral roots. After a short distance these visceral efferent axons diverge from the ventral roots and enter the **communicating (visceral) rami,** which are short, segmented nerves (Fig. 7.8) connecting the thoracolumbar spinal nerves with the **sympathetic trunk.** The paired sympathetic trunks (Fig. 7.9) are longitudinal nerves located ventrolateral to the vertebrae. Situated segmentally along these trunks are **sympathetic trunk ganglia,** also called the chain or paravertebral ganglia. Within the sympathetic trunk ganglia are cell bodies and dendritic processes of sympathetic **second neurons.** While most preganglionic fibers within each communicating ramus synapse upon second neurons in the closest trunk ganglion, others project longitudinally to other segments or else pass through the chain ganglia and join splanchnic nerves. Preganglionic axons in splanchnic nerves then synapse upon second neu-

rons in **abdominal sympathetic ganglia** located near the major abdominal branches of the aorta (celiac, cranial and caudal mesenteric ganglia).

There are several alternate courses that axons projecting from neurons in the sympathetic trunk ganglia can follow: (a) dorsally through communicating rami to join spinal nerves (Fig. 7.8) and reach target tissues in or near the integument, (b) ventrally via splanchnic nerves to abdominal visceral organs, or (c) longitudinally within the sympathetic trunk to exit and join spinal or splanchnic nerves at a different level. Postganglionic axons from the abdominal sympathetic ganglia project to visceral organs.

The embryonic caudal cervical and first three thoracic trunk ganglia fuse to form the **cervicothoracic ganglion.** Cranial to this along the cervical sympathetic trunk are

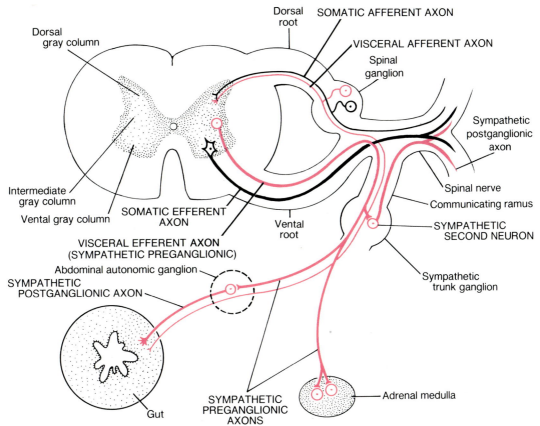

Figure 7.8. Schematic section at the thoracic level of the spinal cord illustrating the anatomical organization of somatic and visceral (*red*) components of the peripheral nervous system.

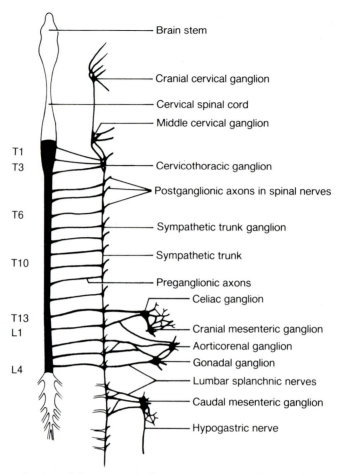

Figure 7.9. Organization of the sympathetic nervous system. Preganglionic axons from the spinal cord leave the ventral roots and enter a sympathetic trunk ganglion via a communicating ramus. These axons may synapse upon a second neuron in the closest trunk ganglion, may travel cranially or caudally along the sympathetic trunk to a different trunk ganglion, or may pass through the ganglion and synapse upon a neuron in an abdominal plexus ganglion. Only ventral roots T_1–L_4 carry preganglionic axons. Trunk ganglia located cranial or caudal to these levels receive their inputs from axons running in the sympathetic trunk.

similar aggregates of second neurons, the **middle cervical** and **cranial cervical ganglia.** Preganglionic axons to these two ganglia travel cranially along the sympathetic trunk from the thoracic spinal region. There are no sympathetic visceral efferent axons emanating from the cervical spinal cord.

The communicating rami between the spinal nerves T_1 through L_4 and the thoracolumbar sympathetic trunk will contain both preganglionic and postganglionic axons. The remainder of the lumbar and the sacral communicating rami will contain only postganglionic sympathetic axons that

project from caudal thoracic and lumbosacral trunk ganglia to the spinal nerves serving the caudal part of the animal.

In the cervical region the **vertebral nerve** serves as a communicating ramus for postganglionic axons coursing from the cervicothoracic ganglion to cervical spinal nerves. This nerve passes with the vertebral artery through the transverse canal, and is closely associated with segmental cervical spinal nerves as they emerge from the intervertebral foramina. Postganglionic axons of the vertebral nerve join these spinal nerves and project to smooth muscles in neck region.

Other branches from the cervicothoracic ganglion pass to the ventral branches of the spinal nerves that form the brachial plexus for distribution to the thoracic limb.

Most of the axons in the cervical part of the sympathetic trunk are preganglionic, arising from neuronal cell bodies in the first four or five thoracic spinal cord segments. These synapse in the cranial cervical ganglion, from which postganglionic axons project in plexuses along blood vessels and via cranial nerve branches to cephalic structures.

The first and second neurons of the sympathetic nervous system utilize different neurotransmitters. Preganglionic telodendria release **acetylcholine,** for which there are specific receptors on the postsynaptic cell. In contrast, most sympathetic second neurons release **norepinephrine** at their distal terminals.

In addition to forming sympathetic second neurons, some midthoracic level neural crest cells form the secretory **chromaffin cells** in the medulla of the **adrenal (suprarenal) gland.** These crest cells are innervated by preganglionic sympathetic neurons, and release norepinephrine and epinephrine upon stimulation. Thus, they are biochemi-

cally similar to the sympathetic second neurons, but lack neuronal processes.

Parasympathetic Components

The **parasympathetic** visceral efferent system is generally concerned with normal homeostatic regulation of visceral functions. Preganglionic cell bodies (first neurons) are located in brain stem nuclei and their fibers emerge with several cranial nerves (n. III, oculomotor; n. VII, facial; n. IX, glossopharyngeal; n. X, vagus; and n. XI, accessory). In addition there are parasympathetic first neurons in the sacral segments of the spinal cord. Because of this arrangement, the parasympathetic system is sometimes referred to as the **craniosacral** component of the autonomic system.

Both the location and biochemical composition of parasympathetic second neurons are different from those of sympathetics. As a rule these neurons are located in or close to the wall of the organ innervated and have very short axons. Most of them are **cholinergic,** i.e. they release acetylcholine at their terminals. Parasympathetic and sympathetic second neurons are both derived from the neural crest.

In the sacral region, shown in Figure 7.10,

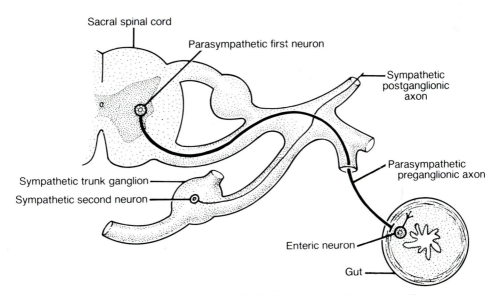

Figure 7.10. Organization of sacral parasympathetic and sympathetic visceral efferent components. The preganglionic component of the sympathetic network would be located in the intermediate gray column of the thoracolumbar spinal cord.

preganglionic neuronal cell bodies derived from the germinal layer of the neural tube are located in the intermediate grey column. Their axons enter segmental ventral roots and spinal nerves. These axons branch off the sacral spinal nerves to form the pelvic nerve, which courses to the urogenital organs and caudal part of the digestive tract.

Parasympathetics are more numerous and diffuse in the head region (Figs. 7.11 and 7.12). The largest component is in the vagus (Xth cranial) nerve, which contains parasympathetic preganglionic visceral efferent axons that terminate on second neurons located in viscera throughout the thoracic and abdominal regions. This large nerve also contains axons having other functions, including many visceral afferent axons plus,

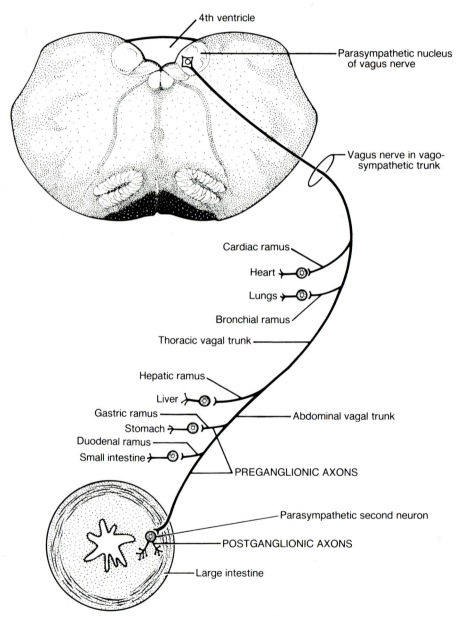

Figure 7.11. Parasympathetic visceral efferent components of the vagus nerve. At the top is shown a schematic transverse section of the medulla.

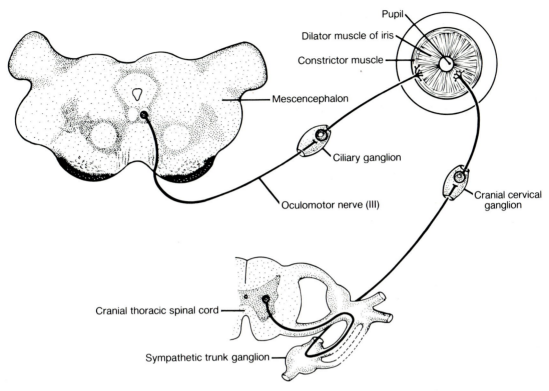

Figure 7.12. Autonomic innervation of the pupillary muscles. In the sympathetic component, the first neurons are located in the intermediate gray column of the cranial thoracic spinal cord. Their axons course through adjacent trunk ganglia and the sympathetic trunk to the cranial cervical ganglion; here they synapse upon second neurons whose postganglionic axons join with other cranial nerves and project to the dilator muscles of the pupil. Parasympathetic first neurons are located within the mesencephalon (oculomotor nucleus). These preganglionic axons project via the oculomotor (IIIrd) cranial nerve to the ciliary ganglion, where they terminate upon second neurons. Axons from the latter project to the constrictor muscles of the pupil.

in the cranial region, somatic efferent axons that innervate muscles of the pharynx, larynx, and esophagus.

The preganglionic neuronal cell bodies associated with the vagus nerve are derived from the germinal layer of the neural tube in the medulla and develop in the region of the mantle layer that corresponds to the intermediate gray column of the thoracolumbar spinal cord. These cell bodies form the **parasympathetic** or visceral motor **nucleus** of the vagus nerve. The preganglionic axons grow out of the medulla in the rootlets of the vagus nerve and course caudally in association with the cervical part of the sympathetic trunk. This nerve segment is called the **vagosympathetic trunk.**

As it passes through the thoracic inlet

branches of the vagus supply the heart. The parasympathetic axons in these branches terminate in telodendria in the wall of the heart at the site of the second order neurons, which are derived from neural crest cells that arose at the levels of somites 1 and 2. This corresponds to the location of the heart primordium at the time of neural crest migration, during the neurula stage. The cell bodies of these second order neurons are clustered in ganglia and have short postganglionic axons that terminate on cardiac muscle cells. The vagus nerves continue through the thorax in close approximation to the esophagus and project caudally, contributing to the plexus of nerves that follow blood vessels to the various organs in the abdomen. In no instances do synapses occur until the preganglionic axons enter the wall of the target.

Enteric System

The neurons located in the wall of the gut are often categorized together with other parasympathetic second neurons. They do share a common embryonic origin, being derived from cranial (myelencephalic) and sacral neural crest cells. Also, some are cholinergic. However, these enteric neurons are unique in many ways.

The wall of the gut has as many neurons (approximately 10^8 in humans) as the spinal cord. Since there are only a few thousand axons in the vagus nerve, very few enteric neurons receive a direct input from the CNS. In fact, most of these neurons project to one another. In addition the enteric ganglia are biochemically extremely heterogeneous, there being over a dozen different neurotransmitters already identified.

The enteric system has two, interconnected subdivisions. Ganglia and axons located circumferentially between the circular and longitudinal muscles of the gut wall constitute the **myenteric ganglion** and **plexus;** those located deep to the muscular layers form the **submucosal ganglion** and **plexus.** The function of these plexuses is to maintain craniocaudal peristaltic waves of contraction. Except in the esophagus this system can operate independent of preganglionic input, which normally serves to coordinate enteric activity with eating and digestion.

Visceral Afferents

All visceral afferent neurons are derived from the neural crest, and their axons often accompany visceral efferent axons to innervate the same tissues. In many cases, especially with respect to sensory innervation of abdominal and thoracic tissues, the afferent cell bodies are located in cranial and spinal ganglia over a considerably greater length of the body than would be predicted from mapping of visceral efferent fiber origins. There are also some visceral afferent cell bodies located in the wall of the gut. Based on their unique functions, afferent axons that innervate chemoreceptors of the olfactory epithelium, tongue, pharynx and palate are sometimes categorized as **special visceral afferents,** even though these target tissues are not of splanchnopleuric origin.

CONTROL OF NEURAL CREST CELL MIGRATION

The translocations of neural crest cell are not random. Rather they are both highly patterned and specific for each axial level of the embryo. For example, crest cells emigrating from the thoracic neural tube migrate metamerically towards the aorta but do not go futher ventrally and do not reach the level of the gut. In contrast many of the crest cells leaving the caudal brain stem or sacral spinal cord levels move to the wall of the gut.

It is possible to analyze how these disparate migratory behaviors are controlled by surgically manipulating either the crest cells or the embryonic tissues around them. For example, when avian premigratory thoracic crest cells are grafted in the place of brain stem (myelencephalic) crest cells, they migrate to and along the gut, where they subsequently form parasympathetic and enteric neurons. Thus, the grafted crest cells move and differentiate in accordance with their new location. These experiments, and many others of a similar design, have proved that it is the **embryonic environment** into and through which crest cells migrate that dictates the course of their movements.

The complete displacements of crest cells are accomplished by two mechanisms: active cell migration and passive translocation. Inert objects such as microscopic latex beads will, if implanted in pathways normally traversed by neural crest cells, partially mimic the apparent movements exhibited by crest cells. These data further indicate the critical role of other cell populations and extracellular matrix components in the morphogenesis of the neural crest (see Fig. 9.4).

The most complex aspect of neural crest distribution is that involved with establishing patterns of pigmentation. Transplantation experiments have shown that crest cell populations from any part of the body placed into a different region of the embryonic integument will form pigment patterns appropriate to their new location (Fig. 7.13). The full expression of individual and species-specific patterns of pigmentation is largely the result of differential expression of crest-derived melanocytes rather than the embryonic distribution of prospective pigment cells. This variable expression of genes responsible for pigment formation and deposition is controlled by the integument. How the somatopleure is programmed to elicit the many striking and unique pigment patterns found in vertebrates is not known.

CONTROL OF AUTONOMIC NEURON DIFFERENTIATION

The development of second neurons of the autonomic nervous system proceeds in three phases. First is **determination,** the committment to develop into an autonomic neuron. The second phase is **cytodifferentiation,** which is the appearance of biochemical characteristics unique to a sympathetic or parasympathetic neuron. This is followed by **maturation,** the elevation of these characteristics to adult levels.

It is not known whether determination occurs before or during migration of crest cells, or possibly, may involve a series of programming events occurring throughout this period. Several experiments have been done in which neural crest cells are excised and grown in culture alone or in combination with other tissues. It was found that when somites were co-cultured with the crest cells many of the latter formed neurons containing norepinephrine, which is the principal neurotransmitter of peripheral sympathetic neurons. In contrast, when crest cells are co-cultured with pieces of the gut they form the various types of neurons normally found in enteric ganglia. These experiments led to the conclusion that tissues encountered during the migratory phase of crest cell development play a causal role in their determination as autonomic neurons. The

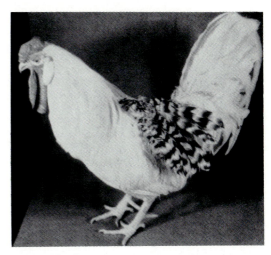

Figure 7.13. A 2½-year-old White Leghorn rooster with an ectopic, pigmented wing. This chimera was created by combining embryonic wing skin from a White Leghorn with peritoneal melanocytes from a Barred Plymouth Rock embryo, and grafting the tissues to the dorsal midline of a Leghorn host embryo. The pattern and colors of pigmentation in the extra wing are characteristic of a normal Barred Rock wing. These data indicate that White Leghorns are colorless because their neural crest cells are unable to form normal melanocytes. Of more importance, this experiment proves that the spatial and temporal expression of melanocytes (i.e. patterns of spots, stripes, barring, etc.) is normally controlled by the integument. (From Rawles ME: Physiol Zool 18:1–16, 1945).

transplant experiments described earlier support this conclusion.

More recent analyses using monoclonal antibodies directed against autonomic neurons have revealed that some crest cells have unique, neural-specific determinants on their surfaces during their initial dispersal from the neural folds. These data raise the possibility that the neural crest is a mosaic of determined subpopulations. However, autonomic neurons are unusual in that some of them can switch from cholinergic to catecholaminergic, and vice versa, even during early postnatal periods. It is not known why the cells remain capable of modulating their phenotype, but these data indicate that early phenotypic expressions of crest cells may be transient.

Even after sympathetic neurons have begun to express their unique biochemical properties, they are dependent upon interactions for their maturation. Figure 7.14 outlines the results of a series of experiments that examined the effect of cutting either the pre- or the postganglionic sympathetic axons on the activity of neurotransmitter-synthesizing enzymes in cranial cervical ganglia. Preganglionic nerve endings in the ganglia contain the enzyme **choline acetyl transferase (CAT),** and cell bodies of the second neurons contain **tyrosine hydroxylase (TOH),** the first enzyme in the synthesis of norepinephrine.

As the data in Figure 7.14C show, cutting either the preganglionic or the postganglionic axons prevents the normal maturation of enzymes in BOTH types of neurons. One component involved in the maturation process is the protein **nerve growth factor (NGF).** It has been known since the early 1950s that all sympathetic and some peripheral sensory neurons are dependent upon NGF for their normal maturation. Adding exogenous NGF can ameliorate the effects of postganglionic axotomy on the maturation of the second neuronal population. Some of this sparing effect is mediated through circulating NGF; some is probably also the result of NGF incorporation at the site of axotomy and intracellular retrograde transport of NGF along the nerve fibers.

PERIPHERAL NERVE—TARGET TISSUE INTERACTIONS

Interactions between nerves and their target tissues play essential roles in the development of somatic efferent and afferent neurons and voluntary muscles. As illustrated in Figure 7.15, more motor neurons are produced during early embryogenesis than survive. This cell death is a programmed feature of many neuronal populations, and the number of neurons that survive is influenced by the size (i.e. number of synaptic sites) of the target tissues. Surgically removing one leg or adding an extra one in the avian embryo markedly alters the pattern of moton neuron cell death (Fig. 7.15).

Conversely, removing the limb-innervating regions of the spinal cord will result in the atrophy of appendicular voluntary muscles and subsequent fusion of the joints (see Chapter 10). Similar effects are seen if motor neurons fail to develop or are destroyed by a disease process in utero, some of which are discussed in the following chapter. These experiments illustrate the necessity of establishing and maintaining contacts between nerves and their target tissues. Comparable interactions occur in the development of visceral efferents and most sensory systems, including the visual system. While these relationships are most important during embryonic development, loss of them at any time in the life of the animal may lead to similar degenerative conditions.

DEVELOPMENT OF THE INNER EAR

The ear is subdivided into external, middle and inner regions, each of which have different embryonic origins. Development of the external and middle ear structures is discussed in Chapters 9 and 14.

The inner ear consists of the **membranous labyrinth** and the vestibular and spiral (acoustic) ganglia associated with the VIIIth cranial nerve. In the embryo these are surrounded by the cartilaginous **otic capsule,** which becomes the ossified petrous and, postnatally, tympanic bulla regions of the temporal bone.

The primordium of the inner ear is first visible at the late neurula stage as a focal thickening of the surface ectoderm, the **otic placode,** located immediately adjacent to the midmyelencephalon. This placode invaginates to form the **otic cup** (Fig. 7.6), which contacts the wall of the myelencephalon. The lips of the cup close, separating the **otic vesicle** (Fig. 1.6 *A* and *B*) from the surface ectoderm. Neuroblasts break away from the ventromedial wall of the otic epithelium; these will form all of the neurons that innervate the inner ear.

Shortly afterwards, a series of outpocketings from the otic vesicle establish the primordia of the endolymphatic, semicircular

A. NEUROTRANSMITTER PRODUCTION IN SYMPATHETIC NEURONS

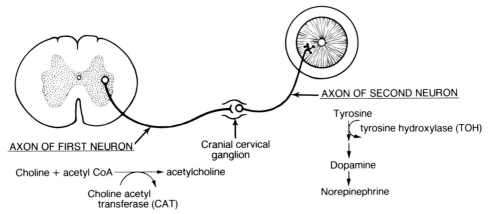

AXON OF SECOND NEURON

Tyrosine

tyrosine hydroxylase (TOH)

Dopamine

Norepinephrine

AXON OF FIRST NEURON

Cranial cervical ganglion

Choline + acetyl CoA ⟶ acetylcholine

Choline acetyl transferase (CAT)

B. POSTNATAL MATURATION OF SYMPATHETIC NEUROTRANSMITTER-SYNTHESIZING ENZYMES

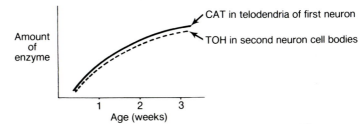

CAT in telodendria of first neuron

TOH in second neuron cell bodies

Amount of enzyme

Age (weeks)

C. EFFECTS OF AXOTOMY ON NEUROTRANSMITTER-SYNTHESIZING ENZYMES

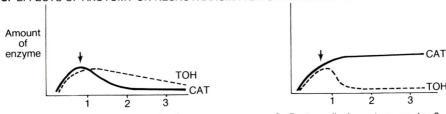

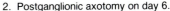

Amount of enzyme

TOH

CAT

1. Preganglionic axotomy on day 6.

CAT

TOH

2. Postganglionic axotomy on day 6.

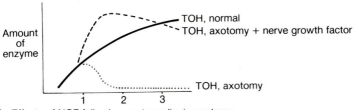

Amount of enzyme

TOH, normal

TOH, axotomy + nerve growth factor

TOH, axotomy

3. Effects of NGF following postganglionic axotomy

Figure 7.14. Control of sympathetic neuron maturation in the cranial cervical ganglion. *A* illustrates the biochemical pathways of acetylcholine and norepinephrine synthesis in the first (preganglionic) and second (postganglionic) components respectively. *B* illustrates the normal maturation of intracellular choline acetyl transferase (CAT) and tyrosine hydroxylase (TOH) in the neonatal mouse. *C* shows the effects on these enzymes of cutting preganglionic or postganglionic axons, or the results of adding nerve growth factor (NGF) following postganglionic axotomy.

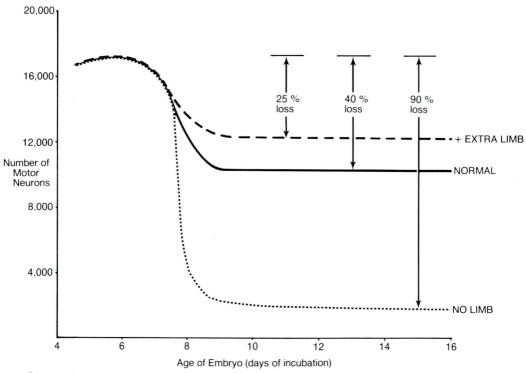

Figure 7.15. Effects of augmenting or deleting avian limb muscles on the embryonic survival of limb-innervating somatic efferent neurons. Note that there is normally a 40% loss of motor neurons in the embryo, and that altering the amount of available target tissues dramatically alters the number of neurons that survive. In some mammals there is a second period of motor neuron degeneration that occurs shortly after birth. (After Hamburger and Oppenheim, 1982.)

and cochlear ducts, as illustrated in Figure 7.16. The central part of each diverticulum for the semicircular ducts closes and degenerates, leaving an epithelial duct connected to the original otic vesicle only at its ends. The sac-like **utricle** and **saccule** form between the semicircular and cochlear ducts (Fig. 7.16 *C* and *E*). One end of each semicircular duct enlarges where it joins the utricle, forming an **ampulla.** Specialized clusters of receptor cells called **cristae** develop within each ampulla; those in the utricle and saccule are called **maculae.**

The cochlear diverticulum is formed from the ventral margin of the otic vesicle. The cochlear duct curls as it elongates, and the epithelial cells on one surface of the duct form specialized hair cells and supporting elements of the spiral organ (organ of Corti).

The embryonic vestibular and cochlear ducts are surrounded by the cartilaginous otic capsule, which undergoes continuous reshaping as the membranous labyrinth grows and later forms the bony labyrinth. The narrow spaces in which the membranous labyrinth develops are the **vestibule, semicircular canals** and the **cochlea,** which are filled with perilymphatic fluid. One surface of the cochlear duct is attached to the connective tissue of the otic capsule via the spiral ligament. Differential reshaping of the cochlea results in the establishment of two chambers beside the cochlear duct. These are the scala vestibuli and scala tympani, which are separated from one another except at the apical tip of the cochlear duct. The scala vestibuli is continuous with the perilymphatic space of the vestibule surrounding the utricle and saccule of the vestibular region of the membranous labyrinth.

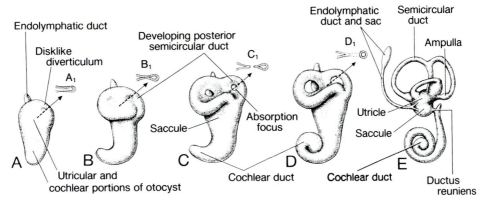

Figure 7.16. Schematic drawings showing in lateral views the sequential formation of the membranous labyrinth in a mammalian embryo of 5- to 20-mm length. (From Moore KA: *The Developing Human*, ed 3. Philadelphia, Saunders, 1982.)

MALFORMATIONS

Aganglionic Large Intestine

All neurons of the enteric plexus are derived from the neural crest, and the integrity of this neural network is essential for normal peristaltic activity of the gut. White foals born from crossing of overo horses show signs of colic within a day of birth and die shortly thereafter. No meconium is present in the bowel of these neonates. Histological examination reveals a complete absence of ganglia in the myenteric plexus in the terminal ileum, cecum and colon. Overo is a spotting pattern in Painted and Pinto ponies in which melanocyte-free areas appear preferentially in the ventral midline of the trunk and the distal aspects of the limbs and snout.

A similar but usually less severe lesion of the enteric nervous system occurs in humans (Hirschsprung's disease) and in two strains of mice (lethal spotted and piebald lethal). In these situations the deficit is restricted to a small region of the colon or rectum.

The correlation between certain pigment patterns and enteric ganglion deficiencies has led to the hypothesis that the primary genetic lesion may affect the neural crest, which is the precursor to both melanocytes and peripheral neurons. However, in vitro experiments using normal and lethal spotted mouse tissues have shown that normal crest cells are prevented from colonizing that re-gion of the gut which, in the mutant strain, is typically aganglionic. Thus, in this situation it is some feature of the gut wall and not of the neural crest population that is abnormal. There are no comparable data on the lethal white foals.

Defects Affecting Schwann Cells

Inherited abnormalities affecting only the peripheral myelin-producing cells are rare, in contrast to the more frequent incidence of CNS myelin abnormalities. Abnormal production or loss of peripheral myelin leads to **hypertrophic neuropathy,** which has been reported as an autosomal recessive in Tibetan Mastiff dogs (see Case History, page 82). It is characterized by generalized weakness beginning between $7\frac{1}{2}$ and 10 weeks postnatally. The weakness is worse in the pelvic limbs and is accompanied by hypotonia and hyporeflexia. If able to walk these dogs display a shuffling, plantigrade gait. Their peripheral nerves have extensive loss of myelin sheaths and slower impulse conduction times. A similar condition has been reported in humans and inbred mice carrying a gene called Trembler.

Congenital Deafness

Congenital deafness occurs infrequently in the dog (less than 0.3% incidence) and cat, and is rare in other domestic animals. In most instances the condition is due to degeneration of the cochlear duct, and signs of hearing impairment are usually evident within a few weeks of birth. Dalmations have the highest incidence of congenital deafness, followed by English Setters, Australian Shepherds, Boston Terriers, Old English Sheepdogs, English Bulldogs, Norwegian Dunkerhunds, and Great Danes.

Despite several attempts, it has not been possible to establish the mode of inheritance of congenital deafness in the Dalmation. In several other breeds it is correlated with the gene for the merle pigmentation pattern. This gene acts as an incomplete dominant and in the heterozygous condition it establishes large areas of bluish gray or dilute tan which often have small black splotches. However, in the homozygous state this gene causes the animal to be almost completely white, with small, blue eyes. Many of these animals have severe visual as well as hearing impairment. The merle traits were originally unique to the collie, and their appearance in several other breeds represents a common collie background. Recently, the incidence of congenital deafness in the collie has dropped considerably as breeders recognize and avoid breeding two merle dogs.

Congenital deafness in cats is also correlated with blue eyes and an absence of pigmentation in the skin. This is the result of a dominant white gene that suppresses the deposition of melanin in the skin and iris.

Spinal Ganglia Hypoplasia

A sensory neuropathy occurs in English Pointers causing loss of pain sensitivity in the paws starting around 3–5 months of age. This leads to self-mutilation of their digits (acral mutilation).

The spinal ganglia are reduced in size due to a deficiency in the number of neuronal cell bodies. Substance P, a neurotransmitter-modulating peptide found in many peripheral nociceptive axons, is reduced in the associated dorsal gray column of the spinal cord. A developmental hypoplasia with slowly progressive postnatal degeneration of somatic afferent neurons is present and an autosomal recessive inheritance is predicted

similar to that described in short-haired pointers. A similar disorder occurs in children with familial dysautonomia and in "mutilated foot" rats.

Bibliography

DEVELOPMENT OF THE PERIPHERAL NERVOUS SYSTEM

Ciba Symposium 83: *Development of the Autonomic Nervous System* London, Pitman Medical Books, 1981.

D'Amico-Martell A, Noden DM: Contributions of placodal and neural crest cells to avian cranial peripheral ganglia. *Am J Anat* 166:445–468, 1983.

de Lahunta A: *Veterinary Neuroanatomy and Clinical Neurology*, ed 2. Philadelphia, Saunders, 1983.

Hamburger V, Oppenheim RW: Naturally occurring cell death in vertebrates. *Neurosci Comment* 1:39–54, 1982.

Le Douarin, NM: *The Neural Crest.* London, Cambridge University Press, 1983.

Noden DM: The migration and cytodifferentiation of neural crest cells. In *Current Research Trends in Prenatal Craniofacial Development.* Pratt RM, Christiansen RL (eds): New York, Elsevier/North Holland, 1980, pp. 3–25.

Patterson, PH: Environmental determination of autonomic neurotransmitter functions. *Annu Rev Neurosci* 1:11–17, 1978.

Weston JA: The migration and differentiation of neural crest cells. *Adv Morphogenesis* 8:41–114, 1970.

PIGMENT CELLS AND PATTERNS

Burns M, Fraser M: *Genetics of the Dog,* ed 2. Philadelphia, Lippincott, 1966.

Geurts R: Hair Colour in the Horse. London, JA Allen, 1977.

Hutt FB: *Genetics for Dog Breeders.* San Francisco, Freeman, 1979.

Jones WE: *Genetics and Horse Breeding.* Philadelphia Lea & Febiger, 1982.

Little CC: *Inheritance of Coat Color in Dogs.* Ithaca, NY, Cornell University Press, 1957.

Rawles ME: Origin of melanophores and their role in the development of color patterns in vertebrates. *Physiol Rev* 28:383–408, 1948.

Robinson, R: *Genetics for Cat Breeders.* Oxford, Pergamon Press, 1977.

Robinson R: *Genetics for Dog Breeders.* Oxford Pergamon Press, 1982.

Searle G: *Comparative Aspects of Coat Color in Mammals.* London, Logos Press, 1968.

Trommerhausen-Smith A: Positive horse identification: 3. Coat color genetics. *Equine Pract* 1:24–35, 1979.

MALFORMATIONS OF THE PERIPHERAL NERVOUS SYSTEM

Brann L, Furtado D, Migliazzo CV, Baxendale J, Wood FD: Secondary effects of aganglionosis in the piebald-lethal mouse model of Hirschsprung's disease. *Lab Anim Sci* 27:946–954, 1977.

Cummings JF, Cooper BJ, de Lahunta A, van Winkle TJ: Canine inherited hypertrophic neuropathy. *Acta Neuropathol* 53:137–143, 1981.

Cummings JF, de Lahunta A, Winn SS: Acral mutilation and nociceptive loss in English Pointer dogs. *Acta Neuropathol* 53:119–127, 1981.

Hultgren BD: Ileocolic aganglionosis in white progeny of overo spotted horses. JAVMA 180:289–292, 1982.

Jacobs JM, Scapavilli F, Duchen LW, Martin J: A new neurological rat mutant "mutilated foot." *J Anat* 132:525–543, 1981.

Jones WE: The overo white foal syndrome. *Equine J Med Surg* 3:54–56, 1979.

Pearson J, Pytel B, Grover-Johnson N, Exelrod F, Dancis J: Quantitative studies of dorsal root ganglia and neuropathologic observations on spinal cords in familial dysautonomia. *J Neurol Sci* 35:77–92, 1978.

Pivnik L: Zur vergleichenden Problematik einiger akrodystrophischer Neuropathien bei Menschen und Hund. *Arch Neurol Neurochir Psychiat* 112:365–371, 1973.

Pulos WL, Hutt FB: Lethal dominant white in horses. *J Hered* 60:50–63, 1969.

Trommershausen-Smith A: Lethal white foals in matings of overo spotted horses. *Theriogenology* 8:308–311, 1977.

Vonderfecht SL, Trommershausen-Smith A, Bowling A, Cohen A: Congenital intestinal aganglionosis in white foals. *Vet Pathol* 20:65–70, 1983.

Webster W: Aganglionic megacolon in piebald-lethal mice. *Arch Pathol* 97:111–117, 1974.

MALFORMATIONS OF THE INNER EAR

Adams FW: Hereditary deafness in a family of Foxhounds. JAVMA 128:302–303, 1956.

Anderson R, Henricson B, Lundquist P-G, Wedenberg E, Wersall J: Genetic impairment in the Dalmation dog. *Acta Otolaryngol* 232:1–34, 1968.

Bergsma DR, Brown KS: White fur, blue eyes and deafness in the domestic cat. *J Hered* 62:171–185, 1971.

Foss I: Development of hearing and vision and morphological examination of the inner ear in hereditary deaf white Norwegian Dunkerhound and normal dogs (black and dappled Norwegian Dunkerhounds) MS Thesis, Cornell University, 1981.

Hayes HM, Wilson GP, Fenner WB, Wyman M: Canine congenital deafness: epidemiological study of 272 cases. *J Am Anim Hosp Assoc* 17:473–476, 1981.

Hudson WR, Ruben RJ: Hereditary deafness in Dalmations. *Arch Otolaryngol* 75:213, 1962.

Lurie MH: The membranous labyrinth in the congenitally deaf Collie and Dalmation dog. *Laryngoscope* 58:279–287, 1948.

Mair IWS: Hereditary deafness in the Dalmation dog. *Arch Oto-Rhino-Laryngologia Italiana* 212:1–4, 1976.

CHAPTER 8

Trunk Muscles and Connective Tissues

TISSUE TYPES

Connective tissues are derived from mesodermal mesenchyme in the trunk, and both mesoderm and ectoderm (the neural crest) in the head. Included in this category are cartilage and bone tissues, which are formed by the processes of **chondrogenesis** and **osteogenesis**. Mesenchymal cells that become **chondroblasts** produce type II collagen fibers and a ground substance whose proteoglycan content varies depending upon the type of cartilage (hyaline, elastic, fibrous) being formed. **Hyaline cartilage** is the most abundant in the embryo and is most often produced in areas of the body where bone will be deposited to replace the cartilage.

Mesenchymal cells that differentiate into **osteoblasts** produce a mixture of fibers and ground substance called osteoid in which calcium and phosphate are precipitated in the process of ossification. **Intramembranous bone** is laid down in mesenchyme without a cartilaginous precursor. The clavicle and roofing bones of the skull are examples of this type of ossification. **Endochondral bone** is produced within and around a hyaline cartilaginous model. The appendicular skeleton, vertebrae and bones forming the floor of the braincase are formed by endochondral ossification.

The other types of connective tissue are heterogeneous, but are all derived from mesenchymal populations and secrete collagenous fibers and ground substances that form an extracellular matrix. Included in this category are tendons, ligaments, dermal and subcutaneous tissues, mesenteries, adipose (fat) cells, and the tissues that ensheath muscle fibers.

The muscular system includes skeletal and visceral muscle. **Skeletal muscle** is voluntary, striated muscle innervated by somatic efferent nerves. **Visceral muscle** includes involuntary muscle of the gut, integument and blood vessels, most of which is nonstriated, and the striated cardiac muscle. These are innervated by visceral efferent peripheral nerves. Their development will be discussed in later chapters.

FORMATION OF VERTEBRAE AND RIBS

Vertebrae are derived from **paraxial mesoderm** that, beginning at the neurula stage, coalesces segmentally to form somites. Each somite has three parts: the **dermatome**, the **myotome** and the **sclerotome** (Fig. 8.1*C*). Myotomes are the source of axial, appendicular and abdominal wall musculature. Sclerotomes form vertebrae and ribs, and dermatomal cells contribute to the dermis.

In the dog there are 40 or more somites. The first four are called **occipital somites**

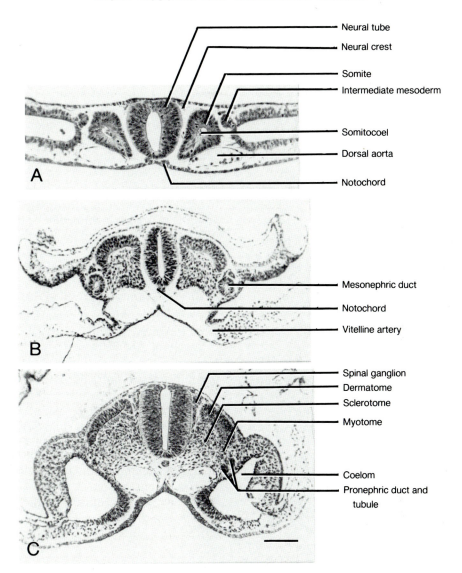

Neural tube
Neural crest
Somite
Intermediate mesoderm
Somitocoel
Dorsal aorta
Notochord

A

Mesonephric duct
Notochord
Vitelline artery

B

Spinal ganglion
Dermatome
Sclerotome
Myotome
Coelom
Pronephric duct and tubule

C

Figure 8.1. Development of somites in the feline embryo. *A* shows the 8th somite from a 14-somite embryo cut in a transverse plane. The somitic mesoderm is epithelial and surrounds a small central cavity, the somitocoel. *B* and *C* illustrate the 14th and 8th somites from a 24-somite embryo, similar to that shown in Figure 1.4. Somites mature in a craniocaudal sequence; thus, the 8th is further developed than the 14th. In *C* the sclerotome has become mesenchymal (*bar*, 0.1 mm).

and mesenchyme from these sclerotomes fuses together to form the occipital cartilages of the skull (see Chapter 9). The remaining sclerotomes all form vertebrae.

The development of sclerotomes proceeds in a craniocaudal sequence as does chondrification of vertebrae. Ossification of the vertebrae is less precise, and in some embryos the thoracic vertebrae may initiate ossification before the cervical segments.

In transverse section each immature somite appears triangular with a small, sometimes indistinct central cavity, the somitocoel, surrounded by mesodermal cells that have formed an epithelium (Fig. 8.1*A*). The ventromedial part of the somite is the first to show signs of further differentiation. These cells become mesenchymal in appearance, marking the initial formation of the sclerotome. This population expands and, concomitantly, the spinal cord and noto-chord enlarge. The net result of these growths is that the ventral part of the spinal cord and the notochord become surrounded by sclerotomal mesenchyme.

Subsequently the sclerotomal cells of each somite form two distinct populations: a cau-dal, more dense population and a cranial, diffuse group. Due largely to differential growth of these parts, the caudal cells of each sclerotome become contiguous with the cra-nial population of the adjacent sclerotome, as illustrated in Figure 8.2. These newly associated populations together form a sin-gle vertebra. This explains why spinal gan-glia and ventral roots are positioned between vertebrae, and myotomes span from one vertebra to another, and the originally inter-somitic arteries are subsequently found en-tering between the pedicles of the vertebral arch.

While there is controversy concerning the precise fates of the two subdivisions of each sclerotome, it is generally accepted that the caudal, dense population gives rise primarily to the neural arch and related parts of each vertebra and also the intervertebral disc. The original cranial, less dense population, which joins with the dense mesenchyme of the adjacent sclerotome, forms most of the body (centrum) of the vertebra.

Chondrification begins within each scler-otomal aggregate at several locations, but these foci soon expand and fuse with one another. The cartilaginous precursor of the centrum surrounds the notochord, uniting left and right vertebral primordia. Within each segment the notochord is almost com-pletely obliterated. However, between ver-tebrae the notochord persists and expands to form a central core, the **nucleus pulposus**, within the **intervertebral disc**. The periph-eral part of each disc, the **anulus fibrosus** (fibrous ring), arises from sclerotomal mes-enchyme. With lateral growth of the trans-verse and costal processes and later fusion of neural arch elements in the dorsal mid-line, the formation of the cartilaginous ver-tebra is complete. This occurs before birth.

Vertebral ossification begins in the 6th week of gestation in the dog, slightly later in larger domestic animals. Primary ossifica-tion centers appear near the middle of each centrum and lateral to the spinal cord in the base of each neural arch (Fig. 8.3). In **altri-cial animals**, which are those like the dog and cat that are born in a relatively imma-ture condition, these ossification centers do

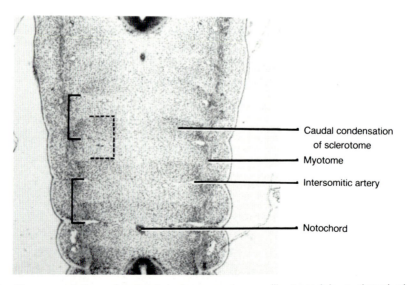

Caudal condensation
of sclerotome

Myotome

Intersomitic artery

Notochord

Figure 8.2. Resegmentation of sclerotomal mesenchyme, illustrated in a dorsal plane section through the cervical region of a 12-mm sheep embryo. Note that within each somitic segment (brackets on left) the sclerotomal mesenchyme has formed two subpopulations; that located cranially is less dense than the caudal subpopulation. *Dashed bracket* indicates one vertebra.

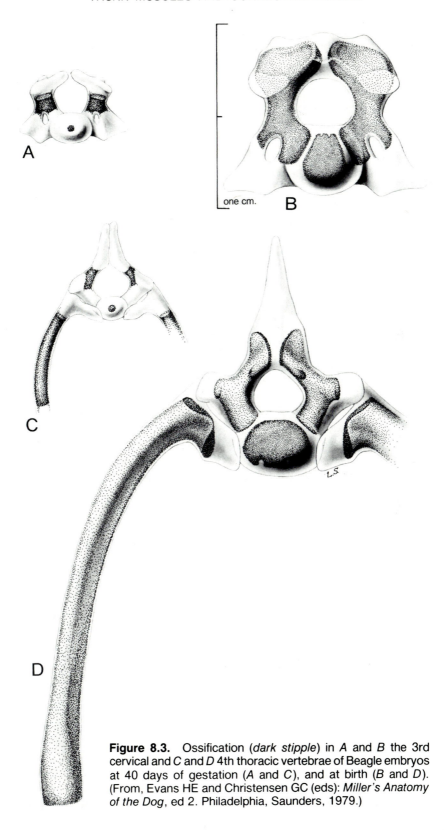

one cm.

A

B

C

D

L.S.

Figure 8.3. Ossification (*dark stipple*) in *A* and *B* the 3rd cervical and *C* and *D* 4th thoracic vertebrae of Beagle embryos at 40 days of gestation (*A* and *C*), and at birth (*B* and *D*). (From, Evans HE and Christensen GC (eds): *Miller's Anatomy of the Dog*, ed 2. Philadelphia, Saunders, 1979.)

not fuse dorsally until after birth. Later in postnatal development, secondary ossification centers will appear on the periphery of the centrum of the vertebra to form the epiphyses and others may form in the distal tips of transverse processes.

At the cranial end of the vertebral column the segmental reorganization of sclerotomal cells deviates from the pattern described above. A mesenchymal aggregate associated with the fifth somite, which based on its position should be the primordial body of the 1st cervical vertebra, the **atlas**, fuses instead with the cranial aspect of the 2nd cervical vertebra, the **axis**, to form part of its cranial articular surface and the **dens**. Thus, the body, cranial articular surface and dens of the axis develop from five ossification centers, while the small body of the atlas forms from only one. The presence of multiple ossification primordia in each segment is not a new condition. Rather, this represents the last vestiges of a situation common to embryonic vertebrae in primitive amphibians and fishes.

Segmental sclerotome-derived condensations lateral to thoracic vertebrae differentiate into cartilaginous ribs located between the developing myotomes. The distal ends of the first nine cartilaginous ribs grow towards the ventral midline, where they contact one of two longitudinal concentrations of somatic mesoderm called **sternal bars** (Fig. 8.4*A*). These two bars fuse in the ventral midline and undergo segmentation to form a series of **sternebrae**. A total of 8 sternebrae normally form, although it is common for the caudal sternebrae to remain paired, as illustrated in Fig. 8.4*B*. Rib pairs 10 through 13 do not reach this ventral level.

It has been shown that contact of sternal bars by the distal tips of each rib (except the first) inhibits the hypertrophy of nearby chondrocytes, which is the initial step in endochondral ossification. As a result the ossification of sternebrae occurs initially be-

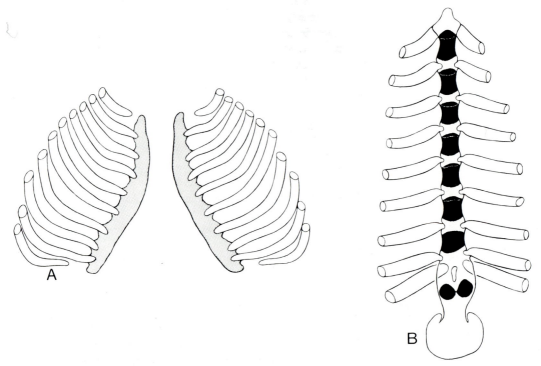

Figure 8.4. Development of the canine sternum. *A* shows the ribs contacting a pair of cartilaginous sternal bars, as would be found in a 25-day embryo. *B* indicates how ossification centers (*black areas*) develop within the fused sternum in between sites of rib apposition. (From Evans HE, Christensen HE (eds): *Miller's Anatomy of the Dog*, ed 2. Philadelphia, Saunders, 1979.)

tween the attachment sites of the ribs (Fig. 8.4B).

INTERACTIONS CONTROLLING AXIAL DEVELOPMENT

The developmental programming of axial structures, including the notochord, neural plate, and paraxial mesoderm, begins during gastrulation, as discussed in Chapter 4. During this stage specific tissue types, especially neurepithelium and somites are determined, and regional differences in axial tissues are established. However, full development of the spinal cord and vertebrae requires many additional interactions.

Chondrogenesis by sclerotomal cells has been well studied. If excised and grown either in vitro or on the avian chorioallantoic membrane, which provides a rich vascular bed, isolated chick embryonic somites usually fail to initiate chondrogenesis (Fig. 8.5A). However, as illustrated, following the addition of pieces of notochord or neural tube to somite cultures, sclerotomal cells do become chondroblasts. This response is specific and does not occur when other, nonaxial tissues are added to somite cultures. These experiments demonstrate that the cytodifferentiation of sclerotomal cells is promoted by adjacent axial tissues.

Does this mean that the notochord *causes* somite cells to become chondroblasts? Probably not. Chondrogenesis occurs if large numbers of somites are cultured together in the absence of other tissues (Fig. 8.5E). Furthermore, biochemical analyses have revealed that both the notochord and sclerotomal cells secrete similar types of extracellular materials, which are identical to the matrix components of embryonic cartilage. Thus, some of the sclerotomal cells are already programmed for the chondrogenic pathway, and interactions with the products released by adjacent structures coordinate and accelerate cytodifferentiation rather than program it.

Most vertebral malformations reflect errors in patterning and growth of sclerotomal tissues. Often as a result of an initial anomaly in somite segmentation, both skeletal

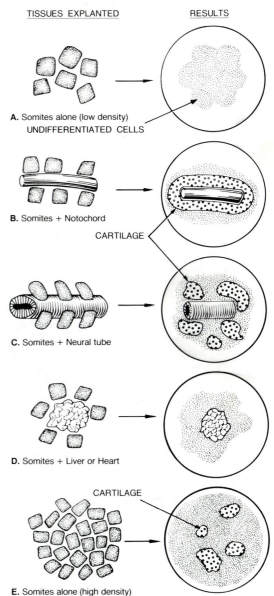

TISSUES EXPLANTED — RESULTS

A. Somites alone (low density)
UNDIFFERENTIATED CELLS

B. Somites + Notochord
CARTILAGE

C. Somites + Neural tube

D. Somites + Liver or Heart

CARTILAGE

E. Somites alone (high density)

Figure 8.5. Summarizes experiments designed to investigate the interactions that promote chondrogenesis within somites. The column on the *left* indicates the embryonic tissues explanted; the drawings on the *right* illustrate the results after several days in tissue culture.

and secondary neuromuscular abnormalities will appear. The normal pattern of vertebral morphogenesis is severely disrupted if either the spinal ganglia or the notochord are not present, as shown in Figure 8.6.

Thus, regardless of the original cause (genetic, teratogenic, idiopathic), once a lesion

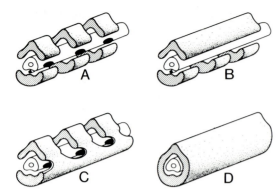

Figure 8.6. Interactions that affect segmentation of vertebrae. *A*, normal pattern. *B*, pattern of development in the absence of spinal ganglia. *C*, development in the absence of the notochord. *D*, effects of removing both notochord and spinal ganglia prior to vertebral development. (From Hall BK: *Developmental and Cellular Skeletal Biology*, New York, © Academic Press, 1978.)

occurs in one part of the developing axial complex it is likely to initiate a cascade of morphogenetic anomalies in adjacent tissues. If peripheral nerves are compromised as a result of the skeletal defect, their target tissues will also be affected.

ORIGINS OF TRUNK AND LIMB MUSCULATURE

While the skeletal derivatives of the somites are well documented, the range of myotome derivatives has until recently been controversial. All axial and body wall musculature in primitive vertebrates is derived from myotomes, as is still readily apparent upon gross examination of body wall in adult fishes. However, the lack of distinct segmental muscles in the body wall and limbs of higher vertebrates, and the inability to find myotome cells moving ventrally to "seed" these areas, has permitted acceptance of the hypothesis that these muscles are formed from lateral somatic mesoderm. Recent experiments in which labeled somites have been transplanted in the place of homologous somites in unlabeled chick embryos have refuted this hypothesis. It is now accepted that all voluntary muscles in the body are derived from paraxial mesoderm. The results of these somite transplantations are summarized in Table 8.1.

Table 8.1.
Embryonic Origins of Avian Trunk and Appendicular Musculoskeletal Tissues

Tissue	Embryonic origin		
	Sclero-tome	Myotome	Somatic mesoderm
Vertebrae	X		
Epaxial muscles		X	
Ribs	X		
Intercostal muscles		X	
Sternum			X
Scapula			X
Clavicle and coracoid			X
Humerus, radius, ulna, carpals, metacarpals, phalanges			X
Extrinsic limb muscles[a]		X	
Intrinsic limb muscles[a]		X	
Pelvis			X
Femur, tibia, fibula, tarsals, metatarsals, phalanges			X
Abdominal wall muscles[a]		X	

[a] Only the muscle fibers are myotomal in origin; connective tissues, including tendons and fascia are formed from somatic mesoderm.

CONTROL OF MYOGENESIS

Mature striated skeletal muscle is a **syncytium**; each muscle cell (myotube) contains many peripherally located nuclei. That this syncytium arises by the fusion of mononucleated cells called myoblasts has been demonstrated both in vitro by direct observation and in vivo through the use of **chimeras**. A chimera is an individual animal that consists of cells derived from more than one embryo. Chimeras can arise naturally, as in the freemartin (Chapter 19), or experimentally by mixing together blastomeres derived from different embryos and then surgically implanting the chimeric morula into a pseudopregnant foster mother.

All murine muscle cells normally have one of two genetically determined isozymic forms of the enzyme isocitrate dehydrogenase (IDH). IDH is a dimer, and the monomers that become linked together in the cytoplasm are products of the same gene. If a chimera is made using blastomeres from mouse strain A, in which the IDH dimer is type *aa*, and strain B, in which the IDH is *bb*, there are two possible outcomes:

1. If only *aa* and *bb* types of IDH are found, then genes from the A and B strains never were present in common cytoplasm; or
2. If *aa*, *bb* and *ab* IDH dimers are detected, then both A and B strain genes must have been present in the same cytoplasm.

The results of these experiments were that all three dimers were found, proving unequivocally that multinucleated skeletal muscle arises as a result of fusion of myoblasts.

The normal development and maintenance of muscle is dependent on its being innervated. Muscle cells that are denervated undergo a progressive shrinkage called **denervation atrophy**. Animals born with local loss of peripheral somatic efferent nerve function have very little muscle in the affected area. For example, if the lumbosacral spinal cord fails to develop, the pelvic limb muscle mass will be very small.

Prior to innervation by motor neurons embryonic muscle cells have many potential receptor areas on their surface. When innervation occurs only a single area ultimately persists as the neuromuscular junction. These extrajunctional receptor areas reappear if the embryonic cell is denervated.

VERTEBRAL MALFORMATIONS

Malformations of the vertebral column that severely compromise the fetal vertebral canal will cause spinal cord compression and the clinical signs will be present at birth or as soon as the animal normally begins to walk. However, many vertebral malformations are less severe at birth, and begin to compromise the vertebral canal and compress the spinal cord later as the musculoskeletal system matures. Therefore, the neurologic signs may not appear until the animal is a few months old, following which they progressively worsen.

Vertebral malformations occasionally occur with no grossly apparent deviation in the vertebral column or compromise of the vertebral canal. For example, failure of sclerotomes to fully segment may result in a **block vertebra**, which is usually the size of two normal vertebrae. This malformation may involve just the vertebral bodies, the arches or all of the vertebra. Other abnormalities in vertebral ossification may produce shortened vertebrae but no abnormal angulation. These usually do not cause any unusual clinical signs.

Alignment Defects

Most vertebral malformations result in a grossly abnormal shape of the vertebral column. A lateral deviation is called **scoliosis**. Deviation of the column in the sagittal plane is called **kyphosis** if vertebrae are fixed in flexed posture (Fig. 8.7) and **lordosis** if they are fixed in an extended posture. Usually in these conditions the vertebral canal is compromised and the spinal cord compressed, resulting in paresis and ataxia in the limbs caudal to the site of the lesion. Except in severe cases, these clinical signs usually do not appear until a few months after birth. An abnormal twisting of the cervical vertebral column is called **torticollis** (twisted neck), popularly termed wryneck.

Many vertebral malformations preferentially occur at a particular axial level and with greater frequency in certain species or breeds. The following discussion is organized according to region, and presents those breeds in which the incidence of specific anomalies is high or known to be heritable.

Cervical Vertebrae

OCCIPITOATLANTOAXIAL
MALFORMATIONS

Abnormal segmentation and development of the caudal occipital and cranial cervical sclerotomes results in an occipitoatlantoaxial malformation. Although this has been observed sporadically in most species, it has been recognized as an autosomal recessive inherited disease in the Arabian horse.

In this malformation the atlas is unilaterally or bilaterally fused to the occipital

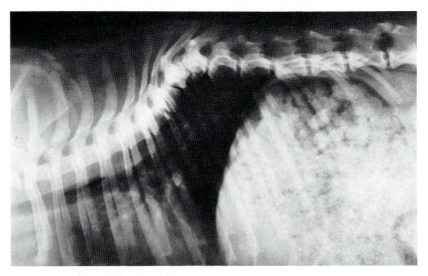

Figure 8.7.   Radiograph illustrating kyphosis at the 8th and 9th thoracic vertebrae in a dog.

bone and its transverse processes (wings) are markedly reduced in size, as shown in Figure 8.8. The atlantal foramen is narrowed and the caudal articular foveae are rounded, resembling occipital condyles. Thus, the atlas appears to have developed partly like the occipital bone. The axis has broad transverse processes which are normally a feature of the atlas. The dens and cranial articular surface of the axis is usually displaced (luxated) beneath the body of the atlas.

Due to the marked narrowing of the foramen magnum and vertebral canal at the atlantoaxial level and concomitant spinal cord compression, these foals usually cannot get up at birth or are very paretic and ataxic. Some foals walk normally at birth but in a few months develop an abnormal gait due to spinal cord compression. The malformation of the atlantooccipital joint can be recognized by an abnormally extended head posture and an inability to manually flex the joint. The abnormal shape of the wings of the atlas can be palpated. In young foals manipulation of this area may elicit a clicking sound due to the subluxation of the axis on the atlas.

HYPOPLASIA OF THE DENS

Atlantoaxial subluxation (Fig. 8.9) is most commonly seen in puppies and young adults of toy breeds of dogs. Subluxation occurs due to absence of the dens and failure of ligamentous support. This causes spinal cord compression that can occur either suddenly, sometimes associated with mild trauma, or progressively. It is not known whether this condition results from a congenital aplasia or hypoplasia of the dens or from a postnatal degeneration.

MIDCERVICAL MALFORMATIONS

A malformation-malarticulation of cervical vertebrae occurs in young, rapidly growing horses of most breeds, with a higher incidence claimed in male thoroughbreds. This most commonly involves the 3rd and 4th cervical vertebrae but may affect vertebrae cranial or caudal to this site. The characteristic feature of this abnormality is a reduction in the size of the cranial or caudal opening of the vertebral foramen, often associated with an excessive flexion of the involved joint. The spinal cord lesion resulting from the associated compression is a focal **myelopathy**. Therefore, this cause of paresis and ataxia is referred to as **cervical stenotic myelopathy**. Both genetic and nutritional factors have been implicated in the appearance and severity of this condition.

Because these horses have an unsteady gait, especially with their pelvic limbs, they

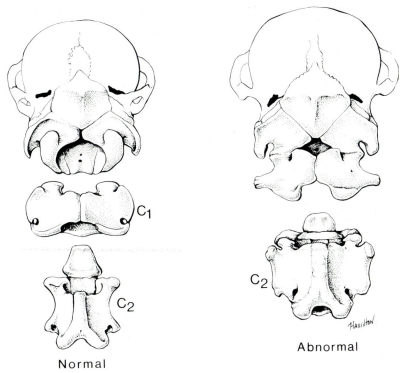

Figure 8.8. Occipitoatlantoaxial malformation in the Arabian foal. *Left*, a normal foal's skull, atlas (C₁) and axis (C₂), disarticulated and viewed from a dorsal perspective. On the *right* is a similar view of an affected Arabian foal in which the atlas is fused to the occipital condyles and is "occipitalized," the axis is "atlantalized," and the foramen magnum is reduced. Note the reduced transverse processes of the atlas.

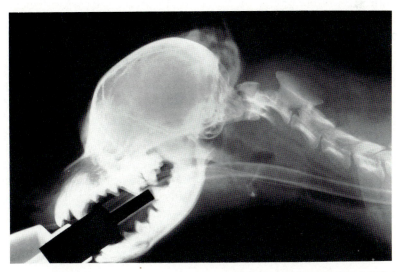

Figure 8.9. Radiograph showing subluxation of the axis in a 9-month-old female Miniature Poodle with absence of the dens. Note particularly the abnormal relationship between C₁ and C₂.

are often called wobblers. However, it is important to recognize that there are many diseases that affect the cervical spinal cord and might cause an animal to wobble.

A sex-linked, recessively inherited malformation affecting the C_2–C_3 or C_3–C_4 articulation has been described in male Bassets. It is characterized by stenosis of the vertebral canal with subsequent spinal cord compression. Clinical signs usually occur by a few months of age and are progressive. We have observed a Basset with this disease in which there was stenosis of the cranial orifice of the second through the fifth cervical vertebrae.

CAUDAL CERVICAL MALFORMATIONS

A caudal cervical vertebral malformation-malarticulation syndrome has been recognized in dogs, most commonly in Doberman Pinschers and Great Danes, and sporadically in other, usually large canine breeds. The 5th, 6th and/or 7th cervical vertebrae are most commonly affected. A narrowing of the cranial orifice into the vertebral foramen is a common finding, as shown in Fig. 8.10, although the spinal cord compression may result from other abnormalities of the vertebra, the intervertebral disks or ligaments associated with these vertebrae. Occasionally, excessive movement of the vertebrae

on flexion of the neck results in a slight subluxation. Some of these abnormalities may result from developmental problems, others are secondary effects of the mild malarticulation that persists as the animal grows.

The cause of the primary abnormality is probably complex. Genetic factors are suspected and nutrition may also be involved, as suggested by the observation that the normal enlargement of the vertebral foramina is retarded due to premature ossification in large breeds of dogs that are overfed.

The onset of clinical signs from spinal cord compression is extremely variable and depends on the severity of the primary malformation and the rate of development of secondary changes at the abnormal articulation, both of which affect the rate and degree of spinal cord compression. These may occur at a few months of age, or not until the dog is 6–8 yr old.

Thoracolumbar Vertebrae

Horses may develop a congenital scoliosis associated with hypoplasia of midthoracic (T_7–T_{10}) vertebral articular processes. In some cases unilateral flexion occurs opposite to the side with the hypoplasia, due to instability of the affected articulation. In addition, horses with congenital lordosis and excessive flexion resulting from bilateral hy-

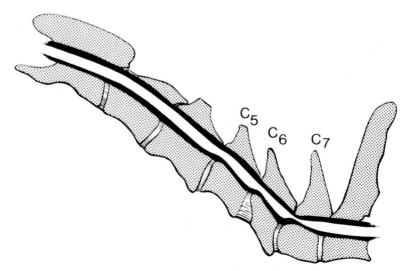

Figure 8.10.   Cervical stenotic myelopathy as found in Great Dane and Doberman Pinscher breeds. The three sites of compression (C_5, C_6, C_7) are illustrated.

poplasia of the articular process of T_5 and T_6 have been described.

A common thoracic-level malformation in dogs involves hypoplasia and incomplete ossification of one or more vertebrae. The vertebral body is shaped like an inverted wedge, and adjacent vertebrae are usually malformed and misaligned, resulting in a marked kyphosis. This condition has been referred to as a "hemivertebra" but is more complex than this term suggests. It is often not recognized until the spinal cord becomes compressed and the dog's gait becomes abnormal, showing paresis and ataxia of the pelvic limbs. This typically does not occur before 3 or 4 months of age and gets progressively worse as the dog grows and compression increases. At that time the vertebral defect can usually be palpated and is obvious on radiographs.

This group of thoracolumbar defects occurs in all breeds of dogs, but is more common in brachycephalic* breeds. It has been reported in the thoracic vertebrae of a line of German Shorthaired Pointers in which an autosomal recessive inheritance has been proposed.

An hereditary "hemivertebra" has been described in mink due to an autosomal recessive gene abnormality. These animals usually develop pelvic limb paresis and ataxia between 8 and 14 weeks of age. The fourth or occasionally the 6th thoracic vertebra is affected by the malformation and subsequent kyphosis and associated spinal cord compression.

---

* Brachycephalic, short head (Boston Terrier, Bulldog, Pug); dolichocephalic, long head (Collie, Russian Wolfhound).

CASE HISTORY

Signalment: A 5-month-old male Dalmation with abnormal hind limb gait.

History: For 1 month this dog had shown difficulty getting up on the hind limbs and his gait was incoordinated in these limbs. These signs progressively worsened, and at times he needed help to get up and try to walk.

Examination: Physical examination was normal except for a palpable dorsal deviation of the midthoracic vertebral column. The dog was very paretic (weak) and ataxic (incoordinated) in the hind limbs and showed spasticity in these limbs. Both were equally affected. Muscle tone and spinal reflexes were normal to exaggerated. Pain perception was normal. Tail and anal reflexes were normal. No muscle atrophy was present in the hind limbs.

Assessment of History and Examination

FACTS	INTERPRETATION
Abnormal hind limb gait	Musculoskeletal or nervous system disease
Normal pelvic limb musculoskeletal examination	Supports nervous system disease
Neurological signs confined to the pelvic limbs	Disease of spinal cord caudal to the second thoracic spinal cord segment or in the peripheral nerves to the pelvic limbs
Clinical signs of spasticity, ataxia, hypertonicity, hyperreflexia, but no atrophy	Suggests a spinal cord lesion between the second thoracic and fourth lumbar spinal cord segment
Normal gait until 5 months old	Not a spinal cord malformation
Progressive signs	Suggests a progressive spinal cord compression, inflammation or degeneration. Does not support an acute injury or spinal cord lesion due to loss of blood supply
Abnormal shape of thoracic vertebrae with dorsal deviation	Vertebral column malformation with kyphosis

Conclusion: Midthoracic spinal cord compression from progressive narrowing of the vertebral canal associated with the vertebral column malformation

The vertebral column malformation is congenital but unaccompanied by a spinal cord malformation or there would be signs of neurological dysfunction present at birth. In this dog, the spinal cord developed normally but became compressed at the site of the vertebral malformation due either to progressive kyphosis or failure of the vertebral canal to enlarge with growth at the site of the malformation or both may be involved. The progressive compression caused the neurologic signs to get worse over the month. Surgical decompression of the spinal cord and careful realignment and stabilization of the vertebral column may stop the spinal cord compression and allow for some improvement in the clinical signs.

In most cases of congenitally abnormal segmentation or articulation with secondary stenosis of the vertebral canal, the exact cause of the defect is unknown. One exception occurs in Siamese cats with a recessively inherited condition called mucopolysaccharidosis VI. This is one of a group of enzyme deficiency diseases that result from abnormal glycosaminoglycan metabolism. These animals are characterized by broad, flattened faces, corneal clouding, and some show progressive hind limb paresis beginning after 4 months of age.

Pathologic examination of the vertebral column in these Siamese reveals fusion of some cervical and thoracic vertebrae without compromise of the vertebral canal. In other regions the thoracolumbar vertebrae are enlarged with secondary compression of the spinal cord. While mucopolysaccharidoses have been described in most domesticated animals, it is only recently that direct methods for their assay have become available. These will permit more ready analysis of possible enzymatic deficiencies in a variety of inherited musculoskeletal defects.

Short-spined dogs result from a compaction of thoracic and lumbar vertebrae with fusion of many of them. This has been reported as an autosomal recessive inherited malformation in the South African Greyhound and in Fox Terriers. These dogs, which have been described since the 17th century, are referred to as "baboon" dogs since they usually sit in a partially upright posture with their pelvis on the ground and hindlimbs extended forward. There is limited movement of the pelvic limbs.

Schistosomus reflexus (clefted body, bent over) is a condition in which the thoracic and abdominal cavities fail to close ventrally. The vertebral column is reflected back upon itself (hyperextended) in the thoracic or thoracolumbar region, resulting in the apposition of the occipital region of the skull to the sacrum. This condition occurs most frequently in cattle, but has been reported in sheep and swine. It may be detected in utero by palpation, and the cow may suffer from **dystocia** (difficult delivery) and require veterinary attention. As a result of impaired innervation, movements of the fetal limbs are reduced, resulting in ankylosis and arthrogryposis.

Lumbosacral Vertebrae

Spina bifida is a failure of the vertebral arch to form dorsally over the vertebral foramen. This can involve part or all of the arch of one vertebra or many adjacent vertebrae. The latter, more extensive condition is called **rachischisis** (rachis = spine; schisis = cleft), and is illustrated in Figure 8.11. If the skin and subcutaneous tissue cover the vertebral defect dorsally so that it is not grossly apparent on physical examination, the defect is termed **spina bifida occulta**. Spina bifida is frequently associated with a spinal cord malformation in which neural tissues and/or meninges protrude through

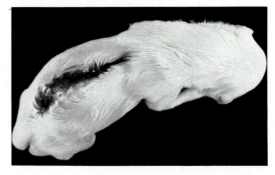

Figure 8.11. Thoracolumbar rachischisis and myeloschisis in a newborn puppy.

the vertebral defect (see Figure 6.18). Although spina bifida can occur at any level of the vertebral column, it is most common in the caudal lumbar and sacral regions.

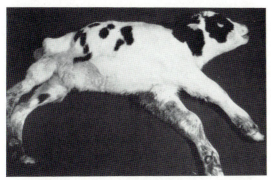

Figure 8.12. Perosomus elumbus in a newborn calf. While all skeletal elements of the hind limbs are present, the joints are fixed (ankylosis) and all of the muscles have degenerated.

Segmentation abnormalities are occasionally observed at the lumbosacral junction. This may involve the first sacral segment acquiring a typical lumbar transverse process or the last lumbar vertebra developing a broad transverse process and articulating with the ilium. Neither condition is associated with clinical signs.

Perosomus elumbus (Fig. 8.12) refers to a deformed body which lacks a lumbosacral and caudal vertebral column and spinal cord. The pelvis and pelvic limbs are present but are rigid (ankylosed), and most associated muscles atrophy early in development.

Caudal Vertebrae

Curled or kinky tails are the result of caudal vertebral malformation. These are common in brachycephalic breeds of dogs,

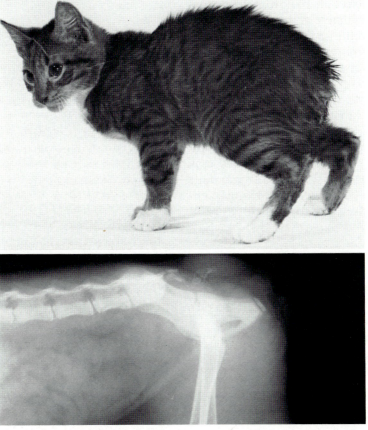

Figure 8.13. The Manx cat. This animal had no perineal sensation, a single cloacal orifice, and showed incontinence. Radiographic examination reveals that the sacral vertebrae are hypoplastic and the caudal vertebrae are missing.

some Manx cats, rodents, and pigs. This defect can occur by itself with no nervous system abnormality. In some brachycephalic dogs and many Manx cats (Fig. 8.13) the caudal vertebral abnormality is associated with more extensive sacral vertebral and neural defects (see Chapter 6).

MALFORMATIONS OF THE STERNUM AND RIBS

Chondrosternal depression (pectus excavatum) is a funnel-like cavitation of the ventral thorax in which the distal, cartilaginous parts of the ribs curve dorsally and attach to a dorsally-displaced sternum. This condition is thought to arise as a result of failure of the normal development of diaphragmatic muscles.

"Swimmer pups" are characterized by an inability of puppies to stand and walk when they normally should. Their muscles are not strong enough relative to their body size and as they struggle to stand their limbs become progressively more abducted, their thorax flattens ventrally and they make lateral swimming movements to move around. The problem is exacerbated if they are kept on a hard, smooth surface. If the situation is recognized early and limb abduction is prevented by tying the limbs together and providing a soft surface, these puppies may recover. A much less severe abduction of the hindlimbs is occasionally seen in kittens, but usually is resolved as their adductor muscles strengthen.

Bibliography

NORMAL DEVELOPMENT AND REVIEWS

Bailey CS: An embryological approach to the clinical significance of congenital vertebral and spinal cord abnormalities. *J Am Anim Hosp Assoc* 11:426–434, 1975.

Chevallier A: Role du mésoderme somitique dans le développement de la cage thoracique de l'embryon d'oiseau. I. Origine du segment sternal et mécanismes de la différenciation des côtes. *J Embryol Exp Morphol* 33:291–311, 1975.

Danilova LV: Somite differentiation in the Karakul sheep embryo. *Fed Proc* 22:T677–T689, 1963.

Ede DA, Hinchliff JR, Balls M: *Vertebrate Limb and Somite Morphogenesis.* Cambridge, Cambridge University Press, 1977.

Evans HE: Reproduction and prenatal development. In Evans HE, Christensen GC (eds): *Miller's Anatomy*
of the Dog, ed 2. Philadelphia, Saunders, 1979.

Gasser RF: Evidence that sclerotomal cells do not migrate medially during normal embryonic development of the rat. *Am J Anat* 154:509–523, 1979.

Hall BK: Chondrogenesis of the Somitic Mesoderm. *Adv Anat Embryol Cell Biol* 53:1–50, 1977.

Hall BK: *Developmental and Cellular Skeletal Biology.* New York, Academic Press, 1978.

Hanson FB: The development of the sternum in Sus scrofa. *Anat Rec* 17:1–21, 1919.

Hodges PC: Ossification of the fetal pig. A radiographic study. *Anat Rec* 116:315–325, 1953.

Holtfreter J, Hamburger V: Embryogenesis: progressive differentiation (amphibians). In Willier BH, Weiss PA, Hamburger V (eds): *Analysis of Development* Philadelphia, Saunders, 1955.

Lindsay FEF: Observations on the loci of ossification in the prenatal and postnatal bovine skeleton. II. The sternum. *Br Vet J* 125:422–428, 1969.

O'Rahilly R, Meyer DB: The timing and sequence of events in the development of the human vertebral column during the embryonic period proper. *Anat Embryol* 157:167–176, 1979.

O'Rahilly R, Muller F, Meyer DB: The human vertebral column at the end of the embryonic period proper. 2. The occipitocervical region. *J Anat* 136:181–195, 1983.

Patten BM: *Embryology of the Pig*, ed 3. New York, Blakiston, 1948.

Strong RM: The order, time and rate of ossification of the albino rat (Mus norvegicus albinus) skeleton. *Am J Anat* 36:313–355, 1925.

Verbout AJ: A critical review of the "neugliederung" concept in relation to the development of the vertebral column. *Acta Biotheor* 25:219–258, 1976.

Wachtler F, Christ B, Jacob HJ: Grafting experiments on determination and migratory behaviour of presomitic, somitic and somatopleural cells in avian embryos. *Anat Embryol* 164:369–378, 1982.

Williams LW: The later development of the notochord in mammals. *Am J Anat* 8:251–291, 1908.

CERVICAL VERTEBRAL ANOMALIES

Cook JR, Oliver JE Jr: Atlantoaxial subluxation in the dog. *Compend Contin Educ* 3:242–248, 1981.

Denny HR, Gibbs C, Gaskell CJ: Cervical spondylopathy in the dog—a review of thirty-five cases. *J Small Anim Pract* 18:117–132, 1977.

Geary JC, Oliver JE, Hoerlein BF: Atlantoaxial subluxation in the canine. *J Small Anim Pract* 8:577–582, 1967.

Lakatos L, Suter M, Baumberger A, Pletscher S: Die Atlantoaxiale Subluxation beim Hund. *Schweiz Arch Tierheilk* 123:455–465, 1981.

Leipold HW, Brandt GW, Guffy MM, Blauch B: Congenital atlantooccipital fusion in a foal. *Vet Med* 692:1312–1316, 1974.

Mason TA: Cervical vertebral instability (Wobbler syndrome) in the dog. *Vet Rec* 104:142–145, 1979.

Mayhew IG, Watson AG, Heissan JA: Congenital occipitoatlantoaxial malformation in the horse. *Equine Vet J* 10:103–113, 1978.

Palmer AC: Deformation of cervical vertebrae in Basset hounds. *Vet Rec* 80:320–433, 1967.

Raffe MR, Knecht CD: Cervical vertebral malformation—a review of 36 cases. *JAAHA* 16:881–883, 1980.

Trotter EJ, deLahunta A, Geary JC, Brasmer TH: Caudal cervical vertebral malformation—malarticulation in Great Danes and Doberman Pinschers. *JAVMA* 168:917–930, 1976.

Wright F, Rest JR, Palmer AC: Ataxia of the Great Dane caused by stenosis of the cervical vertebral canal: comparison in the similar conditions of the Basset Hound, Doberman Pinscher, Ridgeback, and thoroughbred horse. *Vet Rec* 92:1–6, 1973.

Zaki FA: Odontoid process dysplasia in a dog. *J Small Anim Prac* 21:227–234, 1980.

THORACIC VERTEBRAL MALFORMATIONS

Haskins ME, Bingel SA, Northington JW, Newton CD, Sande RD, Jezyk PF, Patterson DF: Spinal cord compression and hindlimb paresis in cats with mucopolysaccharidosis. *JAVMA* 182:983–985, 1983.

Kramer JW, Schiffer SP, Sande RD, Rantanen NW, Whitener EK: Characterization of heritable thoracic hemivertebra of the German Shorthaired Pointer. *JAVMA* 181:814–815, 1982.

Parker AJ, Park RD: Clinical signs associated with hemivertebrae in three dogs. *Can Prac* 1:34–38, 1974.

Rooney JR, Prickett ME: Congenital lordosis of the horse. *Cornell Vet* 52:417–428, 1967.

CHONDROSTERNAL DEPRESSION

Pearson JL: Pectus excavatum in the dog. *Vet Med/Small Anim Clin* 68:125–146, 1973.

Smallwood JE, Beaver BV: Congenital chondrosternal depression (pectus excavatum) in the cat. *J Am Vet Rad Soc* 18:141–146, 1977.

SPINA BIFIDA

James CCM, Lassman LP, Tomlinson BE: Congenital anomalies of the lower spine and spinal cord in Manx cats. *J Pathol* 97:269–276, 1969.

Leathers CW, Wagner PC, Milleson BE: Cervical spina bifida with meningocele in an Appaloosa foal. *J Vet Orthoped* 1:55–58, 1979.

Leipold HW, Huston K, Blauch B, Guffy MM: Congenital defects of the caudal vertebral column and spinal cord in Manx cats. *JAVMA* 164:520–523, 1974.

Mann GE, Stratton J: Dermoid sinus in the Rhodesian Ridgeback. *J Sm An Pract* 7:631–642, 1966.

Martin AH: A congenital defect in the spinal cord of the Manx cat. *Vet Pathol* 8:232–238, 1971.

Morgan JP: Congenital anomalies of the vertebral column of the dog. A study of the incidence and significance based on a radiographic and morphologic study. *J Am Vet Rad Soc* 9:21–29, 1968.

Parker AJ, et al: Spina bifida with protrusion of spinal cord tissue in a dog. *JAVMA* 163:158–160, 1973.

Wilson JW: Spina bifida in the dog and cat. *Comp Cont Ed* 4:626–636, 1982.

CHAPTER 9

Craniofacial Muscles and Connective Tissues

INITIAL ORGANIZATION OF CEPHALIC TISSUES

At the time of neurulation the cranial aspect of the axial system consists of a closing **neural plate,** lateral and ventral to which is **paraxial mesoderm** (see Fig. 6.3). The notochord extends rostrally to the level of the midmesencephalon. Located ventral to the notochord is the **pharyngeal endoderm,** which is covered by lateral mesoderm, including cardiogenic primordia.

As neurulation proceeds caudally, a closed neural tube and pharynx are established. Shortly thereafter the head fold and lateral body folds separate the future head region from extraembryonic tissues. During this period the primordia of the heart are brought together in the ventral midline beneath the pharynx at the level of the rhombencephalon.

At this stage the anatomical organization of cephalic axial tissues (Fig. 9.1) is similar to that of the trunk region and, as will be discussed later, the subsequent development of both these regions is comparable. The exception is the prosencephalic region. The notochord is absent at this rostral level, and paraxial mesoderm is present only as a sparse ventral mesenchyme. The walls and roof of the prosencephalon are directly apposed by surface ectoderm. Ventrally, the rostral tip of the pharynx extends slightly beneath the future diencephalon.

The pharynx differs from the rest of the gut tube in that it is not surrounded by a coelomic cavity. Thus there is no naturally occurring delineation of lateral mesoderm into splanchnic and somatic subpopulations.

DEVELOPMENT OF THE NEURAL CREST

The most unique feature of head development is the presence of a separate, ecto-

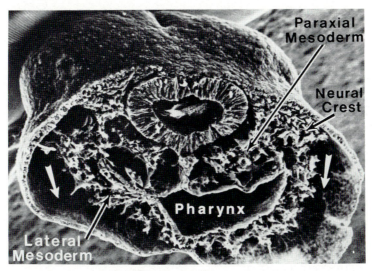

Figure 9.1. Scanning electron micrograph of a late neurula stage avian embryo cut transversely at the level of the mesencephalon. Lateral body folds have completely undercut the head by this stage. Note that paraxial mesoderm, lateral mesoderm (beside and beneath the pharynx), and neural crest cells are contiguous mesenchymal populations. The large *white arrows* indicate pathways of future displacement of crest cells. (Courtesy of K Tosney.)

dermal population of mesenchymal cells that forms all the skeletal and other connective tissues of the facial region. This mesenchymal population is derived from the **neural crest.**

Dispersal of Neural Crest Populations

As described in Chapter 7, neural crest cells are formed from neural folds and subsequently disperse laterally and ventrally from this origin. Unlike the situation in the trunk in which a relatively small number of crest cells proliferate and form peripheral neurons, Schwann cells and melanocytes, the cranial neural crest population is large and is capable of forming all these cell types plus a variety of connective tissues.

Beginning at the junction of the prosencephalon and mesencephalon, the crest cell population shifts laterally and ventrally between the surface ectoderm and underlying mesoderm (Fig. 9.2). The cells pass lateral to the pharynx and then move medially beneath the pharyngeal endoderm. This cephalic neural crest population establishes a continuous, superficial sheet of mesenchyme between the prosencephalic and future laryngeal regions, as shown in Figure 9.3.

From the level of the midbrain caudally, all crest cells leave the dorsal midline, which is subsequently occupied by paraxial mesoderm. This is not the case rostrally. Here the crest population expands to completely envelop the prosencephalon, including the optic vesicles.

In considering the specific derivatives of the neural crest it is easiest to picture them in terms of the interface between the neural crest and mesoderm illustrated in Figure 9.3. This boundary coincides with the pros-mesencephalic junction dorsally, crosses caudal to the adenohypophysis, then runs along the dorsolateral margin of the pharynx to, but not including, the larynx. All of the connective tissue-forming mesenchyme surrounding the prosencephalon and located beside or below the pharynx is derived from the neural crest, whereas the comparable mesenchyme situated immediately ventral and lateral to the mesencephalon and rhombencephalon is derived from paraxial mesoderm. Despite the subsequent flexures of the brain and growth of sense organs, this relationship will not be appreciably altered.

The ventral displacement of the neural crest population is dependent upon three mechanisms. First, individual crest cells are

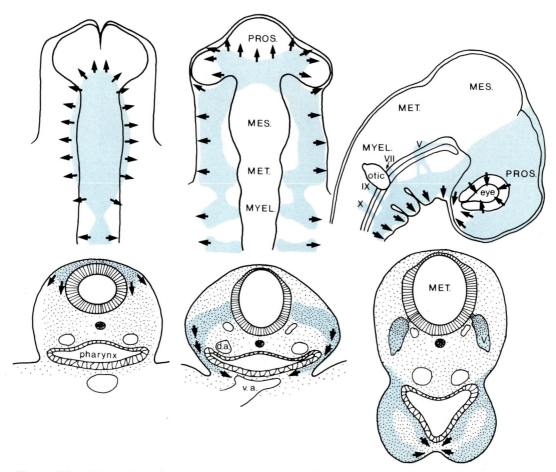

Figure 9.2.   Schematic summary of the translocation of cephalic neural crest cells shown in *blue*. The *top row* shows successive stages in dorsal and right lateral views; the *bottom row* illustrates the same stages in transverse section at the level of the metencephalon (*d.a.* and *v.a.*, dorsal and ventral aorta; *V, VII, IX, X,* cranial sensory ganglia associated with trigeminal, facial, glossopharyngeal, and vagus nerves).

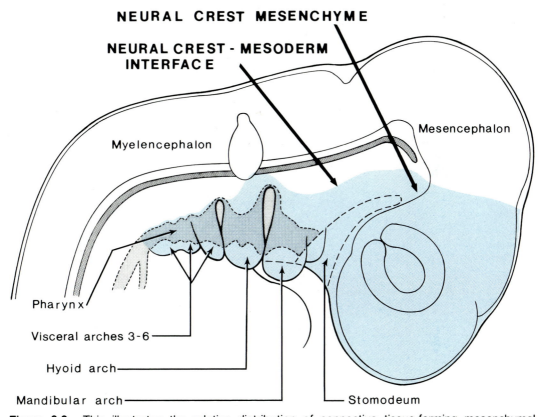

Figure 9.3. This illustrates the relative distribution of connective tissue-forming mesenchymal populations derived from the neural crest (*blue*) and paraxial mesoderm. Subsequently, the location of the interface is altered by further cephalic flexures and growth of the prosencephalon.

highly motile, and the extracellular environment immediately in front of the emigrating crest population changes to promote and orient cell migration. The primary change involves secretion of hyaluronic acid by the surface ectoderm. Once released, these molecules swell due to hydration, causing the surface ectoderm to separate from underlying mesodermal cells (Fig. 9.1). This creates an obstacle-free pathway for crest cell movement. Concomitantly, neural crest cells are

proliferating, which rapidly expands the size of the population.

However, the massive ventral displacement of crest cells is in part the result of a ventral shift in all of the superficial tissues of the embryo at the late neurula stage. As illustrated in Figure 9.4, the surface ectoderm and paraxial mesoderm expand and shift ventrally together with the crest population. Thus, there is a concerted morphogenetic translocation of several cephalic tis-

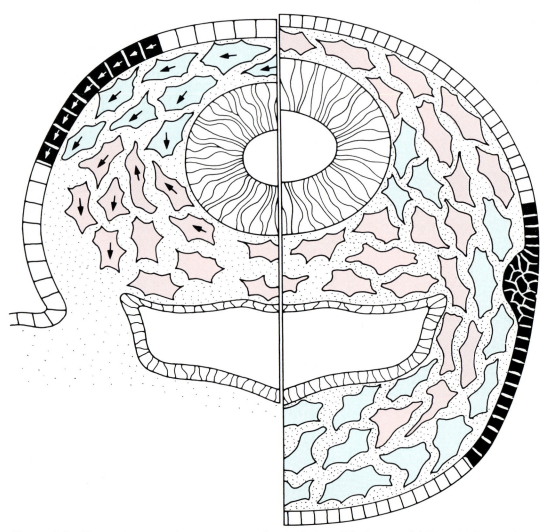

Figure 9.4. The morphogenetic movements of neural crest (*blue*), superficial paraxial mesoderm (*red*), and a patch of surface ectoderm (*black*) following neurulation are illustrated. Note that all three populations shift ventrally in concert, and that this displacement can be accomplished with only slight changes in the relations among them. These movements establish the visceral arches and facial processes. The precise fates of deeper paraxial and lateral mesoderm have not been defined.

sues to establish a new set of ventral cephalic structures.

In summary, craniofacial mesenchymal tissues are derived from two sources. Cephalic paraxial mesoderm develops in close association with most of the otic vesicle and brain similar to the situation described for the trunk. In contrast, connective tissues of the periocular, nasal and oral regions are derived from the neural crest. Although the cartilages and bones of the head have these two disparate origins, they are all biochemically identical.

Formation of Visceral Arches

As neural crest cells move ventrally the pharynx develops a series of bilateral out-pocketings, the **pharyngeal pouches.** The presence of these pouches causes the ventral crest population to become partially segregated into a series of dorsoventrally elongated mesenchymal masses called **visceral arches** (branchial arches). Running through each visceral arch is an aortic arch.

In fishes there are usually five or six fully formed visceral arches, each of which forms a gill arch or, rostrally, contributes to the jaw apparatus. In higher vertebrates there have been both reductions in the number of visceral arches that form, with arches III through VI small and incompletely developed (Fig. 9.5), and major changes in the structures derived from each of the arches.

The **first visceral arch** forms cranial to the first pharyngeal pouch. As shown in Figures 9.6 and 9.7, crest-derived mesenchyme forming this arch separates and grows in two directions: ventromedially to form the **mandibular arch** and rostrally to form the **maxillary process.** The mandibular process continues to expand toward the midline ventral to the pharynx. Eventually the left and right mandibular processes grow together to form the lower jaw (Fig. 9.7). The maxillary process continues to expand beneath the eye; its subsequent growth is discussed in the next section.

The **second visceral arch,** often referred to as the **hyoid arch,** develops in a manner similar to the mandibular arch. It is formed

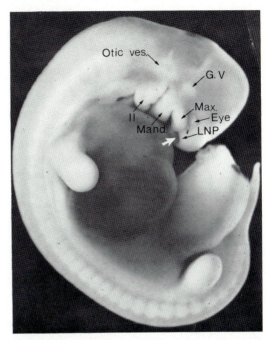

Figure 9.5. Lateral view of an 11-mm calf embryo (approximately 30 days of gestation) showing the early formation of the lateral nasal process (*LNP*), maxillary process (*Max.*), mandibular process (*Mand.*), and hyoid or second visceral arch (*II*). The close relation of these processes to the eye, trigeminal ganglion (*G. V*) and otic vesicle (*Otic ves.*) are apparent. The invaginating nasal pit (*white arrow*) is bounded medially by the median nasal process.

by neural crest cells that emigrated from the cranial myelencephalic neural folds, located immediately rostral to the otic placode. The second arch expands ventrally and then medially beneath the pharynx, eventually fusing with its contralateral counterpart.

Between the 1st and 2nd visceral arches, immediately below the otic vesicle, is a deep furrow called the **first visceral groove.** At one site the surface ectoderm of this groove directly contacts the lateral margin of the first pharyngeal pouch. There is a transient degeneration of both epithelia at this site, forming a **visceral cleft** (opening) between the pharyngeal and the amniotic cavities. In fishes a cleft forms between each of the visceral arches; these openings persist and later become gill slits. However, in mammals there is typically only one cleft established and it closes within a few days.

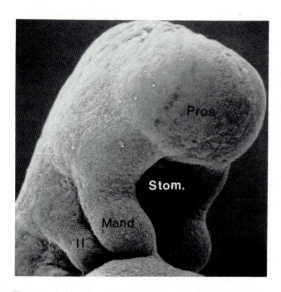

Figure 9.6. A ferret embryo of approximately 16 days of gestation showing the early growth of the mandibular (*Mand.*) and hyoid (*II*) visceral arches. The former circumscribe the stomodeum (*Stom.*), the roof of which is formed by surface ectoderm covering the prosencephalon (*Pros.*). (Courtesy of AJ Steffek.)

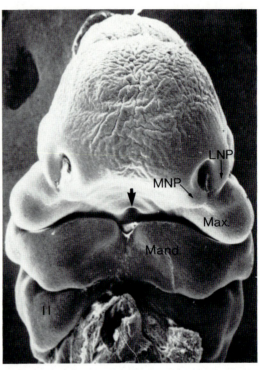

Figure 9.7. Ventral view of an 8-mm dog embryo (approximately 25 days of gestation); the truncus arteriosus has been cut and the heart removed to expose the fusing mandibular processes (*Mand.*) and the elongating hyoid processes (*II*). The maxillary processes (Max.) are growing ventrally and will contact the lateral nasal processes (*LNP*) and, later, the medial nasal processes (*MNP*), which circumscribe the nasal pit. The adenohypophyseal pouch is beginning to form (*arrow*).

Dorsal to the site of cleft formation the surface ectoderm of the first visceral groove and endoderm of the distal first pharyngeal pouch become closely apposed, separated only by a thin layer of mesenchymal cells. This relationship will persist with these tissues forming the tympanic membrane (see Figs. 14.3, 14.5 and 14.6).

The mesenchyme on both sides of the first visceral groove forms a series of small swellings called **auricular hillocks** (Fig. 9.8). The hillocks on the first visceral arch form the tragus and rostral part of the pinna; the rest of the external ear is derived from the second arch. The groove between these hillocks becomes the **external auditory meatus.** During most of fetal development this is filled with an epithelial plug that dissolves close to the time of birth.

As Figure 9.8 illustrates, the external ears initially develop on the ventrolateral surface of the head. The ears do not shift their location. Rather, later growth of the lower jaw and associated muscles greatly expands the volume of tissue ventral to the ear. In animals born with congenital absence of the lower jaw the external ears are located ventrally.

The remaining visceral arches are externally much less prominent, as shown in Figure 9.5, with arches IV through VI indistinguishable. The 2nd visceral arch expands caudoventrally, forming an **opercular fold** that overgrows and covers these caudal arches (see Fig. 14.6).

Establishment of Facial Processes

The development of the face, which includes the orbital, nasal and oral regions, is

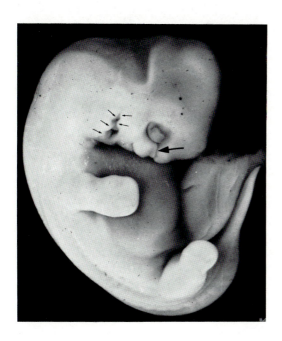

Figure 9.8. 14-mm calf embryo (33 days of gestation). The maxillary and lateral nasal processes are fusing, forming the nasolacrimal furrow (*large arrow*). Mesenchymal growths on both sides of the first visceral groove are establishing auricular hillocks (*small arrows*). Note the ventral location of the presumptive external ear tissues; their apparent dorsal shift later in development is actually due to subsequent elongation of the jaw and growth of ventral neck tissues.

most critically affected by three events: the expansion of subpopulations of rostral neural crest cells, cranial flexure and subsequent growth of the prosencephalon and eyes, and elaboration of the olfactory epithelium. Variations of these account for the many different facial morphologies found among domestic mammals.

The **stomodeum** is the cavity created by the formation of the cranial and lateral body foldings and the subsequent cranial flexure (Fig. 9.9). It is separated from the pharyngeal cavity by the **oropharyngeal membrane (oral plate),** which breaks down following fusion of the left and right mandibular arches. During fetal development the stomodeum becomes greatly elongated as a result of the growth of the mandibular, maxillary and nasal processes. The original site of the oropharyngeal membrane corresponds to the **palatoglossal arch;** thus, the lining of the mouth is largely ectodermal in origin, as is most of the mesenchyme (neural crest) surrounding the oral cavity.

Neural crest mesenchymal cells initially located over the dorsal and rostral surfaces of the prosencephalon are brought to the rostral and ventral surfaces of the head as a result of the >90° cranial flexure. This population, called the **frontonasal mesenchyme,** will form the forehead and nasal regions of the face, and contribute along with other crest cells to the nasal septum and related tissues.

The external nares and epithelial lining of the nasopharynx can all be traced back to a pair of **olfactory (nasal) placodes.** At the time of neural tube closure the presumptive nasal placode-forming ectoderm lies close to the dorsal midline near the rostral tip of the embryo. During cranial flexure formation, these areas shift to a rostroventral position and the ectoderm thickens to form definitive placodes. The formation of these placodes depends upon an interaction between the surface ectoderm and the neuroepithelium of the presumptive telencephalic hemispheres. The establishment of left and right nasal placodes is dependent upon the for-

mation of left and right telencephalic regions of the neuroepithelium.

Each nasal placode invaginates to form the **nasal pit** (Figs. 9.5, 9.7, 9.9), which deepens and subsequently contacts the roof of the stomodeum; this juncture is the **oronasal membrane,** which soon degenerates. Since the palate has not yet formed, there is now present a large oronasal cavity derived from the stomodeum and the nasal pits. Later, the ectoderm lining the nasal pits will expand and, in part, form the **olfactory epithelium.** The ectoderm of the stomodeum, together with that covering the palatine shelves, will form the **mouth;** the endoderm of the pharynx will form the caudal part of the mouth and oropharynx.

As illustrated in Figures 9.9 and 9.10, the nasal pit is circumscribed by two swellings, the **medial nasal process** and the **lateral nasal process,** which are derived from frontonasal mesenchyme. These processes are continuous over the pits dorsally, giving them a horseshoe appearance. The area between the medial nasal processes and extending dorsally over the forebrain is the **frontal prominence.**

Mesenchyme within the **maxillary process** expands rostrally beneath the optic vesicle and contacts the lateral nasal process. The furrow formed at the zone of apposition between these two swellings is the **nasolacrimal groove (furrow),** which is shown in Figures 9.5 and 9.8. As the two processes fuse together, the ectodermal lining of the furrow becomes buried in the mesenchyme as a column of epithelial cells. This will subsequently hollow out to form a duct, the **nasolacrimal duct,** which runs from the conjunctival sac to the **nasal cavity.**

The maxillary process continues to expand medially and rostrally beneath the nasal elevations, eventually fusing near to the midline with the medial nasal process (Fig. 9.11). Together these components form the rostral bones of the upper jaw (maxilla, incisive) and the lip. After establishing their definitive relationships, all of these processes undergo an extensive rostral elongation due

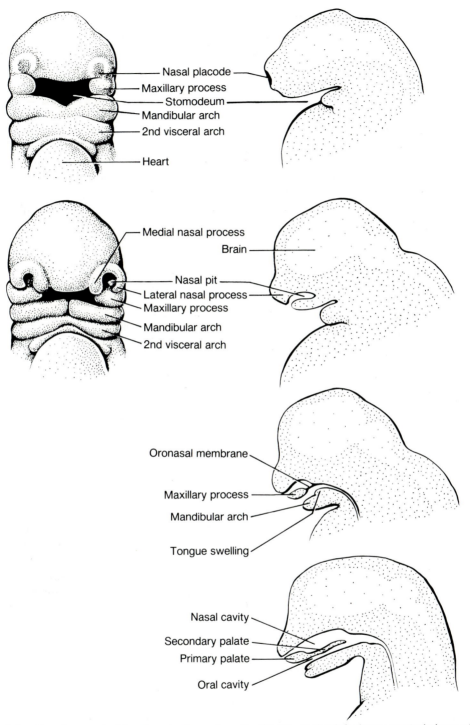

Nasal placode
Maxillary process
Stomodeum
Mandibular arch
2nd visceral arch

Heart

Medial nasal process
Brain

Nasal pit
Lateral nasal process
Maxillary process
Mandibular arch
2nd visceral arch

Oronasal membrane

Maxillary process
Mandibular arch

Tongue swelling

Nasal cavity
Secondary palate
Primary palate
Oral cavity

Figure 9.9. Development of the face and nasal cavity. Series on the *left* shows ventral views of the facial processes; on the *right* are sagittal sections showing the invagination of the nasal (olfactory) placode to form the nasal pit. This contacts the stomodeum at the oronasal membrane, which degenerates to join embryonic nasal and oral cavities. Subsequent formation of the secondary palate (*right, bottom*) will extend the separation between these cavities caudally.

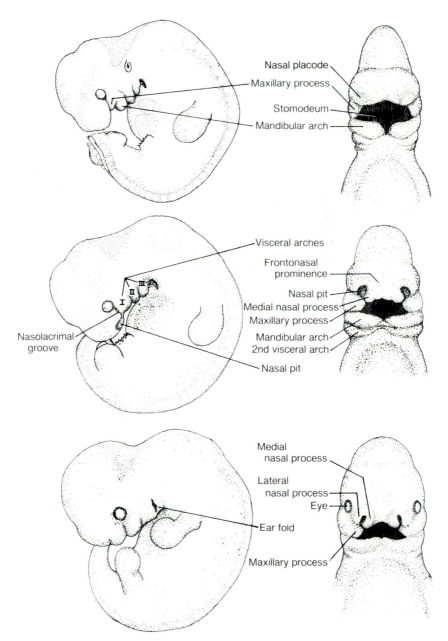

Figure 9.10. Lateral (*left*) and ventral (*right*) views of the formation of the face in a carnivore embryo. These represent stages seen when the embryo is between 6 and 10 mm in length (18–21 days in the cat, 22–26 days in the dog).

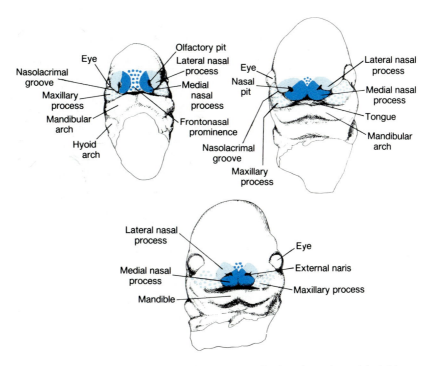

Figure 9.11. Later stages of facial process development in the pig embryo (*dark blue*, medial nasal process; *light blue*, lateral nasal process; *dark blue stipple*, frontonasal prominence; and *light blue stipple*, maxillary process). (Modified from BM Patten (1944)).

to cell proliferation; this is especially exaggerated in horses and cattle and least prominent in brachycephalic breeds of dogs and in cats. Minor variations in the sites of fusion between maxillary and medial nasal processes give rise to the various configurations of folds beneath the external nares of domestic mammals.

PARAXIAL MESODERM DEVELOPMENT

Most of the paraxial mesoderm in vertebrate embryos is segmented, with the first segment (somite) located caudal to the otic placode. The comparable mesodermal tissue located rostral to the first somite forms a continuous mesenchymal population extending rostrally to the optic vesicles and tip of the pharynx. This cephalic paraxial mesoderm is partially segregated into seven pairs of **somitomeres** (Fig. 9.12). Each somitomere is morphologically similar to an immature somite in that it is mesenchymal rather than epithelial and is not separated from adjacent paraxial mesoderm. A somitomere has the same developmental potentials as a somite, although no morphologically distinct myotomal, sclerotomal and dermatomal regions are present.

Paraxial mesoderm adjacent to the mesencephalon and rhombencephalon expands dorsally to completely surround these parts of the brain. Ventrally, this mesenchyme encircles the notochord and, laterally, it encapsulates the otic vesicle. These populations will form skeletal and connective tissues (see Fig. 9.21).

All of the voluntary muscles of the head are derived from paraxial mesodermal cells that cross the crest:mesodermal interface and invade the visceral arches or periocular region. As outlined in Figures 9.13 and 9.14, those mesodermal cells entering the 2nd arch develop into some jaw opening and hyoid muscles, and secondarily expand rostrally and dorsally beneath the surface ectoderm to form the platysma and other facial muscles. Other somitomeres, particularly those located rostrally, send slips around the developing optic vesicle; these later give rise to extrinsic ocular muscles.

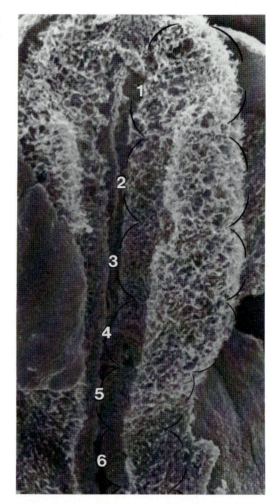

Figure 9.12. Organization of cephalic paraxial mesoderm in a neurula stage avian embryo. In preparing this scanning micrograph, the surface ectoderm and neural tube were removed, exposing the underlying mesoderm. *Brackets* indicate the location of somitomeres. The 8th somitomere (not shown) becomes the first true somite. (Courtesy of S Meier.)

The voluntary muscles associated with visceral arches are traditionally called **branchiomeric muscles.** This is based upon their homology with gill (branchial) and jaw muscles of fishes, but does not accurately describe their embryonic origins. Although these muscles are, like all other voluntary muscles of the vertebrate body, derived from paraxial mesoderm, they are unique in that their connective tissue components (including fascia and tendons) are derived from the

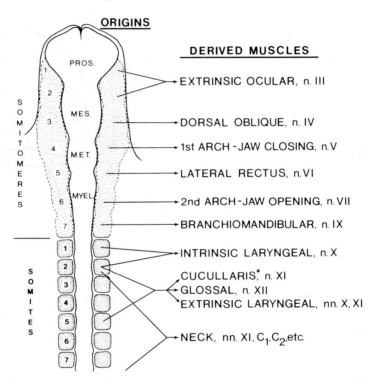

ORIGINS

DERIVED MUSCLES

→ EXTRINSIC OCULAR, n. III

→ DORSAL OBLIQUE, n. IV

→ 1st ARCH - JAW CLOSING, n. V

→ LATERAL RECTUS, n. VI

→ 2nd ARCH - JAW OPENING, n. VII

→ BRANCHIOMANDIBULAR, n. IX

→ INTRINSIC LARYNGEAL, n. X

→ CUCULLARIS,* n. XI
← GLOSSAL, n. XII
→ EXTRINSIC LARYNGEAL, nn. X, XI

→ NECK, nn. XI, C_1, C_2, etc.

Figure 9.13. Summary of the origins of voluntary muscles in the avian head. These origins were established by transplanting each somitomere or occipital somite of a quail embryo in the place of an identical piece of paraxial mesoderm excised from a chick embryo. Quail cells contain an intracellular marker that allows them to be recognized in histological sections. The avian cucullaris is a dorsal, superficial neck muscle that is probably homologous to the mammalian trapezius. Also, in mammals the myogenic cells in the 2nd arch move rostrally and form superficial facial muscles innervated by nerve VII. (From DM Noden (1983b)).

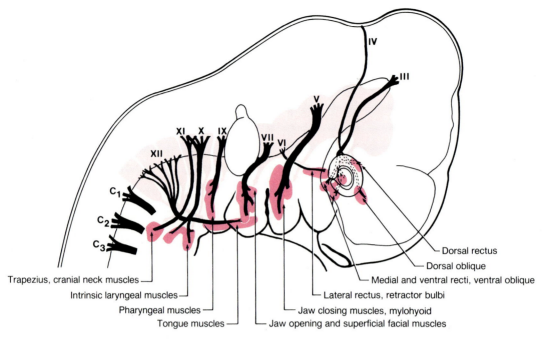

Figure 9.14. Schematic representation of the relation between somatic motor nerves, myogenic precursors (derived from paraxial mesoderm), and visceral arch or periocular regions. *Dark red areas* indicate the locations of voluntary muscle precursors at the time myogenesis begins; *pale red areas* indicate the original locations of these muscle primordia and the directions in which they have moved. III–XII, cranial motor nerves (see Table 9.1); C₁–C₃, cervical nerves.

neural crest. This contrasts with axial and appendicular muscles whose connective tissue components are derived from somitic and lateral somatic mesoderm, respectively.

The paraxial mesoderm located beside the myelencephalon caudal to the otic placode forms true somites. The first five are called **occipital somites** because the sclerotomal portions of these are involved in the formation of the occipital and otic regions of the skull. The myotomal regions of these cranial somites also shift ventrally. Slips from somites one and two move beside the primordia of the laryngeal cartilages and subsequently form laryngeal muscles. Myogenic cells from somites three through five form a large aggregation called the **hypoglossal cord.** This mass moves ventral to the pharynx and enters the neural crest-derived mesenchyme that will form the tongue.

PATTERNS OF INNERVATION

The segmental organization of cranial peripheral nerves is not apparent during gross dissection of the head. This is due in large part to the many shifts and differential growth in location of mesenchymal and surface epithelial tissues that form the target tissues of these nerves. Also, during the evolution of the head the primitive, segmental, organization of the cephalic peripheral nervous system has been altered as parts of the brain and various special sensory organs have undergone major changes. In particular, the segmental appearance of dorsal (afferent) and ventral (efferent) roots described for the trunk is not apparent in the head. However, the organization of these cephalic peripheral nerves and their relation to presumptive target tissues is much less complicated when described in the embryo before the relocation of target tissues has occurred.

Somatic efferent neurons (Table 9.1) project from motor nuclei in the mesencephalon and rhombencephalon and contact the somitomere closest to their site of emergence from the brain, as outlined in Figures 9.13 and 9.14. Their subsequent direction of

Table 9.1.
Distribution of efferent cranial nerves

	Nerve	Function	Embryonic projection	Target[a]
III	Oculomotor	SE	Somitomeres 1, 2	Dorsal, medial, ventral recti; ventral oblique; levator palpebrae muscles
		VE	Parasympathetic 2nd neurons in ciliary ganglion	
IV	Trochlear	SE	Somitomere 3	Dorsal oblique muscle
V	Trigeminal (mandibular ramus)	SE	Somitomere 4 (to 1st visceral arch)	Temporalis, masseter, mylohyoid, rostral digastric, pterygoids, palatines, tensor tympani muscles
VI	Abducent	SE	Somitomere 5	Lateral rectus, retractor bulbi
VII	Facial	SE	Somitomere 6 (to 2nd visceral arch)	Cutaneous facial, auricular, cutaneous cervical, stapedius, caudal digastricus muscles
		VE	Parasympathetic 2nd neurons in pterygopalatine, mandibular and sublingual ganglia	
IX	Glossopharyngeal	SE	Somitomere 7 (to 3rd visceral arch)	Pharyngeal muscles?[b]
		VE	Lateral splanchnic mesoderm	Pharyngeal muscles?[b]
		VE	Parasympathetic 2nd neurons in otic ganglion	
X	Vagus	SE	Somites 1 and 2 (to caudal visceral arches)	Intrinsic laryngeal muscles
		VE	Lateral splanchnic mesoderm	Esophageal muscles
		VE	Parasympathetic 2nd neurons in thoracic and visceral tissues	
XI	Accessory	SE	Occipital somites	Trapezius, cleidomastoid, sternomastoid, cleidocervical muscles
XII	Hypoglossal	SE	Occipital somites 3 to 5	Genioglossal, hyoglossal, styloglossal and intrinsic tongue muscles

[a] Based on data obtained by transplanting labeled somites and somitomeres in avian embryos and extrapolating to homologous muscles in mammals.
[b] Homologies between avian and mammalian systems are not clear; pharyngeal muscles in birds do not arise from somitomeres, and the avian branchiomandibular (3rd arch) complex is derived from somitomere 7.

growth is determined by the morphogenetic movements of each muscle primordium. Thus, cranial nerves III (oculomotor), IV (trochlear) and VI (abducent) grow along with those somitomeres that form extrinsic ocular muscles. Somatic efferent fibers in cranial nerves V (trigeminal), VII (facial), IX (glossopharyngeal) and X (vagus) project to muscle primordia that enter visceral arches I, II, III and IV, respectively. As was discussed in the Introduction, cranial nerve XI (accessory) innervates superficial muscles associated with the shoulder, neck and head (trapezius, cleidocervical, etc.), which are believed to be homologous with gill levator muscles of the caudal visceral arches in fishes. The last of the cranial nerves is XII (hypoglossal), which arises from several roots and contacts those myogenic slips of somites 3-5 that form the hypoglossal cord and invade the tongue.

Visceral efferent neurons belonging to the parasympathetic (craniosacral) component of the autonomic nervous system also emerge with several of the cranial nerves (III, VII, IX, and X). These preganglionic axons project to parasympathetic ganglia located close to the eye (ciliary ganglion) or salivary glands. Second neurons within these ganglia are all of neural crest origin. The preganglionic vagus visceral efferents project to target ganglia associated with thoracic and visceral tissues.

There are postganglionic sympathetic axons associated with many cranial nerves. The cell bodies of these second neurons are located within the cranial cervical ganglion which, although located near the base of the skull, is derived from thoracic neural crest cells.

All **somatic and visceral afferent** functions of the head except vision and olfaction are mediated by cranial sensory ganglia associated with the rhombencephalon. As described in Chapter 7, neurons in these ganglia are derived from two sources, the neural crest and neurogenic placodes. The most rostral of these is the trigeminal ganglion, so named because it has three major projections. The ophthalmic and maxillary nerves are exclusively sensory, and they innervate the regions occupied by frontonasal and maxillary mesenchymal neural crest cells, respectively. The mandibular nerve contains both somatic sensory and motor projections to the mandibular process of the first visceral arch. Figure 9.15 illustrates how the segmental sensory receptive fields of the embryo have become distorted by differential growth of facial processes.

The somatic and visceral afferent components of cranial nerves VII, IX, and X parallel the corresponding motor neurons to individual visceral arches. In addition, the visceral afferents of IX and X are distributed with the vagus nerve to the esophagus and viscera of the thorax and abdomen. The cell bodies of these sensory neurons in VII, IX and X are located in ganglia adjacent to the myelencephalon; these become surrounded by bones forming the skull.

Most of the remaining cranial afferent neurons mediate specialized sensory modalities unique to the head, including olfaction (I, olfactory nerve), vision (II, optic nerve), and taste (nerves VII, IX, X). Hair cells in the membranous labyrinth act as transducers for hearing and vestibular functions; these are innervated by axons of cranial nerve VIII that project from the spiral (cochlear) and vestibular ganglia. Neurons in these two ganglia are derived from the otic vesicle.

Cranial nerves I and II are atypical peripheral nerves. The cell bodies of the olfactory neurons are located in the olfactory epithelium, and are derived from the olfactory placode. Their axons pass from this epithelium through numerous small foramina in the cribriform plate of the ethmoid and enter the olfactory bulbs of the telencephalon. The optic nerve is composed of interneurons of the central nervous system rather than peripheral neurons. These neurons project from ganglion cells within the retina, which is formed from the lateral wall of the diencephalon, to several visual centers in the di- and mesencephalon, especially the lateral geniculate nucleus and rostral colliculus.

PALATOGENESIS

Following the initial growth and fusions of facial mesenchymal populations, the roof of the stomodeum is bounded laterally by the maxillary process and rostrally by the medial nasal process and frontonasal prominence. Entering the roof of the stomodeum are a pair of openings from the short nasal cavities. Thus, as a result of these early morphogenetic movements, a partial separation of nasal and oral cavities is achieved.

The mesenchymal cells located between the nasal cavities initially form the medial nasal processes and ventral aspect of the frontal prominence. These populations aggregate in the rostral midline to form the **medial palatine process,** part of which will become the **primary palate.** Later, the incisive (premaxillary) bone forms within this rostral mesenchyme. The palatine fissures mark the caudal margin of the primary palate. The mesenchyme located superficially between the nasal cavities contributes to the

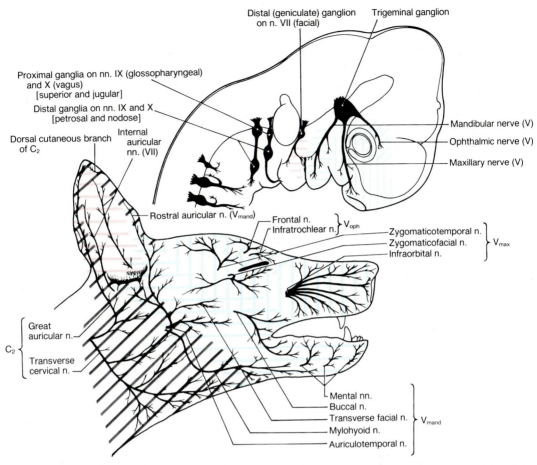

Figure 9.15. Schematic illustration of the relation between somatic sensory nerves, visceral arches, and cutaneous fields of innervation in the embryo (*top*) and adult dog (*bottom*). *Bars* represent areas of skin innervated by branches of trigeminal (*blue*), facial (*red*) and second cervical (*gray*) afferent nerves. Note how the mandibular, maxillary and nasal processes have expanded during fetal and postnatal growth. The embryonic distribution of C_2 axons has not been mapped. $V_{mand, max, oph}$ indicate branches of the mandibular, maxillary and ophthalmic nerves. (Based on HE Evans (1979) and LR Whalen and RL Kitchell (1983).)

rostral cartilages of the snout, the philtrum and the median part of the upper lip.

The **secondary palate** forms later in development (Table 9.2), and results in the nasal and oral cavities being separated to the level of the oropharynx. The **hard palate** contains horizontal wings of the maxillary and palatine bones, while the caudally located **soft palate** has no skeletal elements.

In the embryo the oronasal cavity is partially partitioned by two vertical tissue masses, as shown in Figure 9.16. The **nasal septum** projects from the roof of the cavity ventrally between the two nasal cavities.

Table 9.2.
Time of secondary palate closure

Rat	16 Days
Ferret	27 Days
Cat	32 Days
Dog	33 Days
Pig	33 Days
Horse	7th Week
Cow	8th Week
Human	9th Week

This vertical septum elongates as the nasal cavities enlarge. The tongue grows dorsally from the floor of the stomodeum and rostral pharynx.

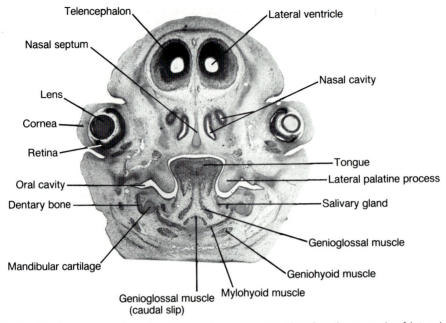

Figure 9.16. Transverse section of a 13-mm feline embryo showing the growth of lateral palatine processes beside the tongue. Note the nasolacrimal furrow beneath the eye.

Broad mesenchymal processes grow into the oronasal cavity from the maxillary processes on both sides. These are the **lateral palatine processes.** Initially these processes extend ventrally on either side of the tongue, as shown in Figures 9.16 and 9.18*A*.

The subsequent two steps, elevation and fusion of the lateral palatine processes, are the most critical events in palatogenesis. For many years it was believed that the elevation of these processes, during which they change from a nearly vertical to a horizontal plane, occurred similar to the movement of a door upon its hinge. This view is no longer tenable. Close examination of lateral palatine mesenchyme during elevation has revealed that this epithelial-covered population flows around and over the tongue. The movement is rapid, and elevation of these palatine shelves is completed within a day.

Concomitant with this morphogenetic rearrangement, the tongue shifts ventrally within the oronasal cavity. In rodents this process has been shown to depend upon an elongation of the **mandibular** (Meckel's) **cartilage** on the day preceding lateral palatine process elevation. Since the tongue is at-tached to the rostral part of the jaw via the genioglossal muscles, elongation of the lower jaw depresses the tongue thereby facilitating palatal process reorientation.

The size of the lateral palatine processes is such that as soon as they assume a horizontal position their margins are apposed, as shown in Figure 9.17. The epithelium covering their medial margin undergoes **autolysis,** and the mesenchymal cores become continuous across the dorsal midline of the oral cavity. This reorientation also brings the paired lateral processes in contact with the medial palatine process (primary palate), rostrally, and all three fuse together. Similarly, the lateral palatine processes fuse with the nasal septum, thereby partitioning the nasal cavity into two separate chambers.

Mesenchyme in the rostral two-thirds of the lateral palatine processes undergoes intramembranous ossification, forming the hard palate; these ossification centers then fuse with large, more laterally situated centers to form the maxillary and palatine bones. Mesenchyme in the caudal third of the lateral palatine processes expands to form the soft palate.

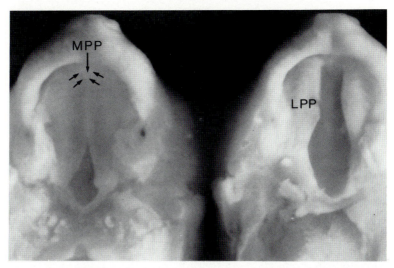

Figure 9.17. Ventral views of the roof of the mouth during closure of the lateral palatal processes in 27-day (22-mm) ferret embryo littermates. Although both are the same age, the shelves of the embryo on the left have elevated and fused over two-thirds of their length, while the shelves of the embryo on the right have not yet apposed. *Arrows* indicate the site of fusion of secondary to primary palate (*MPP* and *LPP*, medial and lateral palatine processes).

ORAL CAVITY

At the time of head folding the roof of the stomodeum is formed by the ventral surface ectoderm, which underlies the prosencephalon. Formation of the maxillary and frontonasal processes expand the cavity rostrally, and formation and elevation of the lateral palatine processes separate oral from nasal cavities. The floor of the oral cavity is initially formed from stomodeal ectoderm and, caudally, from ventral pharyngeal endoderm. The lateral walls of the oral cavity are formed by first visceral arch mesenchyme sandwiched between stomodeal and surface ectodermal layers.

Lips and Gums

On the apposed surfaces of the maxillary and mandibular processes, approximately midway between the midline and the lateral (or rostral) margin of the oral cavity, the stomodeal ectoderm thickens (Fig. 9.18). This thickening is called the **labiogingival (vestibular) lamina.** It extends in the form of an arch along the inner margins of maxillary and mandibular processes, running along both sides and across the rostral margin of these first arch-derived swellings. The band

thickens, and forms a solid cord of epithelial cells which penetrate the underlying mesenchyme. A trough called the **labiogingival groove** (lip sulcus) forms in the band. Expansion of the mandibular labiogingival groove ventrally and the maxillary groove dorsally results in the formation of the **vestibule.** The tissue rostral and, varying with the species, lateral to the labiogingival groove forms the lips.

Teeth

Medial to the labiogingival band there forms a series of focal thickenings of the oral epithelium that are called **dental laminae.** The mesenchyme underlying each dental lamina also develops a dense aggregation. The dental laminae invaginate, forming **dental buds.** The rows of dental laminae in the dog are first apparent at 25 days of development, by which stage the embryo is approximately 14 mm long and externally resembles that shown on the bottom of Figure 9.10.

Continued expansion and branching of the epithelial dental bud results in the formation of a cup-shaped **enamel organ,** which partially encompasses a neural crest-derived

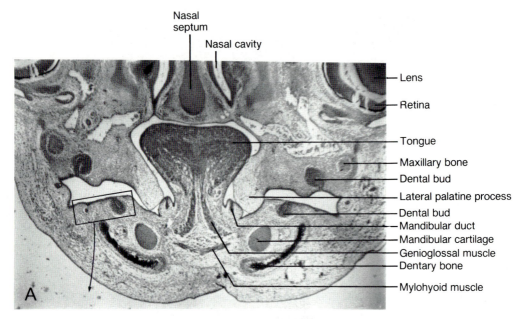

Figure 9.18. *A* shows a transverse section through the oral cavity of a 19-mm (26-day) ferret embryo showing the locations of the labiogingival and dental primordia. The *box* circumscribes the area described in *B–H*, which illustrate stages of tooth and vestibule development.

mesenchymal condensation called the **dental papilla** (Fig. 9.18*F*). This complex will form a **deciduous tooth.** A bud off of the dental lamina between the enamel organ and the surface of the oral cavity will later differentiate into the **permanent tooth.** Domestic animals are **diphyodonts,** which means that they produce two sets of teeth.

Following the cup stage of tooth formation, the inner layer of the enamel organ differentiates into a population of specialized cells called **ameloblasts.** These cells produce **enamel,** which is the material that covers the crown of the tooth. The epithelial cells near the distal (deeper) parts of the cup become **cementoblasts,** which produce **cementum** around the roots of the tooth. In each dental papilla those neural crest cells

located adjacent to the epithelium of the enamel organ differentiate into **odontoblasts.** These cells produce **dentin,** which surrounds the pulp and comprises the major structural material of a tooth.

The earliest tooth to develop is the first mandibular molar. Enamel production begins early in the 8th week of development in the dog, slightly earlier in the cat. Eruption of the teeth occurs postnatally in carnivores but may begin before birth in other domestic animals, as summarized in Table 9.3.

Many of the tissue interactions necessary for the normal development of a tooth are known. Neural crest cells excised from the oral region will differentiate into odontoblasts when placed in tissue culture next to

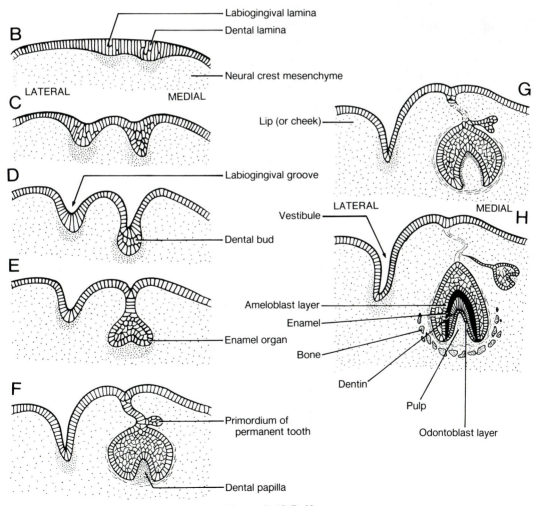

Figure 9.18 B–H.

Table 9.3.
Eruption of teeth in domestic animals[a]

Animal	Deciduous	Permanent
Cat	$2(I_3^3\ C_1^1\ P_2^3)^b$	$2(I_3^3\ C_1^1\ P_2^3\ M_1^1)^b$
	Incisors: 3–4 weeks[c]	Incisors: 3.5–5.5 months[c]
	Canines: 3–4 weeks	Canines: 5.5–6.5 months
	Premolars: 5–6 weeks	Premolars: 4–5 months
		Molars: 5–6 months
Dog	$2(I_3^3\ C_1^1\ P_3^3)$	$2(I_3^3\ C_1^1\ P_4^4\ M_3^2)$
	Incisors: 4–6 weeks	Incisors: 3–5 months
	Canines: 3–5 weeks	Canines: 5–7 months
	Premolars: 5–6 weeks	Premolars: 4–6 months
		Molars: 4–7 months
Pig	$2(I_3^3\ C_1^1\ P_3^3)$	$2(I_3^3\ C_1^1\ P_4^4\ M_3^3)$
	Incisors 1 and 2: 1–3 weeks	Incisors: 8–18 months
	Incisor 3: Before birth	Canines: 8–12 months
	Canine: Before birth	Premolar 1: 3.5–6.5 months
	Premolars: 1–10 weeks	Premolars 2–4: 12–16 months / 4–6 months
		Molar 1: 7–13 months
		Molar 2: 17–22 months
		Molar 3:
Sheep	$2(I_4^0\ C_0^0\ P_3^3)$	$2(I_4^0\ C_0^0\ P_3^3\ M_3^3)$
	Incisors: Before birth—up to 8 days[d]	Incisor 1: 1–1.5 yr
	Before birth—up to 4 weeks[d]	Incisor 2: 1.5–2 yr
	Premolars:	Incisor 3: 2.5–3 yr
		Incisor 4: 3–4 yr
		Premolars: 21–24 months
		Molar 1: 3 months
		Molar 2: 9 months
		Molar 3: 18 months
Ox	$2(I_4^0\ C_0^0\ P_3^3)$	$2(I_4^0\ C_0^0\ P_3^3\ M_3^3)$
	Incisors: Before birth—up to 2–14 days postnatal[d]	Incisor 1: 1.5–2 yr
	Premolars: Before birth—up to 2–3 weeks[d]	Incisor 2: 2–2.5 yr
		Incisor 3: 3 years
		Incisor 4: 3.5–4 yr
		Premolars: 2–3 yr
		Molar 1: 5–6 months
		Molar 2: 15–18 months
		Molar 3: 24–28 months
Horse	$2(I_3^3\ C_1^1\ P_3^3)$	$2(I_3^3\ C_1^1\ P_3^3\ \text{or}\ {}_3^4\ M_3^3)$
	Incisor 1: 1 week	Incisor 1: 2.5 yr
	Incisor 2: 1 month	Incisor 2: 3.5 yr
	Incisor 3: 5–9 months	Incisor 3: 4.5 yr
	Canines: Never erupt	Canine: 4–5 yr
	Premolars: Before birth or 1st week postnatal	Premolar 1: 5–6 months
		Premolar 2: 2.5 yr
		Premolar 3: 3 yr
		Premolar 4: 4 yr
		Molar 1: 1 yr
		Molar 2: 2 yr
		Molar 3: 3.5–4.0 yr

[a] From Habel RE: *Applied Veterinary Anatomy*, Ithaca, NY, Habel, 1973; and Nickel R, Schummer A, Seiferle E, Sack WO: *The Viscera of Domestic Mammals*. Berlin, Verlag-Paul Parey, 1973.
[b] I, C, P, M = incisor, canine, premolar and molar teeth.
[c] All ages postnatal unless otherwise indicated.
[d] Late maturing breeds.

any embryonic epithelium. This includes epithelium from a foot pad, or even that from the **diastemal** region (a nontooth bearing area between the incisors and premolars). However, oral epithelium will form an enamel organ only when cocultured with neural crest mesenchyme from the oral region. Other mesenchymal populations, or even neural crest cells from other regions, will not promote this development. These experiments indicate that perioral neural crest mesenchyme is different from other mesenchymal populations. Research on amphibian tooth development suggests that migrating crest cells become "activated" by the pharyngeal endoderm, and thus acquire the competence to promote tooth development.

The problems of why teeth develop in particular locations and have unique, regionally-specific shapes are more difficult. When presumptive molar epithelium is cultured next to presumptive incisor mesenchyme, the resulting tooth has a distinctive incisorform appearance, indicating again the unique role of the neural crest in odontogenesis.

Salivary Glands

Most of the salivary glands are derived from invaginations of the **ectodermal epithelium** of the oral cavity, although some may come from the adjacent endodermal epithelium of the oropharynx. A cord of epithelial cells grows into the adjacent mesenchyme, extends a variable distance, then begins to branch. On the ends of the branches a solid mass of epithelial cells forms. The entire system subsequently becomes hollowed out. The original site of invagination becomes the external orifice for the exocrine gland. The epithelial cord and its branches become the duct system and the cells on the distal ends of the smallest ducts become the secretory **acini** of the gland. In most cases the duct becomes greatly elongated as a result of the growth of the upper and lower jaws.

For the **mandibular** and monostomatic **sublingual glands** the excretory orifice, marking the site of origin of the gland, is located rostrally on the lower jaw in the **linguogingival groove** near the rostral attachment of the tongue. In the 10- to 12-mm embryo the primordia of these two glands first appear as two linear furrows in the groove between tongue and mandible (see Figure 9.18). The main ducts are separate but the excretory orifice may be common to the two duct systems. The polystomatic sublingual gland consists of multiple microscopic glands whose ducts enter the main excretory duct of the monostomatic gland or open on the floor of the oral cavity adjacent to the tongue.

The excretory ducts of the **zygomatic** and **parotid salivary glands** enter the vestibule lateral to the caudal maxillary teeth. The parenchyma of the zygomatic gland is located in the orbit ventrolateral to the eyeball, while that of the parotid gland is lateral and ventral to the external ear canal. Multiple microscopic salivary glands also develop from the epithelium covering the lips, cheeks, and palate (labial, buccal, and palatine glands).

Tongue

The tongue initially appears as four distinct swellings in the floor of the pharynx and oral cavity (Fig. 9.19). These outpocketings are, in order of their appearance, the **median tongue swelling** (tuberculum impar), which forms on the ventral midline of the pharyngeal floor at the junction of the 1st and 2nd visceral arches, two **distal tongue swellings** (lateral lingual swellings), which are much larger and form in the stomodeum on either side of the ventral midline, and the **proximal tongue swelling** (copula), a large midventral prominence overlapping the distal appositions of the 3rd and 4th visceral arches.

The distal tongue swellings are initially filled by neural crest mesenchymal cells of the first visceral arch. Caudally this mesenchyme underlies the pharynx; thus, the surface of the caudal part of the tongue is formed from endoderm. However, much of the 1st arch is lined by stomodeal ectoderm, which contributes to the rostral part of the tongue (blue area in Fig. 9.19). These distal tongue swellings expand greatly, incorporating the smaller median tongue swellings, and

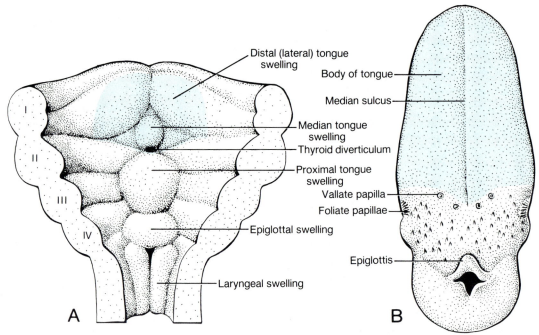

Figure 9.19. Development of the tongue. *A* is a dorsal view of the floor of the stomodeum and pharynx showing the locations of glossal swellings; *B* shows the parts of the adult tongue derived from these swellings. I–IV are visceral arches. *Blue* indicates the region of the glossal surface derived from stomodeal ectoderm.

then fuse in the midline. Together these will form the **body** of the tongue.

The proximal tongue swelling expands and forms the **root** of the tongue. The vallate papillae, which are aligned in a "V" with its apex directed caudally, approximately demarcate the body of the tongue from the root. As discussed earlier, the muscles of the tongue are derived from occipital myotomes that secondarily invade the hypoglossal region.

The afferent innervation of the tongue reflects the early pattern of development of the tongue from several visceral arches. Exteroceptive (tactile, thermal) sensations from the ectodermal epithelium of the first visceral arch are mediated by the lingual branch of the mandibular (Vth) cranial nerve; those from the root, derived from the 3rd and 4th arches are mediated by the lingual branch of the glossopharyngeal (IXth) cranial nerve. Taste is mediated by separate afferent neurons; those from cranial nerve VII project to the body and those from nerve IX to the root of the glossal epithelium.

Like all other parts of the integument, the surface of the tongue is a continually renewing population, with each epithelial cell having a lifespan of 7–10 days. It has been experimentally shown that the appearance, maturation and maintenance of epithelial cells forming each **taste bud** are dependent upon the presence of the gustatory neuron dendritic zones. If the VIIth and IXth nerves are cut, the taste buds are visibly reduced in size within the 1st day after axotomy and are completely gone within a week in rodents. This is another example of a neuron: target tissue interaction, similar to those described in Chapters 7 and 8. Only gustatory neurons will support taste bud development; efferent neurons such as the hypoglossal nerve or somatic afferents such as the auriculotemporal nerve will not suffice.

Pituitary Gland

When the stomodeum is first formed, the ectoderm of the dorsal aspect of this cavity is closely apposed to the ventral neurectoderm of the diencephalon. At the site of apposition the stomodeal ectoderm thickens, forming a placode, and then invaginates. This invagination is paralleled by an evagination of ventral diencephalic neurectoderm, as shown in Figure 9.20. The stomodeal ectodermal evagination forms the **adenohypophyseal pouch** (Rathke's pocket); the neurectodermal evagination forms the **infundibulum.**

This close apposition is maintained even though continued growth of the oral region greatly expands the distance between the floor of the brain and the roof of the oronasal cavity. During this period the adenohypophyseal pouch closes, forming a vesicle completely separated from the stomodeum. The epithelial cells of the adenohypophyseal pouch form the endocrine cells of the **adenohypophysis**, which forms the pars distalis and pars intermedia of the pituitary. The infundibulum expands into the caudal surface of the adenohypophysis. The distal part of this diencephalic evagination develops into the **neurohypophysis.** The lumen of the neurohypophysis is, in fact, an extension of the third ventricle of the hypothalamus.

Occasionally a canal, the adenohypophyseal foramen, is found in the center of the mammalian basisphenoid bone. This results from the persistence of epithelial tissue that formed the stalk of the adenohypophyseal pouch. Unless the stalk remains patent, which is very rare, animals with this canal

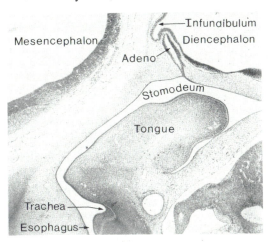

Figure 9.20. Development of the pituitary illustrated in a median section of a 14-mm calf embryo. The adenohypophyseal pouch (*Adeno.*) is a diverticulum of the stomodeum. The floor of the diencephalon evaginates to form the infundibulum that develops into the neurohypophysis.

have no clinical abnormality. It is more commonly seen in brachycephalic breeds of dogs.

CRANIOFACIAL SKELETOGENESIS

The developing head skeleton can be topographically separated into three parts. The **neurocranium** forms a trough in which all parts of the brain except the telencephalon lie; it extends rostrally from the occipital region to the nasal septum. The **dermatocranium** includes the roofing bones of the skull (the **calvaria**) and nose. Finally, the **viscerocranium** (splanchnocranium) is composed of the jaws and other skeletal structures that develop within visceral arch mesenchyme.

The neurocranium initially appears during the 4th week of gestation in the dog as several mesenchymal condensations beneath the brain and around sensory epithelia (olfactory, optic and otic). These begin to chondrify and then grow together (Figs. 9.21 and 9.22) to form a longitudinal cartilaginous trough ventral and rostral to the developing brain. Dorsolateral extensions of this cartilage form lateral processes that follow the changing contours of the brain and sense organs. The periocular mesenchymal condensation does not chondrify in mammals, but forms the fibrous sclera.

Later (7th-week dog), several ossification centers will appear in this cartilage, marking the sites of formation of occipital and sphenoid complexes and the vomer and ethmoid bones (Fig. 9.23). These bones form in close association with the cartilage tissues and are referred to as **endochondral** or replacement bones. Both paraxial mesoderm, caudal to the diencephalon, and neural crest mesenchyme, rostrally, contribute to the neurocranium.

Concomitantly two series of osteogenic foci condense in the mesenchyme between the brain and the dorsal and lateral surface ectoderm. These foci grow rapidly and form the **intramembranous** (dermal) bones of the **calvaria.** Figure 9.24 summarizes the embryonic sequence of skeletogenesis of the canine skull.

The visceroskeleton includes cartilages

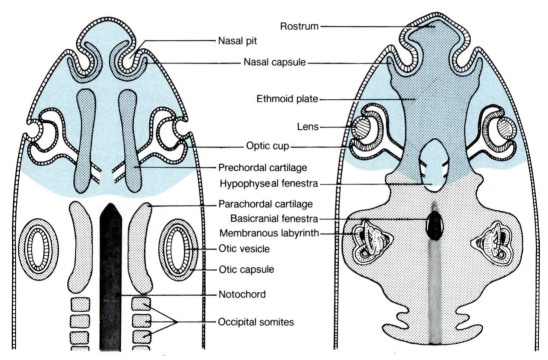

Figure 9.21.   Schematic illustration showing the early embryonic centers of chondrification beneath the brain and associated with special sensory organs. These subsequently fuse together to form the neurocranium. *Blue area* indicates regions derived from the neural crest. (Redrawn after Weichert CK: *Anatomy of the Chordates*, ed 3. New York, McGraw Hill, 1965.)

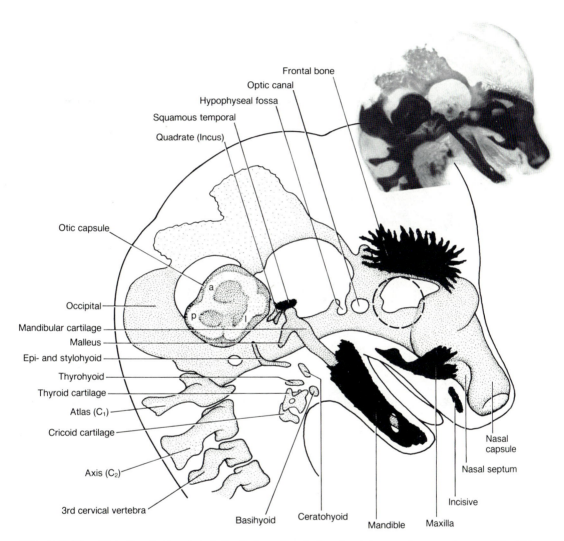

Figure 9.22.   The chondrocranium (*stippled*) and early-forming intramembranous bones (*black*) in a 19-mm (26-day) ferret embryo (*a, p* and *l* indicate the anterior, posterior and lateral semicircular canals). The *insert* is a photomicrograph of the specimen from which this sketch was made.

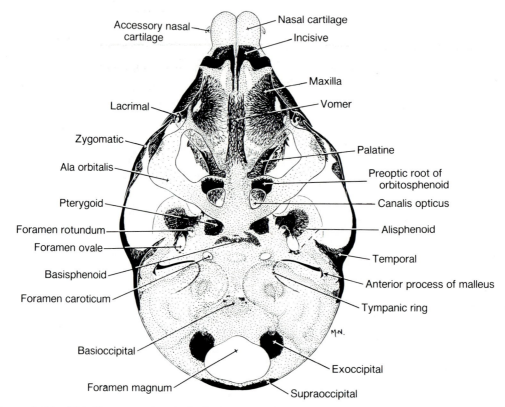

Figure 9.23.   This illustrates the skull of a 71-mm (40-day) Beagle fetus shown in dorsal view with the frontal and parietal bones removed to reveal the floor of the braincase. (From HE Evans (1979).)

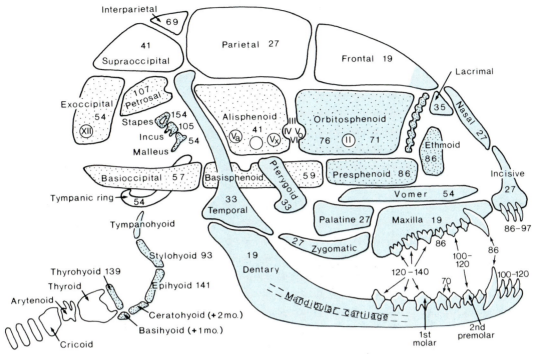

Figure 9.24. Timetable for ossification of bones in the head of the dog. *Numbers* represent size of the fetus in millimeters when deposition of bone matrix or dental enamel is first detectable. Bones formed by endochondral ossification are *stippled;* those derived from the neural crest are *shaded blue*. The nasal capsule, tympanohyoid and laryngeal skeleton do not ossify. Roman numerals indicate foramina of cranial nerves (Redrawn after HE Evans (1979).)

and both endochondral and intramembranous bones, all of which are derived from neural crest mesenchymal cells. Skeletogenesis begins in these processes after they establish the proper relationships with each other, and it is the pattern of growth of these skeletal tissues that largely determines the final shape of the face.

The earliest skeletal element to form in the viscerocranium is a cartilaginous rod in the 1st arch. This **mandibular** (Meckel's) **cartilage** (Fig. 9.22) is subsequently surrounded by intramembranous osteogenic sites that fuse together to form the mandible. The lower jaw articulates with the squamous portion of the temporal bone, which is of neural crest origin. The remainder of the temporal bone is derived from paraxial mesoderm.

Most of the skeletal structures of the remaining visceral arches have been lost or greatly modified during vertebrate evolution, and there is little remaining in mammals of the elaborate piscine gill skeleton. The 2nd (hyoid) arch mesenchyme gives rise to the **basihyoid,** cells in the 3rd arch to the **ceratohyoid** and **epihyoid** endochondral bones, and the 4th arch to the **thyrohyoid.** Based on apparent homologies it is often stated that the laryngeal cartilages are derived from neural crest cells of the rudimentary 5th visceral arch. However, experimental analyses of the distribution of neural crest cells in birds have shown this to be untrue; the **arytenoid** and **cricoid** cartilages are mesodermal in origin, as are all of the tracheal ring cartilages. Since birds do not have a thyroid cartilage, there is no conclusive data regarding the precise embryonic origin of this structure.

The dorsal skeletal primordia within visceral arches 1 and 2 of primitive vertebrates have become highly modified to transmit and amplify vibrations from the tympanic membrane to the perilymphatic fluid surrounding the cochlear duct. Embryonically the mesenchyme of these arches surrounds the 1st pharyngeal pouch, which forms the auditory tube and middle ear chamber.

Neural crest cells in the 2nd visceral arch form part or all (in mammals) of an endochondral bone called the **columella** in birds and reptiles or **stapes** in mammals. This bone abuts upon the **vestibular window** (fenestra ovalis). As shown in Figure 9.25, the stapes is a vestige of the large, jaw-supporting hyomandibular bone of fishes. Other 2nd arch neural crest-derived mesenchyme contributes slightly to the formation of the **otic capsule.** Whether this contribution represents remnants of the more dorsal skeletal components of the hyoid arch of fishes is not known.

The dorsal skeletal components formed from the 1st visceral arch have also changed dramatically during vertebrate evolution. In modern birds and reptiles there is a prominent **quadrate bone** formed by endochondral ossification of these neural crest cells, as illustrated in Figures 9.25 and 9.26A. The lower jaw articulates with this bone, which articulates with the skull at the otic region.

In mammals the lower jaw articulates directly with the squamous part of the temporal bone. The quadrate, freed of involvement with jaw movement, has become reduced in size and transformed into the **incus** of the middle ear (Fig. 9.26). Similarly, another proximal element of the premammalian 1st arch, the **articular** bone, has been modified and forms the **malleus.** The mammalian **tympanic bulla** grows from a ring of dermal bone that is homologous with the angular bone of birds and reptiles (compare Figs. 9.23 and 9.24 with 9.26A).

The shifting of these tissues to the region of the middle ear does not represent a significant change in their original embryonic location. Rather, it is the site of jaw:skull articulation that has shifted rostrally during vertebrate evolution. This example demonstrates how a change in one set of tissue relations can lead to profound morphological and functional alterations in adjacent tissues.

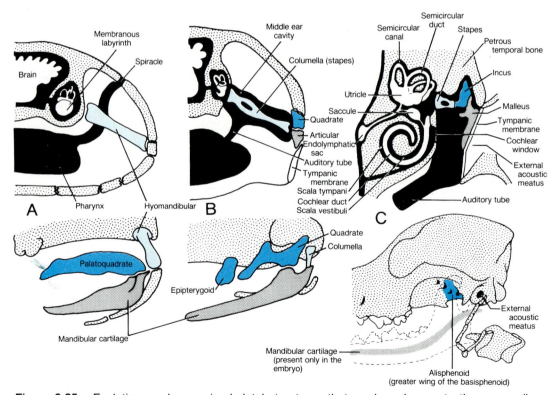

Figure 9.25.   Evolutionary changes in skeletal structures that are homologous to the mammalian middle ear bones, shown schematically in transverse (*top row*) and lateral views. *A*, fish; *B*, primitive reptile; and *C*, mammal. (Adapted from Romer.)

MECHANISMS OF VISCERAL ARCH DEVELOPMENT

Within the visceral arch neural crest populations are cells that form melanocytes, cartilages, bones, tendons, dermis, smooth muscle, and other connective tissues as well as sensory neurons, glia, and Schwann cells within the peripheral ganglia and associated nerves. Not only do the cells have to become programmed and express these diverse, unique phenotypes (i.e. cytodifferentiation), but they have to do so in particular sites in the visceral arch and, together with surrounding cells, form structures that have the appropriate three-dimensional shape. This property is called patterning (refer to Chapter 4).

While numerous experiments provide clues regarding the cytodifferentiation of neural crest cells, they do not explain how the many different skeletal structures found in visceral arches develop in appropriate locations and with characteristic, species-specific shapes and growth potentials, i.e. the problem of patterning. To investigate whether patterning is controlled by interactions emanating extrinsic to the crest population or is programmed within this mesenchyme, neural crest cells that would normally form the 2nd visceral arch were surgically removed from a neurula-stage chick embryo and replaced with a crest population destined to enter the 1st arch. As shown in Figure 9.26*A*, the skeletal structures normally formed in the hyoid and mandibular arches are very different.

The results of these experiments are most dramatic. The transplanted cells entered the second visceral arch but formed skeletal structures typically found in the mandibular arch (Fig. 9.26*B*). These host embryos have two lower jaws! Thus, the spatial pattern of skeletogenesis within a visceral arch is programmed in the neural crest population before it leaves the neuroepithelium. Differences in skeletal morphology between arches are based upon the original location of the crest primordium along the neuraxis.

Although patterning is an essential component in the development of all systems, its expression is most readily apparent in the skeletal system. A comparable, regionally specific programming of the mesenchyme that forms connective tissues in the limbs will be discussed in the next chapter. This process is also a key component in vertebrate evolution, as developmentally minor alterations in the expression of a skeletal pattern may result in a significant change in the adaptive abilities of the animal. Conversely, aberrations of patterning are a major cause of congenital malformations. The molecular basis underlying the acquisition and expression of this spatial programming is unknown.

MALFORMATIONS OF THE HEAD REGION*
Defects Related to Abnormal Brain Development

Abnormal closure of the cephalic neural tube or a failure of the meninges or roofing bones of the skull to develop properly leads to defects similar to those described in Chapters 6 and 8. **Anencephaly** is an absence of brain tissue that results from failure of the cranial neural folds to fuse. As was the case for myeloschisis, it is not possible for the skeletal and connective tissue-forming paraxial mesodermal cells to form dorsal roofing structures without proper neural tube closure. Anencephaly most commonly involves the telencephalic hemispheres.

The appearance of these animals varies depending upon the extent and location of the neural defect. At the lesion site the exposed neuroepithelium degenerates, leaving the floor of the neurocranium visible beneath a layer of vascular and meningeal tissues. When the prosencephalon is involved, growth of the upper facial region is compromised, causing the eyes to protrude from shallow orbital sockets.

An **encephalocele** (cranium bifidum, meningoencephalocele) is a herniation of any part of the brain. This occurs if mesenchyme forming any of the skeletal compo-

---

* Excluding pharyngeal pouch anomalies, Chapter 14.

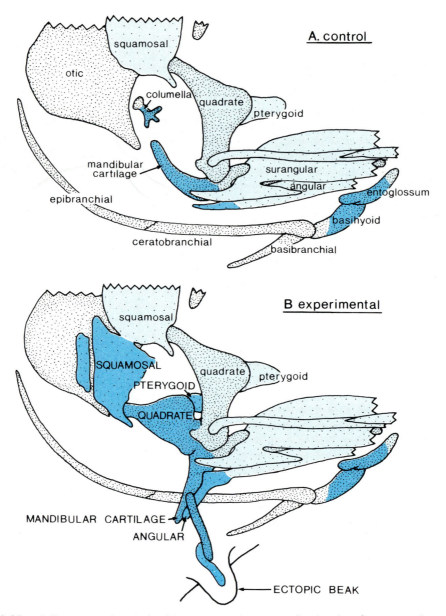

Figure 9.26. *A* illustrates the skeletal structures that normally develop from neural crest cells entering the first (*pale blue*) and second (*dark blue*) visceral arches of the chicken embryo. The results of removing presumptive **2nd** arch neural crest cells and replacing them with a presumptive **1st** arch crest population are shown in *B*. The grafted mesenchymal cells invade the 2nd arch region but many of them form skeletal structures that are appropriate for a 1st arch. This indicates that the population was already programmed with respect to **patterning** of connective tissues at the time of transplantation, i.e. before emigration from the neural folds. Labels for ectopic skeletal structures are in capital letters.

nents of the calvaria fails to develop properly. However, the primary defect can occur in either the developing brain or surrounding mesenchyme. As with partial anencephaly, an encephalocele can occur at occipital, parietal or frontonasal regions, with the last of these usually associated with secondary dysmorphologies of the face. If the protruding brain tissue is not covered by skin, the condition is termed **exencephaly** (Fig. 9.27).

Holoprosencephaly results from any re-

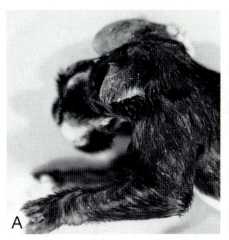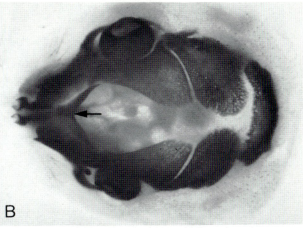

Figure 9.27. *A* illustrates encephalocele in a newborn cat exposed to the drug griseofulvin during gestation. *B* is a dorsal view of a newborn rat pup cleared and stained to show bones; the schisis between the frontal bones indicates the location of the encephalocele. The median bone (*arrow*) rostral to the opening is called an interfrontal. This condition in the rat was induced by administering aspirin to the pregnant female.

duction in the normal separation of the prosencephalon into paired cerebral hemispheres, olfactory system, and optic vesicles. Mild forms of holoprosencephaly, in which only the olfactory system or corpus callosum are affected, have been described in humans and probably occur in domestic animals.

As the severity of the neural defect increases there is greater compromise of facial skeletal structures. The most severe form of holoprosencephaly results in **cyclopia** (circle eye), which was described in the Introduction. Cyclopia is characterized by a single, centrally located orbit (Fig. 9.28*A*) containing a normal or rudimentary eye or various degrees of fusion of two eyeballs. The eyelids are absent or rudimentary, and the nose is absent or exists as a tubular appendage, the **proboscis,** located dorsal to the orbit. There are no nasal cavities. The ethmoid, incisive, and all skeletal structures of the nose are absent. The telencephalon consists of a large, single cerebral lobe with no olfactory bulbs or nerves.

A teratogen present in the plant *Veratrum californicum* causes cyclopia if fed to pregnant sheep on the 14th day of gestation. At this time the ovine embryo is at the early neural plate stage of development. By the 15th day this teratogen will no longer produce craniofacial malformations.

While the exact mechanism of action of this teratogen is not known, analysis of cyclopia produced in amphibian embryos by surgical lesioning has clarified how the facial dysmorphology arises. As discussed in Chapter 4, interactions between the presumptive neural plate and underlying mesoderm are necessary for the region-specific programming of the neurepithelium. As a result of these interactions, paired optic and telencephalic structures are delineated from a single median primordia. The bilateral telencephalic neural tissues then cause overlying surface ectoderm to form paired olfactory placodes. Subsequently, frontonasal mesenchyme derived from the neural crest expands over the rostral surface of the prosencephalon, between the emerging telencephalic lobes and, ventrally, the olfactory invaginations.

If the initial step in this progression is disrupted by lesioning the mesoderm underlying the rostral part of the presumptive neural plate, a cyclopic larva is produced (Fig. 9.27*B*). When the neural plate folds and closes, a single telencephalic lobe is produced, resulting in a single olfactory placode. Instead of being paired and located laterally, the optic primordia are fused into a single optic vesicle that grows from the floor of the diencephalon, and only a single lens placode

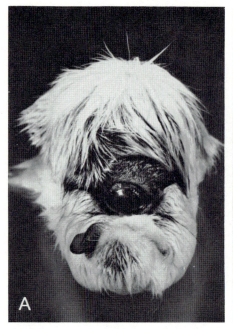
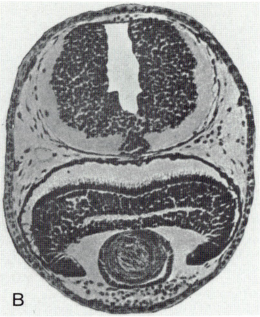

Figure 9.28.   Cyclopia in *A*, a newborn goat and *B*, experimentally induced in an amphibian larva (described in text). Additional examples shown in Figure I.3 of the Introduction.

is induced in these animals. Thus, the normal route of frontonasal neural crest displacement is blocked, and none of the tissues normally derived from this population can develop.

Cebocephaly (monkey face) is a less severe form of holoprosencephaly in which the orbits are abnormally close together and incorrectly oriented so as to open rostrally. Frontonasal structures are present but reduced. Total absence of all prosencephalic, frontonasal, and 1st visceral arch tissues results in **otocephaly** (ear head), so named because the external ears are located at the rostral tip of the head.

Abnormal Development of Facial Mesenchyme

Abnormal development of the nasolacrimal furrow or duct following fusion of the maxillary and lateral nasal processes will result in an animal with lacrimal secretions flowing over the side of the face. Often a minor lesion or blockage of the duct can be corrected.

Failure of these two mesenchymal processes to meet and fuse produces a **facial cleft** (Fig 9.29), which is a schisis from the medial angle of the eyelids to the oronasal cavity. Secondary asymmetries of the face and cleft palate usually are present.

An unusual malformation characterized by encephalocele, anophthalmia and severe facial defects occurs in the "new look" (Eastern) strain of Burmese cats (Fig. 9.30). Be-

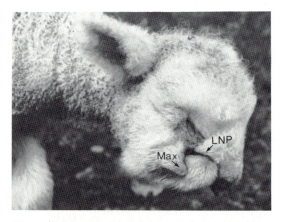

Figure 9.29.   Facial cleft in a newborn lamb. The embryonic maxillary (*Max*) and lateral nasal (*LNP*) processes have failed to fuse, leaving a broad cleft from the eye to the oronasal cavity. The lower jaw is curved to the right, partially obscuring this cleft.

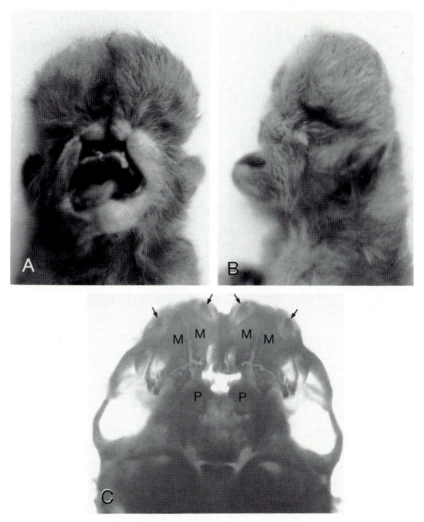

Figure 9.30.   Inherited craniofacial malformations in the Burmese cat. *A* and *B* show the face and profile of an abnormal neonatal kitten with encephalocele, maxillary brachygnathia, four whisker pads, and involution of the eyelids due to hypoplasia of the eyes. *C* illustrates the skeletal defects in the roof of the oral cavity (ventro-dorsal view). Note the presence of four canine teeth (*arrows*) and two pairs of maxillae with palatal shelves (*M*). The palatine bones (*P*) are enlarged but are not duplicated. The incisive bone and teeth are absent.

tween 25 and 40% of these kittens lack incisive, ethmoid, and nasal bones and nasal cartilages, and die shortly after birth. In the rostral midline there is an extra pair of maxillary bones, including lateral palatine processes. The skin covering the abnormal upper jaw has four sets of whisker pads rather than the normal two.

This is a malformation of patterning, in which the frontonasal mesenchyme is deficient and becomes programmed to form maxillary-type structures, presumably as a result of an abnormality in the underlying prosencephalon. The condition is inherited as an autosomal dominant with incomplete expression, and appears to be inseparably linked to the "new look" phenotype in Burmese cats (described in Chapter 5).

Cleft lip (cheiloschisis), and **cleft palate (palatoschisis)** may occur separately or together, unilaterally or bilaterally. Cheiloschisis (Fig. 9.31) results from failure of the medial nasal and maxillary processes to fuse completely; this is frequently accompanied

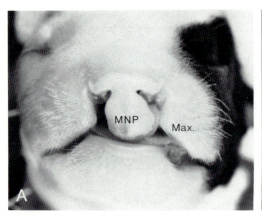 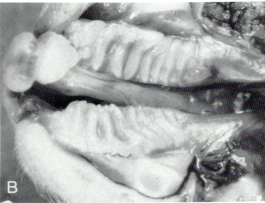

Figure 9.31. Cheiloschisis and palatoschisis in a newborn puppy, shown in *A*, rostral and *B*, ventral views. The lower jaw was removed in *B*. A cleft lip results from failure of the maxillary (*Max.*) and medial nasal (*MNP*) processes to unite. In *B* the nasal septum is visible between the unfused lateral palatine shelves.

by a schisis of the primary palate. Palatoschisis is a failure of the elevation, apposition or fusion of the lateral palatine processes, resulting in an opening between oral and nasal cavities. When the cleft is bilateral, the ventral aspect of the nasal septum is exposed and both nasal cavities communicate along their entire length with the oral cavity.

The frequent occurrence of cleft palate in animal populations (0.6 cases per 1000 births) is due to two factors. First, this series of events happens later in development than most other morphogenetic events; as such, it is possible to interfere with palatal shelf development and not affect other systems. More importantly, there are many relatively independent tissues that must develop normally and synchronously for the palate to form. If the oronasal cavity is too wide or the lateral palatine processes are too short, which can occur if the migration or growth of maxillary neural crest cells are deficient, the shelves will not become apposed when they reach the horizontal plane. The high incidence of cleft palate in brachycephalic breeds of dog, especially the Bulldog, may be due to these factors.

The events associated with fusion are independent of the position of the shelves, and are transient. Thus, if the shelves are not apposed at the same time as breakdown of the marginal epithelium occurs, fusion will not take place. Similarly, disruption of the normal biochemical changes in the extracellular matrix around palatal shelf mesenchymal cells, or a reduction in the straightening and elongation of the mandibular cartilage, which promotes depression of the tongue, can result in palatoschisis.

Numerous specific causes of cleft palate in domestic animals have been reported. There is a significantly higher than average incidence in Abyssinian cats, which suggests a breed disposition. Also, palatoschisis has been reported as a recessive inherited trait in one strain of Hereford cattle. Cleft palate is a common finding in the malformations created by the ingestion of various species of lupine by pregnant cattle. Scoliosis, torticollis, and arthrogyposis often accompany cleft palate in both the inherited and teratogen-induced situations; this syndrome is most common in Charolais cattle.

Many teratogens have been implicated as causes of cleft palates. **Corticosteroids** administered to some inbred strains of pregnant mice between 11.5 and 12.5 days of gestation will consistently produce cleft palates in the offspring. **Hypervitaminosis A** and **folic acid deficiency** will also produce cleft palates in experimental animals. **Griseofulvin,** a ringworm treatment, causes cleft palate along with other cranial malformations in kittens (Fig. 5.6). **Dioxins,** a contaminant of the herbicide Agent Orange and a combustion product of PCBs, are potent inducers of palatoschisis in the ferret at very low (10 parts per billion) levels.

Various sedatives, anesthetics, and tranquilizers taken by pregnant women prior to 12 weeks of gestation have been implicated in the genesis of cleft palates. In utero infections of the developing fetus with the rubella virus, the herpesvirus, or the cytomegalovirus also have produced cleft palates in humans.

Cleft palates occasionally occur in several of the newborn in a litter of dogs or cats. These are usually sporadic in a breeding kennel but the possibility of inheritance must not be overlooked.

Choanal atresia or **stenosis** causes neonatal **dyspnea** (respiratory distress). The choanae are the caudal openings of the nasal cavities into the common nasopharynx dorsal to the soft palate. If these openings fail to form in the development of the nasal cavities, it is termed **atresia** (a = lacking; tresis = a hole). An opening that is patent but more narrow than normal is called **choanal stenosis** (Fig. 9.32).

This condition is most frequently seen in horses. With bilateral atresia or severe stenosis, the foal usually dies shortly after birth due to the inadequacy of respiring through the mouth. Foals may survive if there is less severe stenosis or unilateral atresia, but they will by dyspneic, especially upon exercise.

Embryonic abnormalities of the lower jaw include **agnathia** (gnathos = jaw), which is the complete absence of the lower jaw, and **mandibular brachygnathia** (brachy = short), which is reduction in length of the mandible. This is called an "overshot" jaw. **Maxillary brachygnathia** ("undershot" jaw) is the condition in which the maxillary region is shorter than the mandibles. This is a common feature in the brachycephalic breeds of dogs.

Malformation of Oral Tissues

Abnormalities in the number of teeth are numerous. Complete absence of teeth is **anodontia**. This presumably results from a failure of the dental lamina and neural crest mesenchyme to interact.

Extra or **supernumerary teeth** may occur within the jawbone or in other areas of the head (**heterotopic polydontia**). In horses these occur near the external ear cartilage and are termed "ear teeth" (Fig. 9.33). They are often embedded deep in the tissues with an ectodermal tract (fistula) extending to the surface of the head. Since enamel organs normally develop from 1st visceral arch ectoderm, a normal but misplaced tissue interaction could give rise to supernumerary teeth displaced towards the external ear canal, which is derived from the ectodermal-lined furrow located between visceral arches 1 and 2.

Secretion of ectopic salivary tissue within a cyst around the ectopic teeth may cause a swelling that fluctuates on palpation. This

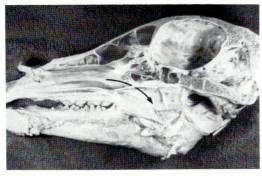

Figure 9.32. Equine choanal stenosis. *Arrow* indicates the obstructed passageway between nasal cavity and nasopharynx.

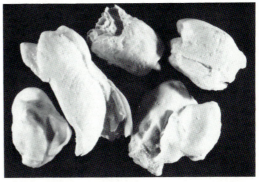

Figure 9.33. Ectopic "ear teeth" removed from an adult horse.

cyst probably arises from ectoderm of the first visceral furrow that was improperly incorporated into the external ear canal and became an inclusion in the adjacent mesenchyme. Ectopic teeth located in other parts of the head, including the adenohypophysis have been described in several species.

Other tissues derived from the oral cavity have also been described in ectopic locations. For example, pituitary endocrine cells can develop in the wall of the nasopharynx. These represent abnormal differentiation of adenohypophyseal pouch cells in the wall of the stomodeal ectoderm rather than in their normal location adjacent to the neurohypophysis. If present in sufficient numbers they can produce hormone imbalances.

Parapituitary epithelial residues are occasionally found around the adenohypophysis. These epithelial vesicles are remnants of the hypophyseal pouch that differentiate as if they were still part of the stomodeal epithelium. They can form cysts or produce neoplasms that grow to occupy a considerable area, and which then embarrass the pituitary or adjacent parts of the brain. When neoplastic these are called **craniopharyngiomas.**

A third example of ectopic differentiation of oral tissues has been reported in cats. This is the formation of a tuft of hair on the surface of the tongue, which represents a normal surface ectoderm—neural crest mesenchyme interaction occurring in an inappropriate location, i.e. an error in patterning. Similar lesions called **dermoids** occur on the anterior surface of the eye, most frequently in cattle and cats.

A lethal hereditary glossopharyngeal defect has been described in the Basset hound. These newborn puppies have an extremely narrow tongue with the lateral, normally fimbriated edges folded medially on the dorsal surface of the tongue. This prevents normal sucking and may interfere with swallowing. The shape of the tongue has given rise to their designation as **"bird-tongue" dogs.** The tongue malformation has a recessive inheritance.

Bibliography

REVIEWS

Bhaskar S: *Orban's Oral Histology and Embryology*, ed 9. St. Louis, Mosby, 1979.

deBeer GR: *The Development of the Vertebrate Skull.* London, Oxford University Press, 1937.

Gans C, Northcutt RG: Neural crest and origin of vertebrates: a new head. *Science* 220:268–274, 1983.

Horstadius S: *The Neural Crest.* London, Oxford University Press, 1950.

Jarvik E: *Basic Structure and Evolution of Vertebrates,* New York, Academic Press, 1980.

Le Douarin NM: *The Neural Crest.* London, Cambridge University Press, 1983.

Moore, WJ: *The Mammalian Skull.* London, Cambridge University Pres, 1981.

Noden DM: Patterns and organization of craniofacial skeletogenic and myogenic mesenchyme: a perspective. In Dixon AD, Sarnat B (eds): *Factors and Mechanisms Influencing Bone Growth.* New York, A. R. Liss, 1982, pp 167–203.

Noden DM: Craniofacial development: new views on old problems. *Anat Rec* 208:1–13, 1984.

Patten BM: *Embryology of the Pig,* ed 3. Philadelphia, Blakiston, 1948.

Slavkin H, Bavetta LA: *Developmental Aspects of Oral Biology.* New York, Academic Press, 1972.

Sperber GH: *Craniofacial Embryology.* Chicago, Year Book Medical Publishers, 1976.

EMBRYOLOGY ARTICLES

Bates MN: The early development of the hypoglossal musculature in the cat. *Am J Anat* 83:329–356, 1948.

Berke JP: The development of the rostral neuraxis and neural crest in the rabbit embryo up to 16 somites. *Bol. Inst. Estud. Med. Biol. Univ. Nac. Mex.* 23:185–212, 1965.

Diewert VM: The role of craniofacial growth in palatal shelf elevation. In Pratt RM, Christianson RL (eds): *Current Research Trends in Craniofacial Development.* New York, Elsevier North Holland, 1980, pp 165–186.

Evans HE: Reproduction and prenatal development. In Evans HE, Christensen GC (eds): *Miller's Anatomy of the Dog.* Philadelphia, Saunders, 1979, pp 13–77.

Hunter RM: The development of the anterior postotic somites in the rabbit. *J Morphol* 57:501–531, 1935.

Mead CS: The chondrocranium of an embryo pig, *Sus scrofa. Am J Anat* 9:167–215, 1909.

Meier S: Development of the chick embryo mesoblast: morphogenesis of the prechordal plate and cranial segments. *Dev Biol* 83:49–61, 1981.

Noden DM: The migration and cytodifferentiation of cranial neural crest cells. In Pratt RM, Christiansen RL (eds): *Current Research Trends in Prenatal Craniofacial Development.* New York, Elsevier/North Holland, 1980, pp 3–25.

Noden DM: The role of the neural crest in patterning of avian cranial skeletal, connective and muscle tissues. *Dev Biol* 96:144–165, 1983a.

Noden DM: The embryonic origins of avian craniofacial muscles and associated connective tissues. *Am J Anat* 168:257–276, 1983b.

Tamarin A: The formation of the primitive choanae

and the junction of the primary and secondary palates in the mouse. *Am J Anat* 165:319–337, 1982.

Whalen RC, Evans HE: Prenatal dental development in the dog, *Canis familiaris:* chronology of tooth germ formation and calcification of deciduous teeth. *Anat Histol Embryol* 7:152–163, 1978.

MALFORMATIONS

Adelmann HB: The problem of cyclopia. *Q Rev Biol* 11:161–182, 284–304, 1936.

Batstone JHF: Cleft palate in a horse. *Br J Plast Surg* 19:327–331, 1966.

Cohen MM Jr: An update on the holoprosencephalic disorders. *J Pediat* 101:865–869, 1982.

Cohen MM Jr: Mutations affecting craniofacial cartilage. In Hall BK (ed): *Cartilage.* New York, Academic Press, 1983, vol 3, pp 191–228.

Cooper HK, Mattern GW: Genetic studies of cleft lip and palate in dogs. *Birth Defects* 7:98–100, 1971.

Dennis SM, Leipold HW: Agnathia in sheep: external observations. *Am J Vet Res* 33:339–347.

Elzay RP, Hughes RD: Adontia in a cat. *JAVMA* 154:667–670, 1969.

Goodman RM, Gorlin RJ: *The Face in Genetic Disorders.* St. Louis, Mosby, 1970.

Gorlin RJ, Cervenka J, Pruzansky S: Facial clefting and its syndromes. *Birth Defects* 8:3–18, 1971.

Heider L, Wyman M, Burt J, Root C, Gardner H: Nasolacrimal duct anomaly in calves. *JAVMA* 167:145–147, 1975.

Hughes EH, Hart H: Defective skulls inherited in swine. *J Hered* 25:111–115, 1934.

Jurkiewiez MJ, Bryant DL: Cleft lip and palate in dogs. *Cleft Palate J* 5:30–36, 1968.

Lauvergne JJ, Blin PC: Fissure palatine hereditaire associee a l'ankylose des membres dans la race Charolais. *Ann Zootech* 18:291–300, 1967.

Loevy HT: Cytogenetic analysis of Siamese cats with cleft palate. *J Dent Res* 53:453–456, 1974.

Mason TA: Atresia of the nasolacrimal orifice in two thoroughbreds. *Equine Vet J* 11:19–20, 1979.

Mulvihill JJ, Mulvihill CG, Priester WA: Cleft palate in domestic animals: epidemiologic features. *Teratology* 21:109–112, 1980.

Noden DM, de Lahunta A, Evans HE: Inherited craniofacial malformations of Burmese cats. *Vet News,* Winter: 4–6, 1983.

Pruzansky S: *Congenital Anomalies of the Face and Associated Structures.* Springfield, Charles C Thomas, 1961.

Ross RB, Johnston MC: *Cleft Lip and Palate.* Baltimore, Williams & Wilkins, 1972.

Scott FW, de Lahunta A, Schultz RD, Bistner S, Riss RC: Teratogenesis in cats associated with griseofulvin therapy. *Teratology* 11:79–86, 1975.

Shupe JL, Jones LE, Binns W, Keeler RF: Cleft palate in cattle. *Cleft Palate J* 1:346–355, 1968.

Stewart RW, Selby LA, Edmonds LD: A survey of cranium bifidum: an inherited defect in swine. *Vet Med Small Anim Clin* 67:677–681, 1972.

Wijeratne WVS, Beaton D, Cuthbertson JC: A field occurrence of congenital meningoencephalocele in pigs. *Vet Rec* 95:81–84, 1974.

Zook BC, Draper DJ, Graf-Webster E: Encephalocele and other congenital craniofacial anomalies in Burmese cats. *Vet Med Small Anim Clin* 78:695–701.

Limb Development

GENERAL PRINCIPLES

Limb abnormalities and dysfunctions are among the most commonly encountered congenital problems in domesticated animals. In part this is because appendicular tissues are particularly sensitive to both genetic (intrinsic) and environmental (extrinsic) perturbations during the stages at which morphogenetic tissue interactions are occurring (Fig. 10.1).

The frequency of observed limb defects is also attributable to the relative autonomy of the developing limb. Except for the limb-innervating regions of the central nervous system, other body tissues develop independent of the limbs. This contrasts with defects involving the notochord, liver, kidney, etc., which are more likely to be lethal in utero or in early postnatal stages, and are less frequently encountered in clinical practice.

In discussing limb development there are several features that must be explained. To begin with it is necessary to define the origins of limb tissues. As was described in Chapter 8, all appendicular connective tissues arise from lateral plate somatic mesoderm, while voluntary muscles are of somitic origin. A second problem is to identify the mechanisms controlling shaping (morphogenesis) and internal organization (patterning) of the nerves, blood vessels, muscles, skeletal and connective tissues in the limb. The critical period of limb development is coincidental with the time at which these processes are occurring.

This stage is followed by a period of rapid growth during which muscles and skeletal tissues mature, tendons and ligaments are formed, and joints develop. For the latter it

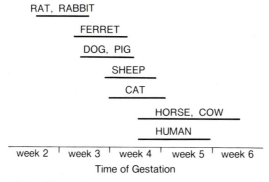

Figure 10.1. The critical period in mammalian limb development.

is necessary that the limb be functionally innervated and moving, otherwise **anky-losis**, which is fixation of a joint, will occur. This stage lasts until the animal has reached its adult size.

EMBRYOLOGY OF THE LIMB

The initial event in limb formation is an aggregation of lateral plate somatic meso-derm beneath the surface ectoderm at four discrete sites. This marks the formation of the **limb buds** (see Fig. 1.6*J*). As each limb bud enlarges, the surface ectoderm thickens in a discrete zone located along the distal margin of the bud. This thickening is called the **apical ectodermal ridge** (AER) (Fig. 10.2). It is found in all tetrapod vertebrates and persists until the digital mesenchyme has condensed. Normal limb development is dependent on the interaction between limb bud mesoderm and the apical ectoder-mal ridge.

The limb bud rapidly elongates distally, as illustrated in the series of stages shown in Figure 10.3. As this occurs, the mesenchyme within the bud forms two morphologically distinct populations. The proximally located mesenchyme is the first to show overt signs of cytodifferentiation, forming chondro-genic condensations that soon develop into the scapula or pelvis, then, later, the hu-merus or femur, etc.

While this is occurring the more distal mesenchyme, which is located immediately beneath the AER, remains cytologically ho-mogeneous. This distal population is the source of cells from which the middle (an-tebrachial, crural), then distal (carpal, tarsal) and, finally, phalangeal structures will se-quentially develop.

The elongating limb becomes flattened in the dorsoventral plane of the embryo, and the distal part acquires a paddle shape (Fig. 10.3 *B* and *C*). As distal outgrowth contin-ues, the limb bends ventrally so that the original ventral surface of the limb bud be-comes the medial surface. Subsequently the limbs rotate, which brings the cranial margin of the distal part of the limb medially (Fig. 10.4). The first digit, then, is derived from tissues originally located in the cranial part

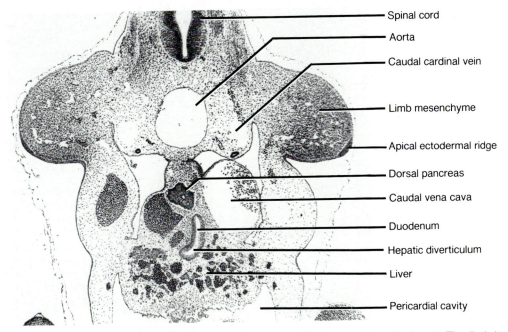

Spinal cord

Aorta

Caudal cardinal vein

Limb mesenchyme

Apical ectodermal ridge

Dorsal pancreas

Caudal vena cava

Duodenum

Hepatic diverticulum

Liver

Pericardial cavity

Figure 10.2. Section through a 6-mm cat embryo immediately caudal to the heart. The limb buds of the forelimbs are well developed, although overt differentiation of the skeletal tissues has not yet begun. Note the prominent apical ectodermal ridge on the distal tip of each bud.

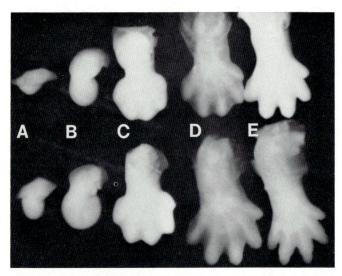

Figure 10.3. Early development of the hind limb (*upper row*) and forelimb (*bottom row*) in a carnivore, as exemplified by the ferret. Note that the forelimb is consistently more advanced than the hind limb. Dog or cat limbs would have a similar appearance at *A*, 8- to 10-mm; *B*, 12- to 13-mm; *C*, 15- to 16-mm; *D*, 18- to 19-mm; and *E*, 21- to 23-mm stages. In the ferret this series represents animals at 19, 21, 24, 26, and 27 days of gestation.

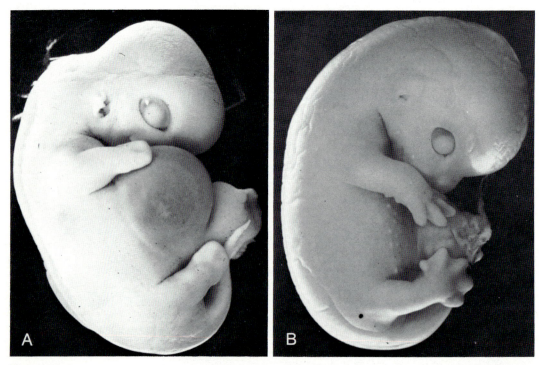

Figure 10.4. *A*, sheep and *B*, cat embryos of 17-mm crown-rump length to illustrate rotation and adduction of the limbs. The large ventral swelling in the sheep is the liver, which is temporarily displaced ventrally by the enlarged mesonephros present in the ruminant fetus.

of the limb bud. The descriptions of limb development in this chapter all refer to these original embryonic axes.

Within the mesenchyme located immediately beneath the cranial and caudal ectoderm are areas of cell death called **necrotic zones**. At later stages similar necrotic zones will appear in the mesenchyme between the digits. Experiments have shown that these mesenchymal cells are programmed to degenerate as a normal terminal stage of their differentiation. This cell death is an important component of the shaping of the limb, especially the digits.

The limb bud is invaded by angiogenic cords, which are the primordia of the endothelial lining of blood vessels, during early outgrowth stages (Fig. 10.2). As will be discussed in detail in the next chapter, these cords are outgrowths from cervical intersegmental arteries. Initially these vessels establish an arteriovenous plexus, with a central artery connected via many small channels to a marginal sinus located along the cranial, distal and caudal margins of the limb. In the thoracic limb the central artery is a distal extension of the subclavian. It subsequently forms the brachial and interosseous arteries. Nerves enter the limb shortly thereafter, well in advance of the onset of myogenesis.

After the myogenic primordia enter the limb bud from the ventral part of adjacent somites, they form two distinct condensations called the **dorsal** and **ventral muscle masses**. These condensations subsequently segregate into the primordia of individual muscles.

MORPHOGENETIC FIELDS

Morphogenetic fields are areas of embryonic tissue that appear morphologically to be undifferentiated but that can be shown experimentally to be committed to particular fates. Because it is readily accessible to surgical manipulation, the embryonic limb primordium is well suited to demonstrate the properties of a morphogenetic field, properties that are common to many developing organs.

If most of the ectoderm and underlying mesenchyme that normally would form a limb are removed at a stage prior to any visible signs of limb bud formation and are implanted in a neutral location, such as the wall of the abdomen, they will form a complete limb in that ectopic site (Fig. 10.5). This indicates that the presumptive limb-forming tissues are capable of **self-differentiation**, in much the same way as were the grafted presumptive axial tissues described in Chapter 4.

More surprisingly, the tissue adjacent to the wound on the donor embryo will also frequently form a complete limb (Fig. 10.5 *B*), even though under normal circumstances this tissue would have participated in the development of only part of a limb. Similarly, if a dorsoventral cut is made through the middle of the limb-forming area at an early stage, dividing it into separate cranial and caudal halves, then two complete limbs will form, one from each half.

Both these experiments demonstrate a property called **embryonic regulation**, which is the ability of embryonic tissues to recognize changes in their size or position and

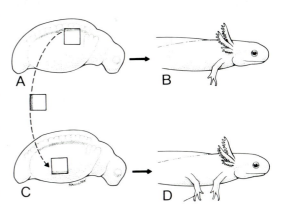

Figure 10.5. Properties of the morphogenetic field, as experimentally demonstrated using amphibian embryos. Removing most of the forelimb field (*A*) does not prevent the normal development of a limb (*B*). This demonstrates the property of embryonic regulation. Rotating the excised tissue 180° and grafting it to an ectopic site (*C*) results in the formation of a misdirected, ectopic limb (*D*). This demonstrates the properties of polarization and self-differentiation.

form a complete, patterned set of appropriate structures. It is different from **regeneration**, in which a lost but previously present differentiated part is replaced. In embryonic regulation a developmental potential, the ability to form a complete and normal structure, is reestablished in what was previously a subpopulation of the original tissue.

Finally, if the potential limb-forming region is rotated 180° around both axes (craniocaudal, dorsoventral) and reimplanted, a limb will develop with a normal dorsoventral orientation but a reversed craniocaudal polarity (Fig. 10.5*D*). Thus, at least in the craniocaudal plane, the presumptive limb-forming tissue is **polarized** early in embryonic development. Rotations at slightly later stages result in both planes being reversed.

Thus, the properties of a **morphogenetic field** are:

1. **Self-differentiation,**
2. **Embryonic regulation, and**
3. **Polarity.**

Many experiments have shown that the limb is not unique in having these properties. There is an area in the median part of the rostral neural plate from which the optic vesicles later develop that displays these properties. In addition to limb and eye fields, there is a heart field, a mouth field, etc. In fact, the entire neural plate and underlying mesoderm exhibit all these same properties. In all these cases the fate of the field, i.e. the fate of the cells considered collectively, is unchangeable; one cannot get cardiac structures from a limb field. However, the precise fates of individual cells are not fixed until later stages.

MECHANISMS OF LIMB DEVELOPMENT

The concept of patterning introduced in Chapter 4 is a fundamental feature in the development of all multicellular organisms. Here again, experimental analyses of limb development provided some of the best insights into how this elusive process occurs during vertebrate embryogenesis. The fol-

lowing four sets of experiments, all performed on avian embryos, illustrate these principles.

QUESTION 1. Are prospective limb-forming tissues different from other tissues?

EXPERIMENT 1: Transplant either (A) limb bud **mesenchyme** beneath flank ectoderm, or (B) limb bud **ectoderm** atop flank mesenchyme.

RESULTS: In (A) an AER develops in the flank ectoderm and a supernumerary limb forms. But, in (B), the AER of the grafted ectoderm regresses and no ectopic limb develops.

CONCLUSION: Limb-forming mesenchyme is unique in its ability both to initiate the formation of an ectodermal AER and to provide for maintenance of the AER. This mesenchyme also specifies the shape and form of the limb, as was shown in Chapter 4 (Fig. 4.2).

QUESTION 2. What is the function of the AER?

EXPERIMENT 2 (Fig. 10.6): Extirpate either (*B*) the AER or (*C*) the non-AER ectoderm from a partially developed limb, in this case the wing of a chick embryo. An additional test of AER function is to (*D*) graft an extra AER onto an otherwise normal limb bud.

RESULTS: In the absence of an AER, limb outgrowth ceases. However, those tissues whose primordia were already formed continue to develop normally. In contrast, removal of non-AER ectoderm does not affect the continued morphogenesis of the limb.

If an extra AER is present, limb development is drastically altered, so that two distal outgrowths form. One of these is the normal one, the other results from the ability of the grafted AER to **reorganize** underlying limb mesenchyme, causing it to form a second set of distal skeletal elements. The results are comparable to the effects of splitting the limb field.

CONCLUSIONS: The AER is essential for continued proximodistal outgrowth of the limb. This ectodermal thickening can ini-

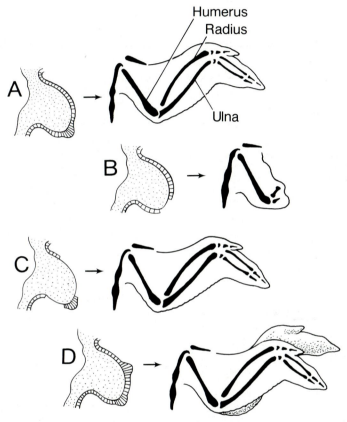

Figure 10.6. Experimental analysis of the role of the AER in avian limb development. *A,* normal limb bud and later limb skeleton. *B* shows the results of AER extirpation, *C* of non-AER ectoderm extirpation, and *D* of grafting an extra AER.

tiate reorganization of underlying limb mesenchyme to produce duplications of distal tissues.

QUESTION 3. What controls the proximodistal patterning of limb structures?

EXPERIMENT 3 (Fig. 10.7): This problem can be examined using **heterochronic** transplantations, i.e. grafting tissues which are of different ages. In the first of these experiments the distal tip of the wing, including the AER and some underlying mesenchyme, was excised from a 3-day chick embryo and transplanted in place of the same tissue on an older, 4-day, wing bud. The reciprocal, old-onto-young, transplantation is also illustrated.

RESULTS: In both cases the transplanted cap developed autonomously. The young cap developed all the structures that normally would have formed from it, even though some of the same structures were already present on the host's limb. Entire segments were always added or lost; there was never a wing with half a radius or ulna. In the old-onto-young series entire limb segments were missing.

CONCLUSIONS: The proximodistal patterning of the limb is programmed within the distal cap, which includes the AER and subjacent mesenchyme, and is independent of proximally located tissues.

Proximodistal patterning occurs only in segmental quanta. Animals may be born with partially developed limb bones, such as only the proximal part of the radius, which appears to contradict the results of these experiments. However, these congenital deficiencies are believed to be the result of a lack of sustained growth of embryonic cartilages.

QUESTION 4. How is the craniocaudal polarity of the limb established?

EXPERIMENT 4: Surgically rotate the distal limb ectoderm and mesenchyme 180° (Fig. 10.8) or, as shown in Figure 10.9, transplant a small piece of caudal mesenchyme immediately beneath the cranial surface ectoderm at either proximal or distal parts of the limb bud.

RESULTS: In the first of these two series, both a normal set of distal limb tissues and a duplicate set with reversed cranio-

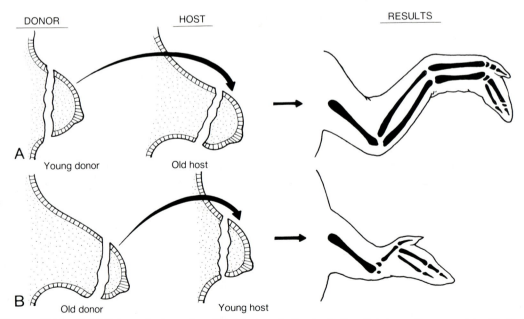

Figure 10.7. Establishment of proximodistal limb polarity. In *A*, the distal cap from an older (4-day) limb bud is removed and replaced with that of a younger (3-day) bud. *B* shows the results of the converse experiment. In the first case an entire extra antebrachial segment is added; in the second case it is missing.

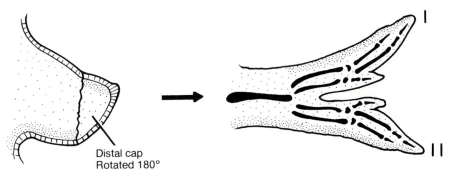

Distal cap
Rotated 180°

Figure 10.8. This experiment demonstrates the effects of rotating distal limb bud mesenchyme and ectoderm, including the AER. The original caudal mesenchyme is *darkly stippled*. Most of the rotated distal cap material forms a rotated distal limb (*I*). However, the nonrotated mesenchyme elicits the formation of a new AER, and together these form a limb having normal polarity (*II*).

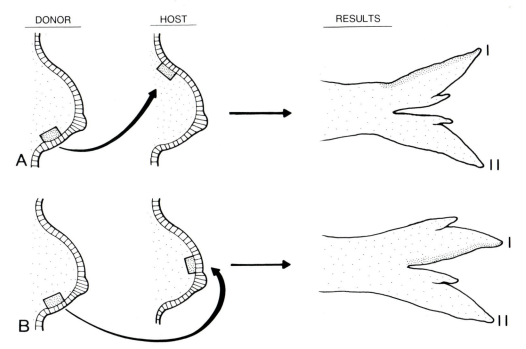

Figure 10.9. Analysis of the role of caudal mesenchyme in the establishment of craniocaudal polarity in the avian limb. Caudal mesenchyme is transplanted to a cranial or distal site. *Heavily stippled areas* indicate tissues transplanted or derived from the graft. In both cases the new limb (*I*) developed with its caudal margin closest to the implanted tissue.

caudal polarity developed. Detailed analyses of these embryos indicated that the caudally located limb outgrowth developed under the control of a new AER, which formed in response to an AER-promoting influence located in the underlying, nonrotated mesenchyme. This is not surprising, given the results of Experiment 1 that showed how prospective limb

mesenchyme can elicit the formation of an AER.

The more cranially located limb outgrowth developed from the rotated mesenchyme and original AER. Its craniocaudal polarity was reversed relative to the host, but was normal for the cap, which had been rotated 180°.

When only small pieces of caudal mesenchyme were grafted, duplicate sets of distal limb structures again formed. Usually the implanted tissue participated along with host mesenchymal cells in the formation of these duplicates. However, the polarity of the duplicate outgrowth varied depending upon the site of graft implantation. If the graft was implanted proximally, the polarity of the duplicated limb was reversed craniocaudally (Fig. 10.9*A*). When it was placed distally, the polarity of the duplicate was normal (Figure 10.9*B*). In all cases, regardless of the site of implantation, the duplicate limb developed *with its caudal margin adjacent to the site of mesenchyme implantation.*

CONCLUSIONS: Caudal limb mesenchyme can initiate a reorganization of adjacent limb mesenchyme and, subsequently, cause the formation of a new AER and development of a complete supernumerary limb. Any extra limb formed will develop with its caudal margin adjacent to the grafted caudal mesenchyme. This region of mesenchyme has been called the **zone of polarizing activity (ZPA)**.

As with most problems in morphogenesis and patterning, the molecular basis for this polarizing activity is not known. Most investigators favor the hypothesis that craniocaudal polarity is established by some biochemical agent produced by ZPA cells that diffuses throughout the limb. In fact, there are some chemicals, vitamin A for example, that can mimic the polarizing function of ZPA cells. However, our understanding of how mesenchymal cells normally interact with each other in a morphogenetic field is too fragmentary to eliminate direct cell-to-cell interactions as a basis for limb polarization.

These experiments have defined at least a few of the basic parameters by which a developing limb becomes patterned. Many of the same errors in patterning that can be experimentally created in amphibian and avian embryos occur in domestic animals, as will be discussed later in this chapter.

GROWTH AND SHAPING OF SKELETAL TISSUES

Once condensation of presumptive cartilage cells has occurred in the limb mesenchyme, the tissue can be grown in organ culture and will develop with its characteristic gross shape. For example, an explant of proximal hind limb bud mesenchyme grown in culture will form a cartilaginous rod capped by a large, eccentric head, which is a unique feature of the femur. However, the formation of the smaller processes, tuberosities, and grooves, as well as maintenance of intrinsically programmed shapes depend on the tensions exerted by muscle (tendon) and ligament attachments.

This stress-dependent reshaping continues through the life of the animal, but is most active prior to closure of the epiphyseal plate. Figure 10.10 illustrates the effects of disrupting the normal set of attachments upon the neonatal growth of the scapula. Considerations of the causes of some limb deformities and also of how to correct them using applied tensions are extremely important in treating defects in which long bones or joints are crooked. **Talipes** (club foot) in humans and **angular limb deformities** in foals are two examples.

APPENDICULAR MALFORMATIONS
Limb Reductions

Many malformations of the limbs involve loss of specific parts. These are named using the particular defect as a descriptive prefix and -melia (melos = limb) or -dactyly (dactylos = digits) as a suffix.

Amelia, (a = lack of) complete absence of a limb;

Ectromelia, partial or complete absence of a limb or its parts (e.g. carpal ectromelia, no carpal bones);

Hemimelia, absence of half of one or more segments of a limb (e.g. radial hemimelia, no radius; the distal structures, such as the medial carpals would be present but may be dislocated, as shown in Fig. 10.11);

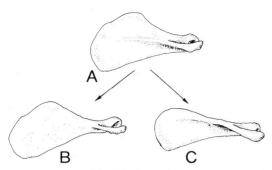

Figure 10.10. Effects of neonatal tenotomy on growth of the rat scapula. *A*, normal scapula. *B*, excision of trapezius and infraspinatus muscles results in reduction of the infraspinous fossa. *C*, excision of supraspinatus muscle results in reduction of the supraspinous fossa.

Meromelia, absence of part of a limb (e.g. crural meromelia, absence of tibia and fibula);

Micromelia, a limb that is reduced in size, smaller than normal but all its component parts are present;

Phocomelia, (phoco = seal) absence or reduction of one or more proximal limb segments, often accompanied by abnormalities of other parts of the limb;

Syndactyly, fused digits;

Brachydactyly, shortened digits; and

Ectrodactyly, absence of one or more digits.

Most of these malformations probably result from interference with the limb field or developing limb bud, similar to the results of the experimental manipulations presented earlier.

Syndactyly, the partial or complete fusion of digits, can be inherited in cattle, in which species it is commonly called **mulefoot**. The right forelimb is most frequently affected and the left hind limb is least often affected, the reasons for which are unknown.

As was discussed in Chapter 5, a range of limb reductions is frequently seen in the same litter or herd. This results from differences in **penetrance** in the case of an inherited malformation, such as occurs in the Dachshund. In these litters the least affected might be normal or have unilateral syndac-

tyly, others could show ectrodactyly or distal ectromelia, and the most severely affected would have complete ectromelia. One line of mixed-Fox Terrier dogs has been described in France in which bilateral thoracic ectromelia was inherited as a single autosomal recessive. In the case of defects resulting from teratogenic insult, a broad spectrum of anomalies can be due to differences in the exact age of each fetus at the time of exposure or to individual differences in fetal metabolism.

Phocomelia is a condition in which the proximal but not the distal parts of the limb are missing or malformed. This condition was rare in humans until the late 1950s, and was subsequently linked to the sedative Thalidomide. This drug is highly teratogenic if ingested between 28 and 50 days of gestation in man.

Limb Duplications

Polydactyly, the presence of one or more extra digits, is common in pigs and cats (Fig. 10.12). In the "double pawed" cat it is inherited as an autosomal dominant. Partial or complete duplication of one limb is called **bimelia**.

As introduced in Chapter 2, whole or partial limbs occasionally are found on ectopic sites. In these cases the malformation

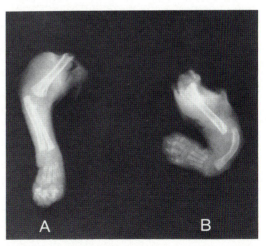

Figure 10.11. Radiograph of *A*, normal forelimb and *B*, contralateral malformed limb from a neonatal kitten with radial hemimelia.

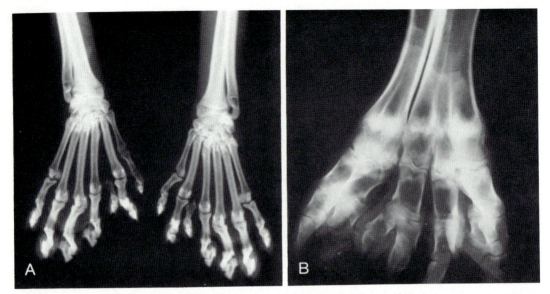

Figure 10.12.   Radiographs showing polydactyly in *A*, a cat and *B*, a calf.

is named according to the location of the supernumerary appendage. **Notomelia** (notos = back) refers to a limb growing from the back of an animal. **Perineomelia**, in which the ectopic limb projects from the perineum, has been found in dogs and cattle (Fig. 10.13). These cases result from the formation of a limb field in the atypical site, and it is common to find all or parts of the pelvis also present. The ectopic limbs are usually devoid of muscle tissues and the joints are fused. Whether this is due to an early absence of myotome-derived cells or a secondary muscle degeneration caused by a lack of innervation is not known.

Limb and Joint Deformities

ARTHROGRYPOSIS

Arthrogryposis means crooked limb (arthro = joint; gryposis = crooked). It is a deformity of the limb characterized by curvature, or retention of a joint in a flexed or extended position. The pathogenesis of this congenital disease is variable. It can result from a primary skeletal-joint malformation, from a muscle dysplasia that produces abnormal tensions on joints and secondarily causes a deformity, or from a disease or lesion of the nervous system that produces denervation, lack of muscle contraction and

secondary abnormal joint formation. Sustained inequalities in muscle tension or immobility in utero will cause modification of joint capsules, ligaments and articular surfaces resulting in permanent fixation of a joint (**ankylosis**). All these systems must be thoroughly examined in attempting to understand the pathogenesis of any one case. The causes are variable and include inheritance, in utero intoxications, in utero infections of the embryo, and manganese deficiencies.

"**Crooked-calf**" **disease** is a form of arthrogryposis that occurs in range cattle raised in the western United States and Alaska, where various species of the **lupine** plant grow in pastures. The malformation includes arthrogryposis of the thoracic limbs and occasionally pelvic limbs, scoliosis, torticollis, and sometimes cleft palate. The elbows are usually fixed in flexion and cannot be extended even after cutting the flexor tendons. A malarticulation of the humerus and ulna is assumed to be the primary defect, since no neural or muscle tissue lesions are seen. The disease can be reproduced by feeding pregnant cows specific lupine species between 40 and 70 days of gestation, but the actual teratogenic agent in the plant has yet to be isolated (see Table 5.4).

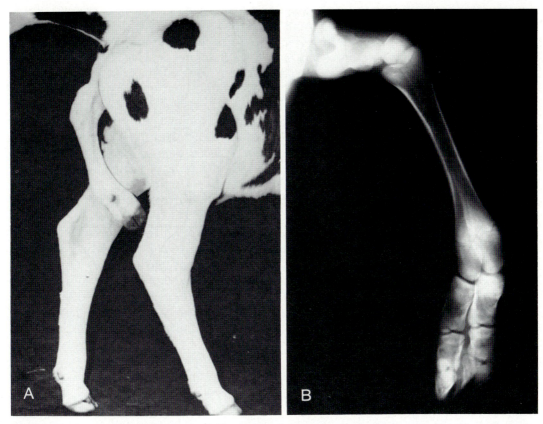

Figure 10.13. Perineomelia in a calf. The distal skeletal structures look normal in this radiograph, but the tarsus is nodular and the tibia shortened. The other proximal elements were reduced to nodules, and there were components of an ectopic pelvis deep to the normal ischium. This animal also had atresia ani, absence of the left kidney, and a patent urachus.

Arthrogryposis can result from in utero Akabane virus infection, which causes denervation of limb muscles and, subsequently, reduced movement of the developing joints. As discussed in Chapter 6, the limb-innervating ventral gray column is one site of destruction by this virus in the bovine fetus. Also, an autosomal recessive gene has been identified which causes arthrogryposis in Charolais calves. These animals have scoliosis and kyphosis, and 40% have cleft palate.

Although much less common, arthrogryposis is also found in foals and is referred to as the **contracted foal syndrome**. Distal limb segments are preferentially effected, with the metacarpo- and metatarsophalangeal joints twisted and usually flexed. Mares delivering these foals frequently suffer dystocia. The range of possible causes is similar in horses and cattle; inheritance, influenza virus and ingestion of locoweed have all been implicated in this equine limb deformity.

An hereditary arthrogryposis occurs in young Swedish Lapland dogs. This autosomal recessive disease manifests its clinical signs at 5–7 weeks of age. These consist of a rapidly progressive weakness and muscle atrophy followed by contractures causing fixation of joints in different degrees of flexion and extension. The inherited abnormality is an **abiotrophy** of neurons in the central nervous system. The inability of neuronal cell bodies to survive is thought to be due to the lack of (a-) some vital substance (-bios-) in the neuron necessary for its growth (-trophy). The rapid, progressive degeneration of somatic efferent neurons in the ventral gray column of the spinal cord accounts for the denervation of skeletal muscle and its subsequent atrophy. When this occurs in the young growing puppy, contractures of muscles produce limb deformity.

HIP DYSPLASIA

Hip Dysplasia is an inherited condition usually associated with large, muscular breeds of dogs. It is characterized by abnormal maturation of the hip joint. Onset of signs may occur at 3–5 months or not until the dog is fully grown. Many young dogs show no evidence of the abnormality, and only 75% of dogs that develop hip dysplasia are identifiable radiographically at 1 year of age; 95% can be identified by 2 years of age.

Initial signs include stiffness and pain upon movement of one or both hind limbs, which may progress to more severe lameness. Anatomic features include a shallow acetabulum and flattened, sometimes subluxated femoral head. The exact pathophysiology is still debated. Some investigators believe the skeletal defects are secondary to a loosening of the joint capsule, which may be due to a disparity in growth rates between

skeletal tissues (rapid) and associated muscles (slower). Others question this hypothesis, since the condition occasionally occurs in medium and smaller sized dogs, such as Cocker Spaniels and Corgis. In addition it is possible to aggravate or ameliorate the degree of dysplasia in many cases by modifying diet, exercise, and hormone levels in pups during the postweaning period of rapid growth. These data suggest that hip dysplasia is a multifactorial condition.

Whatever the mechanisms, there is no doubt that hip dysplasia has a heritable component and that transmission is polygenic. As such it is more difficult to eliminate from a breed than would be a single gene-based condition. The breeding of two unaffected dogs is no guarantee that all offspring will be normal. However, by *not* breeding moderately to severely affected animals it is possible to significantly reduce the incidence (Fig. 10.14). For example, by selective breeding it has been possible in one study to reduce the incidence of hip dysplasia in German Shepherds from 44.3 to 12.4% over a 7-yr period, with less than half of the affected progeny showing moderate to severe symptoms.

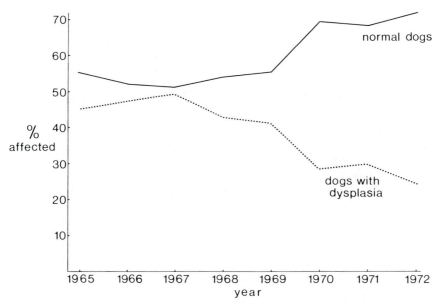

Figure 10.14. Hip dysplasia in young German Shepherd dogs in Switzerland during an 8-year campaign in which affected animals were not bred. (After Freudiger et al., 1973, from Hutt FB: *Genetics for Dog Breeders*. San Francisco, WH Freeman, 1979.)

Hip dysplasia has been reported in most large breeds of dogs but is most frequently associated with the following: Bull Mastiff, English Springer Spaniel, German Shepherd, Gordon Setter, Newfoundland, Norwegian Elkhound, Old English Sheepdog, Retrievers (Chesapeake Bay and Golden), and Saint Bernard.

Elbow dysplasia is much less common and is also a polygenic inherited malformation found in the German Shepherd breed, and occasionally in Pekingese and other breeds. In some dogs it results from a failure of the anconeal process to ossify as part of the ulna. In others with luxations the supporting ligaments may be abnormal. Osteochondrosis may also be involved in the pathogenesis. These dogs show thoracic limb lameness beginning usually at 4–6 months. Unlike hip dysplasia, this condition in German Sheperds responds well to surgical removal of the affected anconeal process.

Bibliography

MORPHOGENETIC FIELDS AND MECHANISMS OF LIMB DEVELOPMENT

Bergsma D, Lenz W: Morphogenesis and malformation of the limb. In *Birth Defects Original Article Series*, New York, AR Liss, 1977, vol 13.

Bryant SV, Holder N: Principles and problems of pattern formation in animals. *Am Zool* 22:1–220, 1982.

Cairns J: The function of the ectodermal apical ridge and distinctive characteristics of adjacent mesoderm in the avian wing bud. *J Embryol Exp Morph* 34:155–168, 1975.

Ede DA: Cell interactions in vertebrate limb development. In Poste G, Nicholson G (eds): *The Cell Surface in Animal Embryogenesis and Development*. Amsterdam, North-Holland Elsevier, 1976, pp 495–543.

Ede DA, Hinchliff JR, Balls M: *Vertebrate Limb and Somite Morphogenesis*. Cambridge, Cambridge University Press, 1977.

Fallon JF, Caplan AI (eds): *Limb Development and Regeneration. Part A. Cell Interactions, Malformations and Regeneration. Progress in Clinical Biological Research*, New York, AR Liss, 1982, vol 110A.

Harrison RG: *Organization and Development of the Embryo.* New Haven, CT, Yale University Press, 1969.

Iten LE, Murphy DJ: Pattern regulation in the embryonic chick limb: supernumerary limb formation with anterior (non-ZPA) limb bud tissues. *Dev Biol* 75:373–385, 1980.

Kelley RO, Goetinck PF, MacCabe JA (eds): *Limb Development and Regeneration. Part B. Extracellular Matrix; Cartilage, Bone and Muscle Development. Progress in Clinical Biological Research*, New York, AR Liss, 1982, vol 110B.

Summerbill D: Interaction between proximodistal and anterioposterior positional coordinates during chick limb development. *J Embryol Exp Morphol* 36:227–237, 1976.

Stocum DL, Fallon JF: Control of pattern formation in urodele limb ontogeny: a review and a hypothesis. *J Embryol Exp Morphol* 69:7–36, 1982.

Zwilling E: Genetic mechanism in limb development. *Cold Spring Harbor Symp Quant Biol* 21:349–354, 1956.

Zwilling E: Effects of contact between mutant (wingless) limb buds and those of genetically normal chick embryos: confirmation of a hypothesis. *Dev Biol* 39:37–48, 1974.

LIMB REDUCTIONS AND DUPLICATIONS

Arnbjerg J: Congenital partial hemimelia tibia in a kitten. *Zbl Vet Med* 26:73–77, 1979.

Behrens E, et al: Polydactylism in a foal. *JAVMA* 174:266–268, 1979.

Dallman MJ, Brown RE: Syndactyly in the dog. *Canine Pract* 1:21–24, 1980.

Gruneberg H, Huston K: The development of bovine syndactylism. *J Embryol Exp Morph* 19:251–259, 1965.

Johnson JL, Leipold HW, Snider GW, Baker RD: Progeny testing for bovine syndactyly. *JAVMA* 176:549–550, 1980.

Johnson JL, Leipold HW, Guffy MM, Dennis SM, Schalles RR, Mueller RE: Characterization of bovine polydactyly. *Bovine Pract* 3:7–14, 1982.

Leipold HW, Dennis SM, Huston K: Syndactyly in cattle. *Vet Bull* 43:39–403, 1973.

O'Rahilly R: Morphological patterns in limb deficiencies and duplications. *Am J Anat* 89:135–193, 1951.

Prentiss CW: Polydactylism in man and the domestic animals, with special reference to digital variations in swine. *Bull Mus Comp Zool Harvard Univ* 15:245–314, 1903.

ARTHROGRYPOSIS

Crowe MW, Pike HT: Congenital arthrogryposis associated with ingestion of tobacco stalks by pregnant sows. *JAVMA* 182:453–455, 1973.

Finocchio EJ: A case of contracted foal syndrome. *Vet Med Small Anim Clin* 682:1254–1255, 1973.

Greene HJ, Leipold HW, Huston K, Guffy MM: Bovine congenital defects: arthrogryposis and associated defects in calves. *Am J Vet Res* 34:87–891, 1973.

Leipold HW, Cates WF, Radostits OM, Howell WE: Arthrogryposis and associated deficits in newborn calves. *Am J Vet Res* 31:1367–1374, 1970.

McIlwraith CW: Limb deformities in foals associated with ingestion of locoweed by mares. *JAVMA* 181:255–258, 1982.

Nawrot PS, Howell WE, Leipold HW: Arthrogryposis: an inherited defect in newborn calves. *Aust Vet J* 56:359–364, 1980.

Rooney JR: Contracted foals. *Cornell Vet* 56:172–187, 1966.

Shupe JL, Binns W: Lupine, a cause of crooked calf disease. *JAVMA* 151:198–203, 1967.

Shupe JL, James LF, Binns W: Observations on crooked calf disease. *JAVMA* 151:191–197, 1967.

Swinyard CA: Concepts of multiple congenital contractures (arthrogryposis) in man and animals. *Teratology* 25:247–258, 1982.

Whittem JH: Congenital abnormalities in calves: arthrogryposis and hydranencephaly. *J Pathol Bacteriol* 73:375–387, 1957.

DYSPLASIAS AND ANGULAR LIMB DEFORMITIES

Allhands RV, Kallfelz FA, Lust G: Radionuclide joint imaging: an ancillary technique in the diagnosis of canine hip dysplasia. *Am J Vet Res* 41:230–233, 1980.

Auck JA, Martens RJ, Morris EL: Angular limb deformities in foals. Part I. Congenital factors. *Compend Cont Ed* 4:5330–5338, 1982.

Auck JA, Martens RJ, Morris EL: Angular limb deformities in foals. Part II. Developmental factors. *Compend Cont Ed* 5:527–535, 1982.

Cawley AJ, Archibald J: Ununited anconeal process of the dog. *JAVMA* 134:454–458, 1959.

Corley EA, Sutherland TM, Carlson WD: Genetic aspects of canine elbow dysplasia. *JAVMA* 153:543–547, 1968.

Fisher TM: The inheritance of canine hip dysplasia. *Mod Vet Pract* 60:897–900, 1979.

Hayes HM, Jr, Wilson GP, Burt JK: Feline hip dysplasia. *J Am Anim Hosp Assoc* 14:447–448, 1979.

Hedhammar A, et al: Canine hip dysplasia: study of heritability in 401 litters of German Shepherd dogs. *JAVMA* 174:1012–1016, 1979.

Henricson B, Norberg I, Olsson S-E: On the etiology and pathogenesis of hip dysplasia: a comparative review. *J Small Anim Pract* 7:673–688, 1966.

Herron MR: Ununited anconeal process in the dog. *Vet Clin North Am* 1:417–428, 1971.

Hutt FB: Genetics for Dog Breeders. San Francisco, WH Freeman, 1979.

Hutt FB, Rasmusen BA: *Animal Genetics*, ed 2. New York, Wiley, 1982.

Ihemelandu EC, Cardinet GH, III, Guffy MM, Wallace LJ: Canine hip dysplasia: differences in pectineal muscles of healthy and dysplastic German Shepherd dogs when two months old. *Am J Vet Res* 44:411–417, 1983.

Kene ROC, Lee R, Bennett D: The radiological features of congenital elbow luxation subluxation in the dog. *J Small Anim Pract* 23:621–631, 1982.

Lust G, Beilman WT, Rendano VT: A relationship between degree of laxity and synovial fluid volume in coxofemoral joints of dogs predisposed for hip dysplasia. *Am J Vet Res* 41:55–60, 1980.

McLaughlin BG: Carpal bone lesions associated with angular limb deformities in foals. *JAVMA* 178:224–230, 1981.

Milton JL, et al: Congenital elbow luxation in the dog. *JAVMA* 175:572–582, 1969.

Olsson S-E: Canine hip dysplasia. In Kirk RW (ed): *Current Veterinary Therapy VII Small Animal Practice.* Philadelphia, Saunders, 1980.

Pharr JW: Radiographic findings in foals with angular limb deformities. *JAVMA* 179:812–817, 1981.

Riser WH, Cohen D, Lindquist S, Mansson J, Chen S: Influence of early rapid growth and weight gain on hip dysplasia in the German Shepherd dog. *JAVMA* 145:661–668, 1964.

Riser WH, Shirer JF: Correlation between canine hip dysplasia and pelvic muscle mass: a study of 95 dogs. *Am J Vet Res* 28:769–777, 1967.

Riser WH: Canine hip dysplasia: cause and control. *JAVMA* 164:360–362, 1974.

Van Sickle DC: The relationship of ossification to canine elbow dysplasia. *Anim Hosp* 2:24–31, 1966.

CHAPTER 11

Cardiovascular System I: Blood and Arteries

HEMATOPOIESIS

Hematopoiesis is the process of blood tissue formation, of which **erythropoiesis**, red blood cell formation, is one component. These processes continue throughout the life of the animal, with new blood cells continually being produced from **stem cells**.

Developmentally, the first blood cells are formed in **blood islands** (Fig. 11.1), which are aggregates of splanchnic mesoderm on the surface of the yolk sac and the allantois.

The peripheral mesenchymal cells of blood islands join together to form vesicles, the lining of which will become **vascular endothelium**. These vesicles coalesce to form vascular channels that subsequently form the vitelline and allantoic vessels.

The central cells of blood islands are called **hemocytoblasts** and will differentiate into blood cells in the early embryo. When the liver subsequently develops, it assumes the function of blood cell production; other tissues, including the mesonephros and the spleen, act as minor hematopoietic sites. During the last third of fetal development, hematopoiesis occurs primarily in bone marrow.

Until recently the prevailing hypothesis concerning the formation of hematopoietic cells in the liver has been that they are derived from stem cells originating in yolk sac mesoderm. This has been proven incorrect in birds by experiments in which the entire embryo-producing region of the neu-

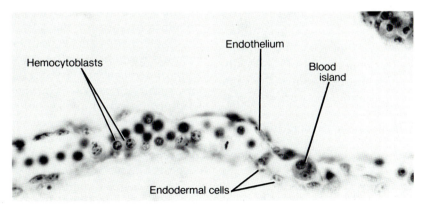

Figure 11.1. Blood islands and extraembryonic blood vessels filled with hemocytoblasts (from a 4-mm feline embryo).

rula-stage blastodisk was excised from a chick embryo and replaced with homologous tissue cut from a quail embryo. As expected, all the early blood cells were of host (chick) origin, having migrated into the grafted embryo from blood islands. However, within a few days this population was replaced with circulating quail blood cells that arose independently in the grafted tissue. Similarly, later forming lymphoid cells are formed intraembryonically, within or near to the organs they will populate (e.g. thymus, bursa).

Correlated with these shifts in sites of red blood cell production are changes in the peptide subunits which, along with heme, form the **hemoglobin** molecule. The pattern of change is similar in all higher vertebrates, although the names given to specific peptides vary according to species. Table 11.1 describes the situation in the mouse.

ANGIOGENESIS

The process of blood vessel formation is **angiogenesis**. As already described, angiogenesis begins extraembryonically during or shortly after gastrulation. At the same time **angiogenic cords** appear within the lateral mesenchyme of the embryo. These solid strands of splanchnic mesodermal cells are first visible lateral to the cardiogenic mesoderm. The cords elongate, grow into the head mesenchyme, and then become patent. They form the aortic arches and dorsal aortae. It is not known whether all other arteries are derived from extensions of these cords, nor has the origin of veins been established.

The mechanisms that control the timing of outgrowth and patterning of embryonic angiogenic cords are not known. In some adult tissues and tumors there are angiogenesis-promoting factors that stimulate the growth of blood vessels. However, comparable factors have not been found in young embryos.

AORTIC ARCH TRANSFORMATION

The early embryonic circulatory system, outlined in Chapter 1, consists of a single tubular heart continuous cranially with paired ventral aortae and aortic arches that empty into dorsal aortae. The two dorsal aortae fuse caudal to the heart but separate again in the abdomen of young embryos. A pair of **vitelline arteries** to the yolk sac and, later, a pair of **umbilical arteries** to the allantois branch from the dorsal aortae at the midthoracic and caudal lumbar levels.

There are five pairs of aortic arches connecting the ventral to the dorsal aortae in higher vertebrates. Each aortic arch passes through the mesenchyme of a visceral arch cranial to the corresponding pharyngeal pouch (Fig. 11.2; see also Figs. 1.5 and 1.6*D*). Primitive vertebrates have six (or more), but the 5th aortic arch is absent in birds and mammals.

All five pairs are never present at the same time in higher vertebrate embryos. This is because aortic arches 1 and 2 degenerate during the formation of the more caudal arches. Originally, there are two separate ventral aortae. However, as aortic arches 3, 4 and 6 develop, the ventral aortae fuse to form a single ventral aortic root or **aortic sac**. This serves as a common chamber delivering blood to aortic arches.

Transformation of the aortic arches includes all those changes that result in the eventual formation of the carotid, pulmonary, and subclavian arteries, and the thoracic part of the aorta, as outlined in Figure I.1 of the Introduction. The major processes operating during these events are **degeneration** of certain vessels and **differential growth** of portions of others. Most of these changes occur during weeks 3 and 4 of development in dogs, weeks 3–7 in horses, and weeks 4–7 in man. At this period the embryo grows from a 2- to 3-mm long neurula to an embryo of approximately 10 mm. These arterial

Table 11.1. Hemoglobin development in the mouse

Hemoglobin type	Composition	Source
Embryonic	$x_2 y_2$	Yolk sac
Fetal$_I$	$a_2 x_2$	(Yolk sac), liver
Fetal$_{II}$	$a_2 Y_2$	(Yolk sac), liver
Adult	$a_2 b_2$	Bone marrow

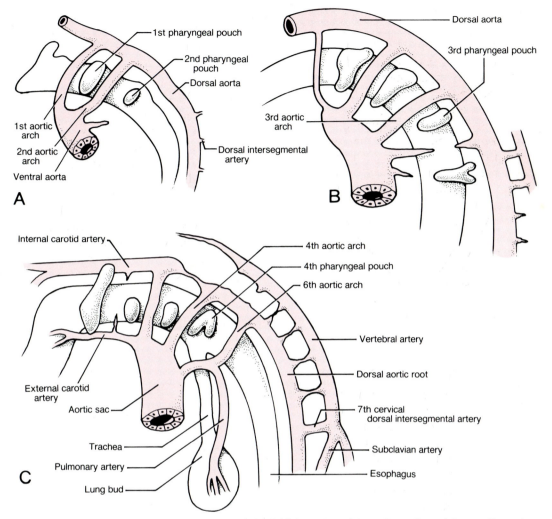

Figure 11.2. Schematic left lateral view of the initial stages of transformation of the aortic arches and formation of the vertebral artery.

changes occur simultaneous with the separation of pulmonary and systemic channels and the partitioning of the heart (see Table 12.1).

The sequence of events during transformation of the aortic arches in mammalian embryos includes the following:

1. Aortic arches 1 and 2 degenerate following a relatively short (3–5 days) period of function, soon after the formation of arches 3 and 4 (Fig. 11.2 *A* and *B*). However, the rostral parts of the dorsal aortae, which were associated with arches 1 and 2, are retained and establish the **internal carotid arteries**.

2. The segment of each dorsal aorta located between the 3rd and 4th aortic arch degenerates (Fig. 11.2*C*). This leaves the 3rd aortic arches as the major arterial channels from the heart to the head, and the 4th aortic arches as the principal channels to the trunk. The paired dorsal aortae extending caudally from the 4th arches to the single, median aorta are called the **dorsal aortic roots** (Fig. 11.3*A*).

As the facial tissues develop, a vessel arises from the proximal (ventral) part of each 3rd arch to deliver blood to them (Fig. 11.2*C*). Indications are that in domestic animals the proximal part of this vessel, which is the

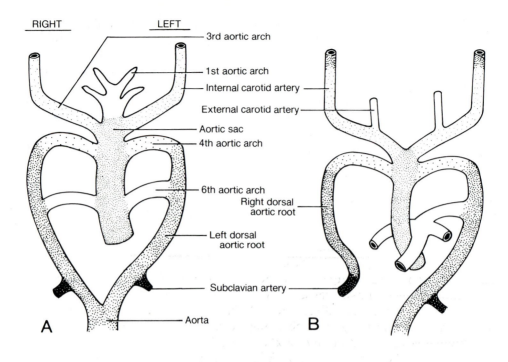

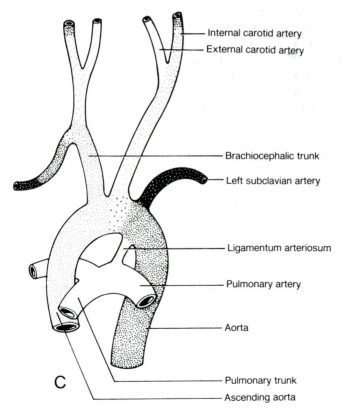

Figure 11.3. *A*, Schematic ventral view showing the later stages of aortic arch transformation. The asymmetric changes in the dorsal aortic roots and subclavian arteries are evident in *B* and *C*.

external carotid artery, is formed from remnants of the cranial ventral aorta and part of the second aortic arch.

3. Each **pulmonary artery** arises as a branch from the 6th aortic arch (Fig. 11.2C). Later, the distal (dorsal) part of the RIGHT 6th aortic arch degenerates between the pulmonary artery and the right dorsal aortic root. On the left the homologous segment persists and becomes the **ductus arteriosus** (refer to Fig. I.1).

4. A series of **cervical dorsal intersegmental arteries** branch from both dorsal aortic roots. Initially these small segmental arteries grow dorsally between the somites (refer to Figs. 1.5 and 8.2). Later, each forms a dorsal, intersomitic branch supplying epaxial tissues and a ventral branch to hypaxial structures. Anastomoses form between adjacent dorsal branches in the cervical region, establishing a longitudinal vessel called the **vertebral artery** on each side of the embryo (Fig. 11.2C). All but the most caudal of the cervical intersegmental arteries, usually the 7th, then degenerate. On both sides of the embryo this remaining intersegmental artery forms a ventral branch that enters the base of the thoracic limb bud. This will become the distal part of the **subclavian artery** (Table 11.2).

5. The **right** and **left subclavian arteries** initially form symmetrically. However, asymmetries in patterns of vascular degeneration and growth result in their assuming quite different appearances, as shown in Figures 11.3 and 11.4. The RIGHT dorsal aortic root degenerates CAUDAL to the origin

of the last dorsal cervical intersegmental artery (the 7th). As a result there is no direct connection between the right aortic arch complex and the dorsal aorta serving the trunk region. The vessel on the right side consisting of the right 4th aortic arch, the remaining part of the right dorsal aortic root, the right caudal dorsal cervical intersegmental artery and its ventral branch is the **right subclavian artery**.

The **left subclavian artery** is initially formed similarly, as a branch of the left caudal dorsal cervical intersegmental artery. However, on the left side the entire dorsal aortic root persists as the thoracic segment of the definitive **aorta**.

Shortly after the arterial branches to the forelimb buds are established, the body of the embryo undergoes a rapid elongation, causing the heart to be displaced from the neck region into the thorax. During this elongation the distance between the first rib and the caudal part of the dorsal aortic roots increases greatly.

The base of the left subclavian artery is attached to the left dorsal aortic root, caudally, and on its way to the forelimb it passes cranially around the 1st rib. Rather than become stretched during elongation of the neck and thorax, there is a cranial shift in the site at which this artery branches from the left dorsal aortic root, as shown in Figures 11.3 and 11.4. The shift is greatest in the horse and ruminants (Fig. 11.5), in which the left subclavian shifts cranially onto the brachiocephalic trunk.

The proximal part of the **right subclavian**

Table 11.2.
Transformation of the aortic arches

Adult artery	Embryonic origins
Common carotid artery	The proximal (ventral) part of the 3rd arch
External carotid artery	A branch off the 3rd arch to facial tissues
Internal carotid artery	The 3rd arch distal to the external carotid artery and the cranial dorsal aorta
Pulmonary artery	Proximal 6th aortic arch and branch to lung tissue
Ductus arteriosus	Distal left 6th aortic arch
Vertebral artery	7th dorsal cervical intersegmental and longitudinal anastomoses between dorsal cervical intersegmental arteries
Subclavian	4th aortic arch, dorsal aortic root (right side only) and ventral branch of the caudal dorsal cervical intersegmental artery

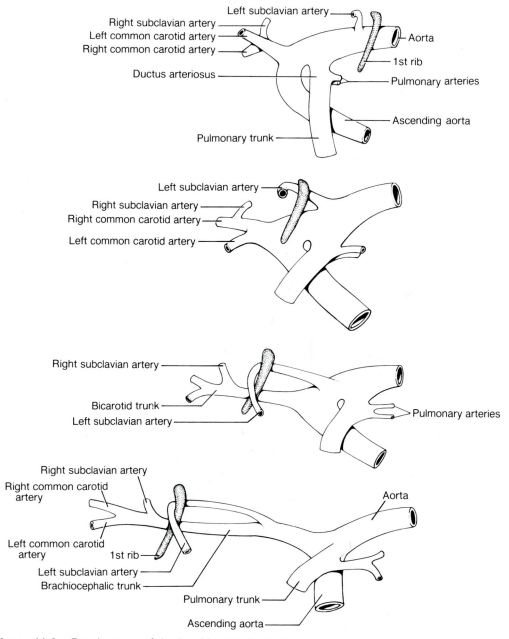

Figure 11.4. Development of the brachiocephalic trunk and subclavian arteries in the horse. Note especially the changes in the position of the origin of the left subclavian relative to that of the 1st rib. These shifts occur during the 8th week of equine gestation (16- to 20-mm crown-rump length). (After Vitums, 1969.)

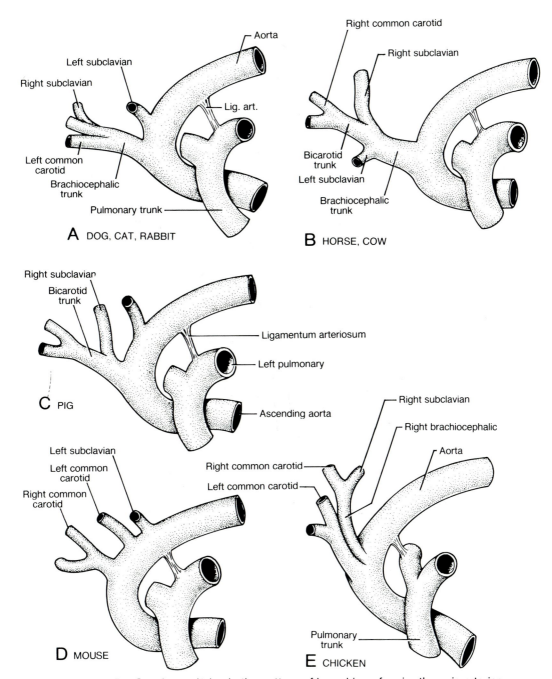

Figure 11.5. Species variation in the pattern of branching of major thoracic arteries.

artery, which was formerly the right 4th aortic arch, also shifts cranially (Fig. 11.3). It usually becomes a branch of the brachiocephalic trunk.

6. The **brachiocephalic trunk** develops from the remodeling of the aortic sac and the proximal part of the left and right 3rd and 4th aortic arches. This transformation results in it being the first extracardiac branch off of the aorta. From it arise the **common carotid** and **right subclavian arteries**. In the horse, cow and pig the common carotids fuse, forming a **bicarotid trunk** (Fig. 11.5). Deviations from the typical pattern of great vessel branching can also occur among members of the same species, especially in the smaller domestic and laboratory animals (Fig. 11.6). These usually are not associated with clinical signs.

Transformation of the aortic arches occurs simultaneously with the partitioning of the heart into its four chambers, which allows for separate pulmonary and systemic

circulation. Critical to this separation is the formation of a partition, the **aorticopulmonary septum**, in the aortic sac between the origin of the 4th and 6th arches. Later, this partition fuses with a septum that bisects the truncus arteriosus (see Fig. 12.9), and together these segregate pulmonary from systemic cardiac outflow channels.

Postnatally, blood leaving the right side of the heart passes through the proximal part of the 6th aortic arches on its way to the lungs, where gas exchange occurs. In contrast, blood entering these arches in the fetus is already oxygen-rich, having come from the placenta to the right side of the heart. While some fetal blood does flow to the lungs, most passes directly into the left dorsal aortic root via the **ductus arteriosus**, which is the distal part of the left 6th aortic arch. Following the translocation of the left subclavian artery, the ductus arteriosus enters the aorta caudal to both the brachiocephalic trunk and the left subclavian artery. In some

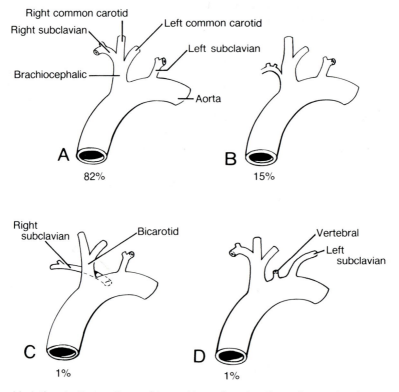

Figure 11.6. Variation in the pattern of branching of major thoracic arteries in one species, the rabbit. (After Alberch, 1980.)

species, notably cattle, the ductus arteriosus is larger than the proximal segment of the aorta; this narrowed segment of the aorta between the ductus and the brachiocephalic trunk is called the aortic isthmus. During the 1st week after birth, the ductus arteriosus closes. However, a fibrous remnant, the **ligamentum arteriosum** persists.

The relation between the 6th aortic arches and the recurrent laryngeal nerves, which are branches of the vagus nerve that innervate the laryngeal muscles, was described in the Introduction. As the neck and thorax elongate, these nerves are pulled caudally by the shifting 6th aortic arches. The left recurrent laryngeal nerve remains caught behind the ductus arteriosus. However, after the distal part of the right 6th aortic arch atrophies, the right recurrent laryngeal nerve slips forward until it reaches the right 4th aortic arch, which has become the proximal part of the right subclavian artery. In adult horses the long, circuitous pathways of these nerves are thought to be important in the pathogenesis of a disease called **roaring**, in which the laryngeal muscles on the left side are paralyzed.

BRANCHES OF THE DORSAL AORTA

Dorsal, lateral, and ventral branches arise from the aorta (Fig. 11.7). The dorsal branches are segmentally arranged in pairs between embryonic somites. The lateral branches are paired but irregularly segmen-

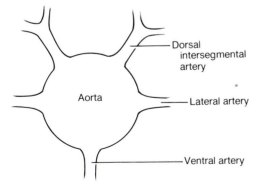

Figure 11.7. Schematic transverse section of the aorta showing all possible embryonic branches. Ventral branches may be initially paired, but only one, usually the right, persists.

tal. The ventral branches occur singly and are irregularly segmented.

Dorsal Intersegmental Arteries

These vessels arise bilaterally between the somites along the full length of the aorta and its roots, and supply many of the derivatives of somitic mesoderm. A dorsal branch supplies the neural tube and epaxial tissues (Fig. 8.2), while a ventral branch supplies hypaxial tissues.

The occipital dorsal intersegmental arteries regress soon after their formation. Most of the cervical dorsal intersegmental arteries are similarly transient, except for the most caudal that is retained as part of the subclavian and vertebral arteries. Branches of the thoracic dorsal intersegmental arteries form the bilateral **intercostal arteries**, and the abdominal dorsal intersegmental arteries form the paired **lumbar arteries**. Derivatives of the 7th lumbar dorsal intersegmental artery that grows into the pelvic limb bud will be discussed in the section on Ventral Aortic Branches, below.

Lateral Aortic Branches

For the most part these paired, irregularly segmented branches supply the derivatives of the intermediate mesoderm including the adrenal gland and the urogenital system. The definitive vessels formed from these lateral branches are the paired phrenicoabdominal, renal, ovarian or testicular, and the deep circumflex iliac arteries. Multiple lateral branches that supply the mesonephros in the fetus atrophy as the mesonephros degenerates.

Ventral Aortic Branches

These large, irregularly segmented arteries grow and branch throughout the dorsal mesentery to supply the splanchnic mesodermal and endodermal tissues of the thoracic and abdominal cavities. Although initially paired, the left ventral branches usually degenerate early in development. The **vitelline arteries** are embryonic ventral branches that supply the yolk sac. Normally only the right persists, forming the **cranial mesenteric ar-**

tery. The other permanent ventral branches include the **bronchoesophageal, celiac** and **caudal mesenteric arteries**.

The **umbilical arteries** initially arise as several pairs of ventral branches from the caudal dorsal aortae to supply the allantois. In the embryo and fetus these arteries course cranioventrally along the urachus, which is the intraembryonic stalk of the allantois, and through the umbilicus to supply the mesoderm of the chorioallantois. The multiple roots of the umbilical arteries degenerate, and a large anastomosis forms linking each of these large vessels with a 7th lumbar dorsal intersegmental artery (Fig. 11.8).

The umbilical arteries also send branches into the nearby pelvic limb buds. After the **external iliac arteries** develop, the appendicular branches of the umbilicals partially degenerate. The distal parts of these vessels are retained and incorporated into the definitive vasculature (popliteal and tibial arteries) of the hind limb. The **internal iliac arteries** also arise as branches of the umbilical arteries. As illustrated in Figure 11.9, the definitive branching patterns of these pelvic arteries

are formed by fusion of the paired dorsal aortae and proximal umbilical arteries.

At birth the umbilical arteries collapse distally from contraction of the muscles in their wall. The segment located between the bladder and the umbilicus in the median ligament of the bladder completely degenerates, but a remnant does persist between the internal iliac artery and the bladder. Coursing through the edge of the lateral ligaments of the bladder, these vessel remnants and their mesenteries form the **round ligaments of the bladder**. In some individuals part of the umbilical arteries remain patent and supply blood to the apex of the bladder by small branches, the **cranial vesical arteries**. The proximal part of the original umbilical arteries is retained as the common and proximal internal iliac arteries.

AORTIC ARCH MALFORMATIONS
Patent Ductus Arteriosus (PDA)

Closure of the ductus arteriosus (Figs. 11.10 and 11.11) must occur at birth so that

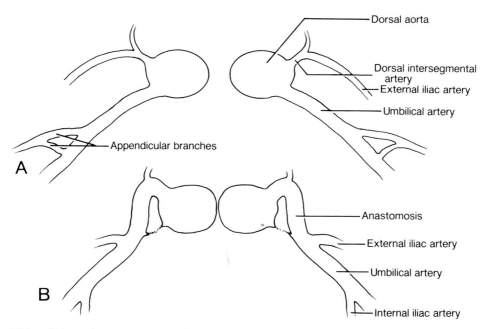

Figure 11.8. Schematic transverse sections through the aortae at the lumbar region showing how the umbilical arteries, which are initially ventral branches, anastomose with lumbar dorsal intersegmental arteries. The early appendicular branches of the umbilical are transient, and are largely replaced by the external iliac arteries.

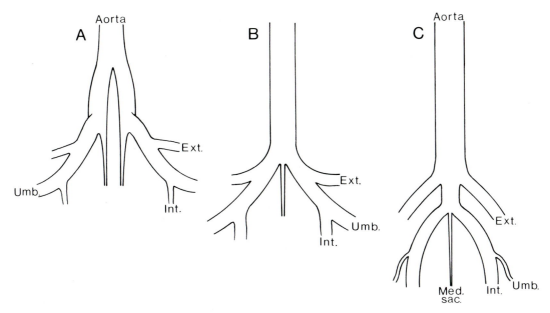

Figure 11.9. Schematic dorsal views showing the progressive fusion of the caudal dorsal aortae and shift in branching sites of the external iliac arteries.

the lungs will receive an adequate flow of unoxygenated blood from the pulmonary trunk. This closure involves functional and anatomical phases. The wall of the ductus arteriosus, unlike the aorta, has a large amount of smooth muscle that contracts when exposed to increased levels of oxygen in the blood, as occurs at birth upon the initiation of respiration. This contraction and functional closure of the ductus occur within a few hours or days of birth. Published data give variable times depending on the species studied and the method of analysis. Beginning a week after birth the lumen of the ductus is slowly obliterated by proliferation of connective tissue. This completes the conversion of the ductus into the ligamentum arteriosum.

The mechanisms of closure are not fully known. If the newborn is **hypoxic**, i.e. deprived of oxygen, closure is delayed. Also, administration of prostaglandin E maintains patency. This prostaglandin has been used in human neonates born with certain heart malformations, in order to retain sufficient mixing of oxygenated with venous blood until corrective surgery can be performed. Conversely, antagonists of prostaglandin ac-

tion, including aspirin and indomethacin, have been used to facilitate or augment closure of the ductus arteriosus.

Simultaneous with this closure there occur a number of important changes in blood pressure and flow as the neonate adapts to its new environment. These also affect the closure of the ductus and the direction of flow should it remain patent. In the fetus the right side of the heart receives a large flow of umbilical blood via the caudal vena cava and is pumping part of this blood throughout the abdominal and caudal circulation via the ductus arteriosus and aorta. The pressure on the right side of the heart (right ventricle + pulmonary trunk) is similar to or slightly greater than that of the left side (left ventricle + aorta). There is a relatively high resistance to blood flow through the developing lungs because vessels forming the pulmonary vascular bed do not expand until after birth. Thus the blood flows through the ductus **from right to left** (pulmonary trunk to aorta) in the fetus.

At birth, with the onset of respiration, there is a sudden decrease in pulmonary vascular resistance resulting from the expansion of the lungs and concommitant vaso-

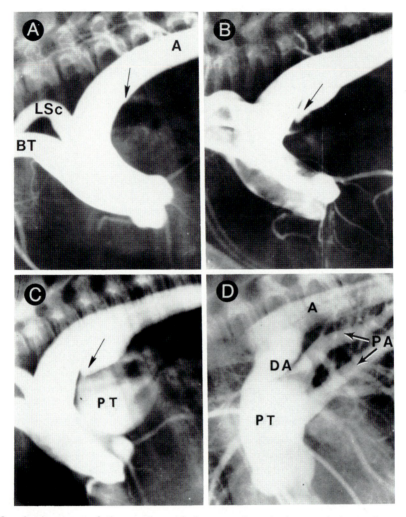

Figure 11.10. Angiograms of the aortic arch in normal and abnormal dogs. *A*, normal aortic angiogram, with contrast material filling the brachiocephalic trunk (*BT*) and left subclavian artery (*LSc*) as well as the aorta (*A*). The site of ductal closure is evident as a small indentation in the ventral aortic wall (*arrow*). *B*, Ductus diverticulum. The ductus arteriosus remains open over part of its length, producing a funnel-shaped ductus diverticulum (*arrow*). *C*, Patent ductus arteriosus with left-to-right shunt. Contrast medium injected into the ascending aorta passes to the pulmonary trunk (*PT*) through a funnel-shaped PDA (*arrow*). *D*, Patent ductus arteriosus with right-to-left shunt. Injection of contrast medium into the right ventricle results in simultaneous opacification of the pulmonary trunk (*PT*), pulmonary arteries (*PA*), ductus arteriosus (*DA*), and descending aorta (*A*). (From Patterson DF: In Rosenquist GC and Bergsma D (eds); *Morphogenesis and Malformation of the Cardiovascular System.* New York, AR Liss, 1978.

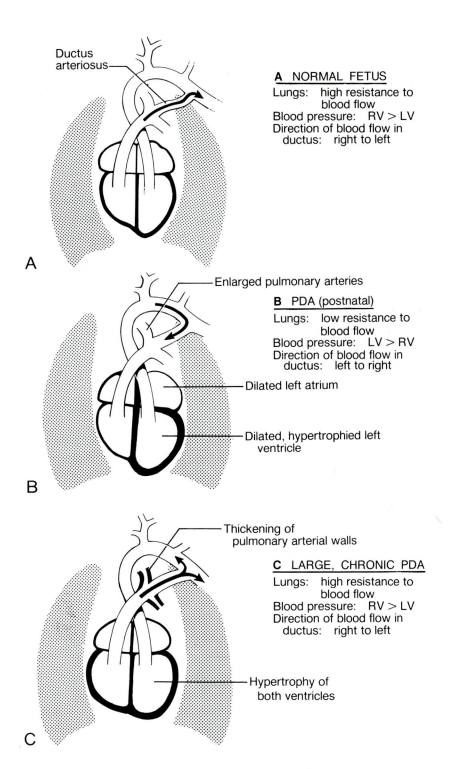

Ductus arteriosus

A NORMAL FETUS

Lungs: high resistance to
             blood flow
Blood pressure: RV > LV
Direction of blood flow in
   ductus: right to left

A

Enlarged pulmonary arteries

B PDA (postnatal)

Lungs: low resistance to
             blood flow
Blood pressure: LV > RV
Direction of blood flow in
   ductus: left to right

Dilated left atrium

Dilated, hypertrophied left
ventricle

B

Thickening of
pulmonary arterial walls

C LARGE, CHRONIC PDA

Lungs: high resistance to
             blood flow
Blood pressure: RV > LV
Direction of blood flow in
   ductus: right to left

Hypertrophy of
both ventricles

C

Figure 11.11.   Patent ductus arteriosus.

dilation of the vascular bed. With this simultaneous decrease in pulmonary resistance and loss of umbilical venous flow at birth, the pressure on the right side of the heart drops. Left heart pressure increases from the increased volume of blood entering from the pulmonary veins, the increased peripheral resistance due to collapse of the umbilical arterial circulation and the necessity for the left heart to supply all of the blood to the systemic circulation. Once pressure in the right heart drops below that in the left heart, the direction of blood flow through the ductus arteriosus is reversed, going now from left to right (aorta to pulmonary trunk). Occasionally this regurgitation of blood through the still patent ductus arteriosus is audible for a few days after birth. This is especially true in sheep, cattle, horses and, less often, pigs. It is difficult to hear in puppies and kittens.

Most abnormal heart sounds are called **murmurs**, and they result from an increased fluid turbulence within the heart or great vessels. The PDA murmur is normal at birth but quickly disappears as functional closure occurs. When the ductus arteriosus fails to close, the murmur persists and this characteristic sound is helpful in the diagnosis of this abnormality.

PDA is the most common cardiovascular malformation in dogs (see Tables 12.2 and 12.4). In one study 0.5% of all canine patients studied had congenital heart disease, and 28% of these were cases of PDA. There is a breed predisposition with Miniature and Toy Poodles, Collies, Pomeranians, Cocker Spaniels and German Shepherds more frequently afflicted. A hereditary basis has been established in the Miniature and Toy Poodles (see Table 12.3). This may involve an abnormality in the smooth muscle of the ductus, perhaps owing to lack of responsiveness to oxygen or antiprostaglandin stimulation. Hypoxia at birth may be contributory. In humans PDA is occasionally associated with in utero rubella (German measles) infections.

Signs of this disease are extremely variable. The condition is often recognized by the presence of the characteristic murmur in an otherwise normal dog presented for routine vaccination. The abnormal sound most frequently associated with PDA is called a **machinery murmur** since it is continuous through all phases of the cardiac cycle. This is because the aortic pressure exceeds pulmonic pressure throughout the entire cardiac cycle. Thus, flow through the PDA is continuous and the accompanying turbulence of the blood causes the murmur. Poor growth resulting in a stunted animal, rapid and labored respirations (**dyspnea**) and abnormal lung sounds (**rales**) may develop as heart failure occurs due to the abnormality in circulation. **Heart failure** simply means an inability of one or both sides of the heart to meet the minimal requirements of peripheral tissues or to accommodate venous inflow.

As a rule the aortic (left side) pressure exceeds pulmonic (right side) pressure, thus blood flows through the ductus from left to right (Figs. 11.10*C* and 11.11*B*). This overloads the pulmonary vasculature and increases pulmonary venous flow to the left atrium, causing it to enlarge. The left ventricle ultimately dilates and hypertrophies due to the increased volume of blood entering from the left atrium and also the increased demands of the systemic circulation for oxygenated blood. When the left heart cannot keep up with this overload, pulmonary congestion occurs. Inadequate draining causes fluid to be lost into the lungs and signs of respiratory failure occur.

Surgical ligation of the PDA will prevent this left-sided heart failure from occurring and is often recommended even in the patient who is physically normal but has the characteristic murmur. The untreated animal has a high susceptibility to congestive heart failure as a young dog. The degree of recovery following surgery in the dog already in heart failure depends on the severity of the cardiac malfunction and the health of the animal.

Occasionally a different manifestation of cardiopulmonary response occurs to a PDA. This is especially true if the ductus arteriosus remains very dilated so that a large volume of blood shunts from aorta to pulmonary trunk. This constant overload on the pulmonary vasculature may induce the formation of fibrotic tissue in the wall of small arterioles of the pulmonary vasculature (Figs. 11.10*D* and 11.11*C*). This restricts flow through the pulmonary vascular bed and thus creates a marked resistance to the flow of blood in the pulmonary trunk, a condition called **pulmonary hypertension**. The right ventricle hypertrophies to accommodate to this increased pulmonary resistance.

Ultimately pressure exerted by the right side of the heart exceeds that of the left and blood begins to flow through the PDA from right to left (pulmonary trunk to aorta). Thus, unoxygenated blood is shunted into the aorta caudal to the great vessels that supply the head. This usually results in pelvic limb weakness and collapse, especially upon exercise. The case presented in the Introduction was typical of this condition. **Cyanosis**, which is the appearance of a blue color in normally pink mucous membranes and extremities, and occasionally total collapse with loss of consciousness (fainting/syncope) will follow as the degree of hypertension and reversal of flow through the PDA worsens. Heart failure is of a right ventricular type, which results in systemic edema. These cases are usually refractory to surgical treatment.

Another possible basis for the pulmonary hypertension associated with a large PDA is a postnatal failure of the pulmonary vascular bed to undergo vasodilation upon initial respiration. As a result the resistance to blood flow through the lungs is maintained at high (fetal) levels. Subsequently, the right ventricle dilates and hypertrophies from pulmonary hypertension, leading eventually to a right-to-left flow of blood through the ductus arteriosus.

Vascular Ring Anomalies

There are several combinations of abnormalities in aortic arch transformation that result in a complete or partial vascular ring being formed around the esophagus and trachea (Figs. 11.12 and 11.13). The key to understanding how this can happen lies in the relation of embryonic aortic arches to the gut tube. Recall that each aortic arch originates midventrally and then passes around the foregut to one of the paired dorsal aortae. Each 3rd arch enters a separate, left or right dorsal aorta, a condition which is retained in the adult. However, the 4th and 6th aortic arches enter dorsal aortic roots which fuse in the midline dorsal to the gut, forming the aorta.

Normally only the left 4th and left 6th aortic arches retain this ventral-to-dorsal connection. However, if either the 4th or the 6th arch retains a ventrodorsal connection around the RIGHT side of the gut (esophagus) while the other is around the left, the esophagus will become constricted between them. Any malformation of this type is called a **vascular ring anomaly**.

The signs of a vascular ring malformation typically begin when the animal is weaned and begins to consume solid foods. Postprandial (after eating) regurgitation of undigested food occurs. The esophagus secondarily dilates cranial to the stricture producing a **megaesophagus** cranial to the base of the heart. Radiography after feeding the animal an emulsion of barium sulfate (Fig. 11.12*B*) will demonstrate the site of the megaesophagus and differentiate this condition, which is produced by a vascular ring anomaly, from a neuromuscular esophageal defect, which causes the entire thoracic esophagus to enlarge.

Vascular ring anomalies occur most commonly in German Shepherds, Weimaraners, and Irish Setters, but have been reported occasionally in all domestic animals.

CASE HISTORY

Signalment: Ten-week-old male German shepherd with vomiting and reduced weight gain.

History: Following weaning the puppy often vomited his meal shortly after eating; the vomitus was undigested and often tubular shaped.

Physical Exam: Physical examination was normal.

Assessment of History:

FACTS	INTERPRETATION
Postprandial regurgitation of undigested food; onset at time of weaning.	Suggests that solid food was unable to enter the stomach. Could be constriction of the esophagus due to (a) a congenital vascular ring defect, (b) a neuromuscular defect, or (c) a focal hypoplasia. An acquired disease (abscess, inflammation, injury) is uncommon at this age, although obstruction by a foreign body is possible.
Other signs normal	Other acquired neuromuscular diseases affecting the esophagus (botulism, myasthenia gravis, and polymyositis) are unusual at this age and normally cause signs of weakness in other muscles.

Radiological Exam: A thoracic radiograph showed a ventral displacement of the trachea in the cranial mediastinum. Following feeding of barium sulfate, radiographs revealed a dilated esophagus cranial to the base of the heart and only a small amount of barium sulfate had reached the stomach (Fig. 11.12).

Assessment of Radiological Exam:

FACT	INTERPRETATION
Ventral deviation of trachea in cranial mediastinum	The trachea may be displaced by a megaesophagus
Esophagus enlarged cranial to the heart	Highly suggestive of a vascular ring malformation which constricts the esophagus over the base of the heart causing megaesophagus cranial to it. A congenital neuromuscular defect of the esophagus would cause dilation of the esophagus to the level of the diaphragm.

Conclusion: The presumptive diagnosis is a vascular ring malformation causing megaesophagus and regurgitation of solid food. Additional angiographic analyses would be necessary to determine precisely which vessels were abnormally formed and causing a constriction. Surgical correction of the vascular ring malformation will usually alleviate the condition, although if the megaesophagus is extensive some dilatation will always remain.

Most of these vascular ring anomalies are associated with a persistent right 4th aortic arch. If the RIGHT 4th aortic arch becomes the arch of the aorta and the RIGHT 6th aortic arch persists as the ductus arteriosus, there is no vascular ring. However, if the LEFT 6th aortic arch persists as the ductus arteriosus with a RIGHT 4th aortic arch for the aorta, then a complete vascular ring is created around the esophagus (Fig. 11.13B). Postnatally this 6th aortic arch may be patent or converted into the ligamentum arteriosum. The vascular circle includes the base of the heart ventrally, the arch of the aorta on the right (right 4th aortic arch and right dorsal aortic root), and the ductus or ligamentum arteriosum (left 6th aortic arch and left dorsal aortic root) on the left. Frequently an anomalous left cranial vena cava accompanies this anomaly (see Fig. 13.5).

This is the most common form of vascular ring malformation. Surgical removal of the offending ductus or ligamentum and dissection of the fibrous tissue in the wall of the esophagus at the site of the stricture will usually relieve the condition.

Many other combinations of vascular anomalies can cause a partial or severe esophageal stricture. For example, if the right subclavian artery is aberrant and remains attached to the aorta by the caudal part of the right dorsal aortic root, this will create a partial vascular ring over the esophagus and usually cause obstruction (Fig.

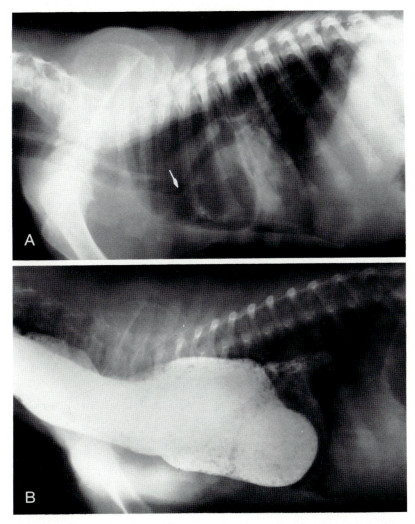

Figure 11.12. Radiographs of a dog with a vascular ring anomaly, taken A, before and B, after being fed a meal of radiopaque material. A shows a ventrally displaced trachea (*arrow*). In B, the megaesophagus is clearly demonstrated.

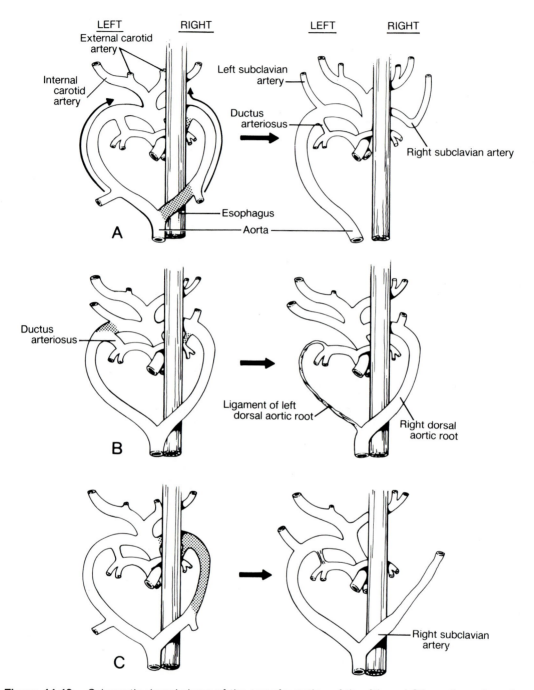

Figure 11.13. Schematic dorsal views of the transformation of the 4th and 6th aortic arches. *A*, a normal dog; *B*, an animal with persistent right 4th arch forming the aorta and left 6th arch as the ductus (ligamentum) arteriosus; and *C*, a case of anomalous branching of the right subclavian artery. *B* and *C* both cause constriction of the esophagus.

11.13*C*). In this malformation the right dorsal aortic root atrophies cranial to the right caudal dorsal cervical intersegmental artery rather than caudal to it.

Although the ring is incomplete, the retroesophageal right subclavian artery is fixed cranially in its course around the first rib. The tension this produces in a cranioventral direction pulls the aorta towards the right and compresses the esophagus. Occasionally the left and right subclavian arteries arise from a common trunk in this anomaly. The mirror image of this partial vascular ring occurs if the right 4th aortic arch persists as the aortic arch and proximal descending aorta and the left subclavian artery is aberrant and remains attached to the aorta instead of becoming a branch of the brachiocephalic trunk.

Both of these conditions involving an aberrant subclavian artery are amenable to treatment by surgery. The aberrant subclavian artery can be ligated and removed from its attachment to the aorta. By collateral circulation involving the vertebral and costocervical arteries the affected thoracic limb will usually receive sufficient blood supply to remain functional. Blood can flow from the normal side to the deprived side and course backwards to fill the subclavian artery. The internal thoracic artery can be filled in a similar manner from the multiple anastomoses with the dorsal intercostal arteries arising from the thoracic aorta.

In rare cases a double aortic arch will persist from the failure of the dorsal aortic root to atrophy on the right side. The ring produced involves both 4th aortic arches and both dorsal aortic roots to the level of the single aorta.

Bibliography

NORMAL

Barone R, Bidaud M: Le developpement du systeme arterial du bassin et du membre pelvien chez le Cheval. *Bull Soc Sci Vet Med Comp* 69:165–175, 1967.

Coulter CB: The early development of the aortic arches of the cat, with special reference to the presence of a fifth arch. *Anat Rec* 3:578–592, 1909.

Hammond WS: The developmental transformation of the aortic arches in the calf (*Bos taurus*), with special reference to the formation of the arch of the aorta. *Am J Anat* 62:149–177, 1937.

Heuser CH: The branchial vessels and their derivatives in the pig. *Carnegie Inst Wash Contrib Embryol* 15:121–139, 1923.

Lehman H: On the embryonic history of the aortic arches in mammals. *Anat Anz* 26:406–424, 1905.

Martin EW: The development of the vascular system in 5-21 somite dog embryos. *Anat Rec* 137:378, 1960.

Moffat DB: Developmental changes in the aortic arch system of the rat. *Am J Anat* 105:1–35, 1959.

Rosenquist GC: Aortic arches in the chick embryo: origin of the cells as determined by radioautographic mapping. *Anat Rec* 168:351–359, 1970.

Sabin FR: Origin and development of the primitive vessels of the chick and pig. *Carnegie Inst Wash Contrib Embryol* 6:61–124, 1917.

Stephan F: Contribution experimentale a l'etude du developpement du systeme circulatoire chez l'embryon de poulet. *Bull Biol Fr Belg* 86:217–308, 1952.

Vitums A: Development and transformation of the aortic arches in the equine embryos with special attention to the formation of the definitive arch of the aorta and the common brachiocephalic trunk. *Z Anat Entwicklungsgesch* 128:243–270, 1969.

PATENT DUCTUS ARTERIOSUS (PDA)

Buchanan JW, Soma LR, Patterson DF: Patent ductus arteriosus surgery in small dogs. *JAVMA* 151:7, 1965.

Carmichael JA, Buergelt CD, Lord PF, Tashjian RJ: Diagnosis of patent ductus arteriosus in a horse. *JAVMA* 158:767–775, 1971.

Legendre AM et al: Secondary polycythemia and seizures due to right-to-left shunting patent ductus arteriosus in a dog. *JAVMA* 164:1198–1201, 1974.

Patterson DF et al: Hereditary patent ductus arteriosus and its sequelae in the dog. *Circ Res* 29:1–13, 1971.

Pyle RL, Park RD, Alexander AF, Hill BL: Patent ductus arteriosus with pulmonary hypertension in the dog. *JAVMA* 178:565–571, 1981.

Scott EA et al: Closure of ductus arteriosus determined by cardiac catheterization and angiography in newborn foals. *Am J Vet Res* 36:1021–1024, 1975.

Smetzer DL, Breznok EM: Auscultatory diagnosis of patent ductus arteriosus in the dog. *JAVMA* 160:80–84, 1972.

VASCULAR RING ANOMALIES

Bartels JE, Vaughan JT: Persistent right aortic arch in the horse. *JAVMA* 154:406–409, 1969.

Buergelt CD, Wheaton LG: Dextroaorta, atopic left subclavian artery, and persistent left cephalic vena cava in a dog. *JAVMA* 156:1026, 1970.

Coward TG: Persistent right aortic arch in two Great Dane litter mates. *J Small Anim Pract* 5:245–247, 1964.

Detweiler DK, Allam MW: Persistent right aortic arch with associated esophageal dilation in dogs. *Cornell Vet* 45:209–229, 1955.

Hathaway JE: Persistent right aortic arch in a cat. *JAVMA* 147:255–259, 1965.

Henwood JK, Green RA: Section of the right subclavian artery to relieve associated regurgitation of food in the dog. *Vet Rec* 76:1155–1160, 1964.

Klotz AP, Brewer NR: Double aortic arch in a dog. *North Am Vet* 33:867–868, 1952.

Lawson DD, Piris HM: Conditions of the canine esophagus. II. Vascular rings, achalasia, tumor, and periesophageal lesions. *J Small Anim Pract* 7:117–127, 1966.

Linde-Sipman JS vander, van der Gaag I: Vascular ring caused by a left aortic arch, right ligamentum arteriosum and part of the right dorsal aorta malarticulation. *Zbl Vet Med* A28:569–573, 1981.

Richmond BT: A case of persistent right aortic arch in the cat. *Vet Rec* 83:169, 1968.

Roberts SJ, Kennedy PC, Delahanty DD: A persistent right aortic arch in a Guernsey bull. *Cornell Vet* 43:537–541, 1953.

Uhrich SJ: Report of a persistent right aortic arch and its surgical correction in a cat. *J Small Anim Pract* 4:337–339, 1963.

Van den Ingh TSGAM, Van der Linde-Sipman JS: Vascular rings in dogs. *JAVMA* 164:939–941, 1974.

Vitums A: Anomalous origin of the right subclavian and common carotid arteries in the dog. *Cornell Vet* 52:5–15, 1962.

Walker RC, Littlewort MCG: Angiography in the preoperative assessment of vascular ring obstruction of the oesophagus in the dog. *Vet Rec* 76:215–219, 1964.

Review

Elison GW: Vascular ring anomalies in the dog and cat. *Compend Cont Ed* 2:693–705, 1980.

Cardiovascular System II: Heart

The heart is the first embryonic organ to undergo functional differentiation. Shortly after the formation of a closed cephalic neural tube, and during the period of formation of somites 10 through 20, the ventromedian tubular heart is formed and begins to contract rhythmically. This organ serves as a peristaltic pump, moving blood from extraembryonic vessels into and through the primitive embryonic circulatory system.

The formation of the **cardiogenic plate**, which is the mesodermal primordium of the heart, is the first stage of heart development. Subsequently, the subcephalic pocket and lateral body folds develop, bringing the left and right cardiogenic primordia together ventrally to form a single median **heart tube**. The third stage of cardiogenesis is the formation of the **cardiac loop**, during which the atrium becomes located cranial to the ventricle. Finally the septa are formed, separating the right, pulmonary outflow, from the left, systemic outflow, and valves develop to prevent the backflow of blood. It is a remarkable feat of embryonic engineering that these processes occur without any interruption in the movement of blood.

During the critical period of cardiogenesis, when the fusion, folding and septation of cardiac tissues occur, the embryo grows from approximately 4 mm to 10–12 mm in length (summarized in Table 12-1). Although the heart enlarges 4- to 5-fold during this brief period, its actual size is extremely small, growing from approximately 1 to 5 mm as measured from ventricular apex to the ventral aorta. Thus, the changes in shape and formation of septa between chambers involve growth and morphogenetic movements over much slighter distances than might be apparent from the sketches in this chapter.

CARDIOGENIC PLATE AND HEART TUBE FORMATION

The first indication of cardiac development occurs in the splanchnic mesoderm cranial and lateral to the site of head folding. A series of vesicles form and then coalesce to create a cavity within the mesoderm. This

Table 12.1.
Critical periods in mammalian cardiogenesis[a]

Event	Timing (shown as dotted bar over the scale below)
Fusion	▪▪▪▪▪▪▪▪▪▪
Onset of contractions	▪▪▪▪▪
1st and 2nd aortic arches present	▪▪▪▪▪▪▪▪▪▪
Formation of septum primum	▪▪▪▪▪▪▪▪▪▪▪▪▪▪▪▪
Presence of foramen primum	▪▪▪▪▪▪▪▪▪▪▪▪▪▪
Appearance of foramen secundum	▪▪▪▪▪
A-V endocardial cushions form and fuse	▪▪▪▪▪▪▪▪▪▪▪▪▪▪▪▪
Bulbar endocardial cushions fuse	▪▪▪▪▪▪▪▪▪▪▪▪▪▪▪▪▪▪
Truncal endocardial cushions fuse	▪▪▪▪▪▪▪▪▪▪▪▪

Number of Somites:	1	10	20	30					
Length (mm):			3 mm	4 mm	5 mm	6 mm	7 mm	9 mm	12 mm	16 mm

[a] Although the embryos of domesticated mammals are very similar at these stages of development, cardiogenesis in the dog and in humans is slightly precocious and equine cardiogenesis is slightly delayed relative to the others.

cavity is elongated transversely and located in front of the site of head folding; it is the precursor of the **pleuropericardial cavity.** On both sides the cavity extends caudally and becomes continuous with the embryonic coelom.

The **cardiogenic plate** is formed by splanchnic mesoderm ventral to the presumptive pleuropericardial cavity, as shown in Figure 12.1*A*. Several vesicles develop from loose aggregates of cardiogenic plate mesoderm and then coalesce to form the precursor of the **endocardial tube.** The mesoderm located cranial to the cardiogenic plate proliferates and thickens. This marks the initial formation of the **septum transversum,** which subsequently will form the central part of the **diaphragm** (see Chapter 15).

The above events occur simultaneously with the process of head folding. During this folding all of the tissues located immediately in front of the neural plate are inverted 180° and brought beneath the cranial parts of the head, as shown in figure 12.1*B* (see also Fig. 2.20). Thus, the primordium of the septum transversum becomes situated caudal to the cardiac tube, and the pericardial cavity is located ventrally.

Concomitantly, lateral body folding and closure of the pharynx begin, bringing right and left cardiac primordia together (Fig. 12.2). This proceeds craniocaudally, forming the primordium of the **truncus arteriosus** first, then the **bulboventricle, atrium** and, lastly, the **sinus venosus.** The primordia of the sinus venosus initially appear as a vascular plexus within the septum transversum together with the presumptive hepatic parenchyma. Later, these three tissues separate.

The endocardial tube is surrounded by a thick layer of mesoderm called the **myocardium,** which later forms cardiac muscle. Outside of this is a thin epicardial layer. Between the myocardial and endocardial layers is a viscous fluid called **cardiac jelly** (Fig. 12.3). Rich in collagen and glycoproteins, this fluid matrix serves two essential functions. First, it permits slight contractions of the myocardium to affect closure of

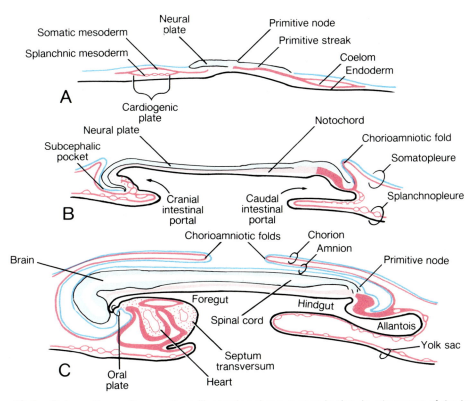

Figure 12.1. Schematic median sections illustrating three stages in the development of the heart in the pig embryo. *A*, early neurula stage, showing formation of the cardiogenic plate. *B*, head fold stage, by which time the cardiac primordium has been brought ventral to the head. *C*, 15-somite stage, after heart looping has begun. (Redrawn after Patten, 1948.)

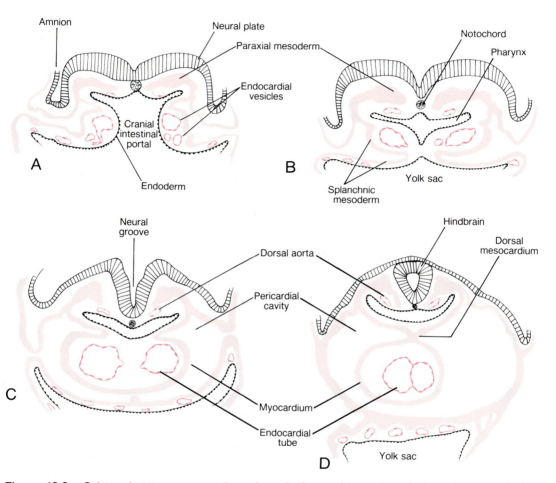

Figure 12.2. Schematic transverse sections through the cardiac region of pig embryos at *A*, 5-somite; *B*, 7-somite; *C*, 10-somite; and *D*, 13-somite stages of development. (Redrawn after Patten and Carlson, 1974.)

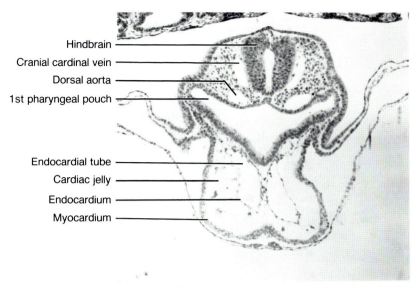

Hindbrain
Cranial cardinal vein
Dorsal aorta
1st pharyngeal pouch

Endocardial tube
Cardiac jelly
Endocardium
Myocardium

Figure 12.3. Transverse section through the hindbrain of a 14-somite cat embryo, near the cranial end of the cardiac tube. The endocardial tubes have not yet fused in the midline ventral to the pharynx.

the endocardial lumen, thus enabling the simple tubular heart to act as a peristaltic pump. Second, cardiac jelly serves as a matrix through which mesenchymal cells derived from the endocardium can migrate. These cells form connective tissues in the septa and valves of the heart.

The mesodermal sheets that suspend the cardiac tube dorsally are thin, and degenerate along most of the heart tube. As a result the heart is free to bend and loop because it is suspended only at its cranial (truncus arteriosus) and future caudal (sinus venosus) ends.

By the time the embryo is 4–5 mm in length (Fig. 12.4A) the heart primordium is located ventral to the hindbrain and pharynx. Subsequently, differential growth of dorsal head and body structures plus cranial and cervical flexures result in the heart becoming located progressively farther caudally.

Cardiac contractions and circulation begin at 35–38 hr of incubation in the chick, at 18–19 days of gestation in the dog, and late in the 4th week of human development. The beat is initially slow, but increases as the atrium and then sinus venosus form. This is because the pacemaker cells that

develop in each newly formed part of the heart have an inherently faster contraction rhythm, and the most rapidly beating population drives the rest of the cardiac muscle cells. Partitioning occurs at 5–8 days in the chick, during the 4th week in the dog, and between 5 and 7 weeks of gestation in humans.

EXTERNAL MORPHOGENESIS

Shortly after its formation, the middle region of the tubular heart, the **bulboventricle**, elongates and forms a C-shaped loop. This initially expands to the right side of the embryo. Continued rapid growth brings it ventral to the rest of the tube (Fig. 12.4).

A deep fold, the bulboventricular sulcus (flange), appears cranioventrally in the bulboventricular loop. This demarcates the subsequent zone of separation of this large chamber into **bulbus cordis** on the right and the **left ventricle**. As the bulboventricular loop grows, the atrium expands towards the left; the sinus venosus and truncus arteriosus are held close to the midline by the **dorsal mesocardium**. As illustrated in Figures 12.4 and 12.5, at this stage blood flows from the vitelline and common cardinal veins into the sinus venosus, then passes cranioven-

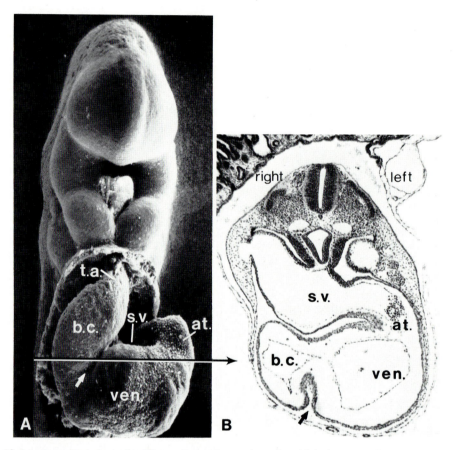

Figure 12.4. *A*, ventral view of a 19-somite canine embryo in which the ventral pericardial and body wall tissues have been removed to reveal the heart loop. *B*, transverse section through the heart loop of a 22-somite feline embryo at the level of the 4th somite, indicated by the *bar/arrow* in *A*. Blood flows from the sinus venosus (*s.v.*) to the atrium (*at.*), ventricle (*ven.*), bulbus cordis (*b.c.*), and leaves the heart through the truncus arteriosus (*t.a.*). The *small arrows* point to the bulboventricular sulcus.

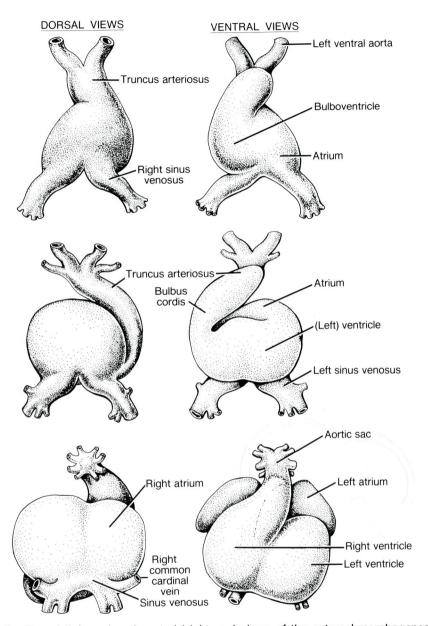

DORSAL VIEWS

VENTRAL VIEWS

Left ventral aorta

Truncus arteriosus

Bulboventricle

Atrium

Right sinus
venosus

Truncus arteriosus

Bulbus
cordis

Atrium

(Left) ventricle

Left sinus venosus

Aortic sac

Right atrium

Left atrium

Right
common
cardinal
vein
Sinus venosus

Right ventricle

Left ventricle

Figure 12.5.   Dorsal (*left row*) and ventral (*right row*) views of the external morphogenesis of the heart at the neurula, 15-somite and 4-mm stages. 1, 2, 3, 4 indicate aortic arches. (Redrawn with modifications after Patten and Carlson, 1974.)

trally and slightly to the left to enter the atrium. The blood is redirected caudoventrally, then from the left to the right side as it passes through the loop of the bulboventricle. It leaves this large chamber flowing craniodorsally. Finally blood returns to the midline of the embryo via the truncus arteriosus and exits the heart.

These initial patterns of cardiac folding and constriction are the result of intrinsic asymmetries in proliferative activity of myocardial cells. This has been shown by excising pieces of the embryonic cardiac tube and maintaining them in organ cultures. The constrictions and bendings occur normally, even in these isolated fragments.

INTERNAL MORPHOGENESIS

Internal partitioning of the heart and the cardiac outflow must occur in the atrium, the atrioventricular canal, the bulboventricular loop and the truncus arteriosus. Division of the aortic sac into pulmonary and systemic compartments by the formation of the aorticopulmonary septum occurs concomitantly with these events. All of these partitionings are influenced by the direction of blood flow, which must continue without interruption throughout the formation of these septal partitions. Also, these events are interdependent, and failure of any one septum to develop properly may secondarily alter the others.

Sinus Venosus, Atrium, Atrioventricular Canal; Endocardial Cushions

During the later stages of bulboventricular loop expansion, the flow of venous blood entering the heart, both from the liver and the head, becomes asymmetrical, with the right side predominating and the flow into the left part of the sinus venosus diminishing. This shift in venous inflow is coincidental with the beginning of internal partitioning, and progresses until the systemic venous input is entirely to the right side.

The right horn of the sinus venosus becomes completely incorporated into the dorsal wall of the expanding right atrium (Fig. 12.6). In the mature animal this region, the **sinus venarum**, has a smooth internal appearance. It is bounded approximately by the cranial and caudal caval veins, by the orifice of the coronary sinus and, laterally, by the crista terminalis and sulcus terminalis. The left horn of the sinus venosus does not become fully incorporated into the wall of the heart, and forms the **coronary sinus**.

Pulmonary veins initially form as a single evagination from the wall of the left atrium. The evagination becomes subdivided into several branches which enter the pulmonary mesenchyme. Later, when the left atrium expands, this original venous diverticulum and the proximal part of several of the branches become incorporated into the atrial wall. The smooth, dorsal wall of the mature left atrium, into which the pulmonary veins enter, is thought to be derived from this early evagination.

As the cardiac loop forms, the constriction between bulboventricle and atrium becomes more pronounced, delineating the **atrioventricular (A-V) canal**. Externally this marks the future waist of the heart. The mesoderm in this constricted region proliferates, resulting in the growth of a circumferential ridge protruding into and partially constricting the A-V canal. This mesenchymal proliferation is not uniform around the orifice, but is greatest in the two regions located in the median plane.

These protrusions into the lumen of the orifice are called the **A-V endocardial cushions**, and are illustrated in Figure 12.7. The two cushions meet and fuse together, forming a single **A-V endocardial cushion** (Fig. 12.7 *D* and *F*). This closure creates two separate channels, the **left** and **right atrioventricular orifices**.

Once the A-V endocardial cushions fuse, this bridge across the A-V canal is permanent and inelastic. Thus, throughout the period when the fetal heart grows rapidly, these initial sites of cushion fusion bind opposite walls together. The same is true for cushions in the truncus and bulbus, which will be described under Partitioning of Truncus Arteriosis and Bulbus Cordis. Later in

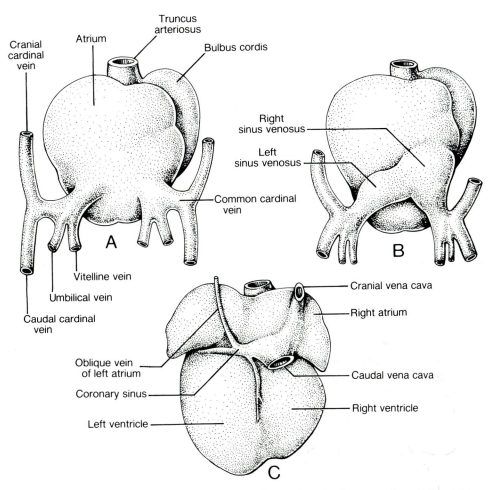

Figure 12.6. Schematic dorsal views of the heart illustrating the incorporation of the right part of the sinus venosus into the wall of the atrium.

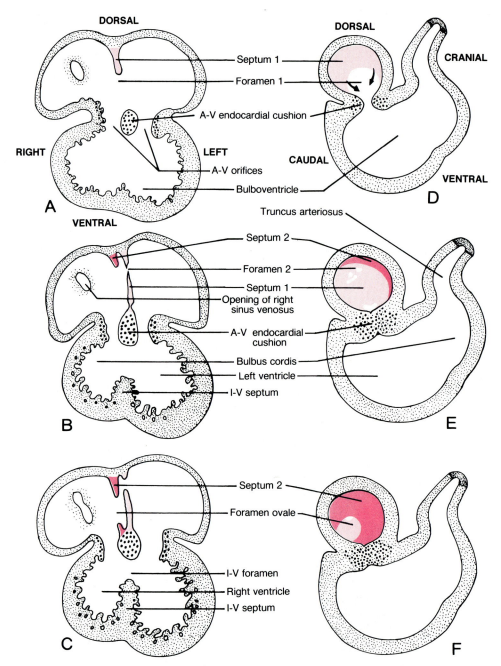

Figure 12.7. Sequential compartmentalization of the heart. *A–C*, heart cut in a transverse plane and viewed from a cranial perspective. *D–F*, heart cut in a paramedian plane and viewed from the right side. These show the formation of the septum primum, septum secundum, interventricular septum (*I-V septum*), and atrioventricular (*A-V*) endocardial cushions.

development, concomitant with the formation of papillary muscles and chordae tendineae, growth of cardiac mesenchyme surrounding the A-V orifices combined with differential expansion of the ventricles results in the formation of the **left** and **right A-V valves.**

Interatrial Septa

Simultaneous with the growth of the A-V endocardial cushions, the left and right sides of the atrium become separated by the **septum primum**. This is a mesenchymal sheet (labeled Septum 1 in Figure 12.7 *A* and *D*) that appears initially on the dorsal wall of the atrium in the median plane. It is relatively thin and expands **ventrally** across the lumen of the atrium towards the growing A-V endocardial cushions. The inner rim of the septum primum is in the shape of a horseshoe, with the two limbs directed toward the enlarging A-V cushions.

The opening between the ventral limbs of the septum primum lies dorsal to the cushions. This opening, called the **foramen primum**, allows blood to flow from the right side of the atrium to the left. As the A-V endocardial cushions meet and fuse, the septum completes its expansion by fusing in the median plane along the entire dorsal surface of the endocardial cushions, thus obliterating the foramen primum.

In order to maintain the flow of blood from right into left atrial chambers a second opening, the **foramen secundum** (labeled Foramen 2 in figure 12.7 *B* and *E*), develops dorsocranially in the septum primum. This occurs prior to the closure of the foramen primum by the coalescence of many small perforations into a single window.

Later, a second membranous sheet, the **septum secundum**, develops to the **right** of the septum primum. It is thicker, and grows **caudally** from the cranial margin of the atrium (Figure 12.7 *D* and *F*). One limb of the septum secundum extends caudally along the dorsal wall of the atrium in the median plane adjacent to the septum primum. The other limb extends caudally along the fused A-V endocardial cushions (i.e. along the ventromedial surface of the atrium), also adjacent to the right side of the septum primum. The two limbs are directed toward the caudal vena cava, which has become incorporated into the wall of the right atrium along with the sinus venosus.

The septum secundum does not grow completely across the atrium. Its caudal, concave edge remains free and is directed toward the opening of the caudal vena cava. The window that remains as a result of incomplete formation of the septum secundum is the **foramen ovale**.

The septum secundum is adjacent to the septum primum, but the two remain separate throughout fetal development. This permits blood to pass from the right atrium through the foramen ovale, then between the two interatrial septa and into the left atrium via the foramen secundum. Because the foramen ovale is directed toward the caudal vena cava, it receives much of the blood entering the heart from that vein, including oxygenated blood from the placenta. The pressure created by this inflow keeps these septa separated by pushing the thinner septum primum towards the left. From the left atrium this oxygenated blood enters the left ventricle then exits the heart via the ascending aorta, from which the brachiocephalic trunk and left subclavian artery branch. The rest of the blood entering the right atrium passes to the right ventricle and then to the pulmonary trunk, where most of it is shunted via the ductus arteriosus into the aorta.

At birth the septa primum and secundum become tightly apposed, largely as a result of diminution in the pressure within the right atrium and elevation of pressure in the left atrium due to pulmonary venous inflow. These combined septa are now called the **interatrial septum**. It is important to visualize that the foramen secundum and the foramen ovale are not overlapping; the former is situated craniodorsally in the septum primum while the latter is located caudally in the septum secundum. Thus, when the two septa become apposed there is no longer a passageway between the right and left atrial chambers.

Apposition of these septa occurs within minutes of birth. Although complete fusion may take several weeks or occasionally never occurs, the higher pressure of the pulmonic input keeps the passageway functionally closed.

Occasionally during postmortem examination, the septa primum and secundum are found to be not fully fused together, so that a blunt probe can be passed from the **fossa ovalis**, which demarcates the former site of the foramen ovale, craniodorsally into the left atrium. This situation is especially frequent in cattle. However, so long as systemic and pulmonic venous inputs to the heart were normal, the differential pressures in the right and left atria would have prevented these septa from separating.

Partitioning of Truncus Arteriosus and Bulbus Cordis

While the A-V endocardial cushions and septum primum are segregating blood entering the common ventricle into left and right channels, the cardiac outflow via truncus and bulbar regions of the heart are also being separated into two channels. This is accomplished by the formation of paired endocardial cushions (ridges) within the truncus arteriosus and bulbar (conal) part of the bulboventricle.

The **truncal cushions** are the first to form (Fig. 12.8). These endocardial cushions expand into the lumen of the truncus from the left and right sides, beginning at the 3- to 4-mm stage while the bulboventricular loop is forming. Within 2–3 days in the dog, 5–6 days in most other domestic animals, these opposing cushions fuse to form the **truncal septum** (Fig. 12.9). There is a slight spiral to this septum, so that the plane at which it bisects the truncus rotates clockwise at progressively more distal (cranial) levels, when viewed from a caudal perspective. This is shown schematically in Figure 12.10. Similar ridges form in the bulbar region of the bulboventricle. However, these **bulbar cushions** arise from the right dorsal and left ventral margins of the heart wall.

The endocardial cushions in the bulbus and truncus grow together and join with the aorticopulmonary septum. This results in a separation of the cardiac outflow into two channels. Because each pair of cushions and aorticopulmonary septum. This results in a separation of the cardiac outflow into two channels. Because each pair of cushions and broad, clockwise spiral ascending from the middle of the bulbus to the roots of the

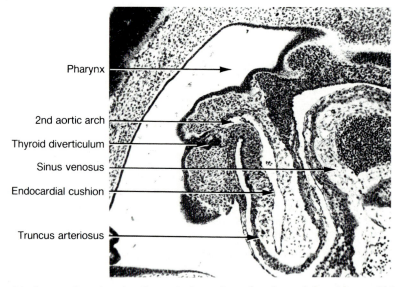

Pharynx

2nd aortic arch

Thyroid diverticulum

Sinus venosus

Endocardial cushion

Truncus arteriosus

Figure 12.8. Median section showing the early formation of endocardial cushions within the truncus arteriosus of a 4-mm guinea pig.

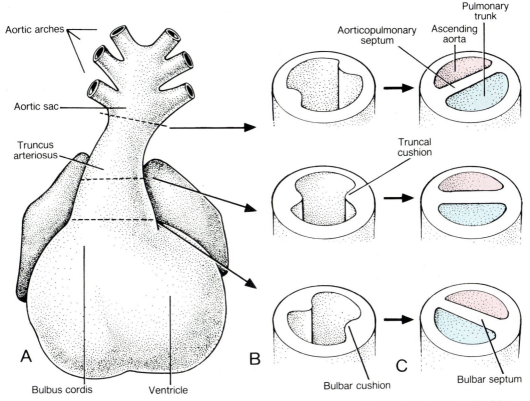

Figure 12.9. Development of the spiral septum. *A*, ventral view of the canine heart at 22–23 days of gestation (5- to 6-mm crown-rump length). Columns *B* and *C* illustrate the formation and fusion (3–4 days later) of aorticopulmonary, truncal and bulbar cushions.

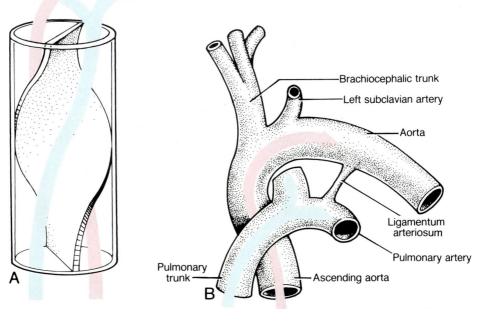

Figure 12.10. *A*, schematic representation of the spiral septum. *B*, ventral view of the pulmonary trunk and ascending aorta.

pulmonary (6th aortic arch) and systemic (3rd and 4th arches) arteries. This partition is the **spiral septum**.

Later in development the two lumina and walls of the bulbus and truncus expand greatly, obscuring the original site of spiral septum formation. Cranially, the two channels become completely separated, forming the pulmonary trunk and ascending aorta (Fig. 12.10*B*). The site of branching of the pulmonary arteries from the pulmonary trunk demarcates the original level of the aorticopulmonary septum. The bulbus cordis and bulbar septum become fully incorporated into the heart.

Interventricular Septum, Cardiac Valves

Growth of the ventricle, which is located on the left ventral side of the heart following looping of the bulboventricle, results in a shift in the position of the single A-V canal from the left side to the center (median plane) of the heart (Fig. 12.11 *A* and *B*). Once the A-V and truncobulbar cushions form and fuse, all that remains is to connect the right A-V canal with the right ventricle and pulmonary trunk, and join the left A-V orifice via the left ventricle to the opening of the aortic root.

The formation and growth of the **interven-**

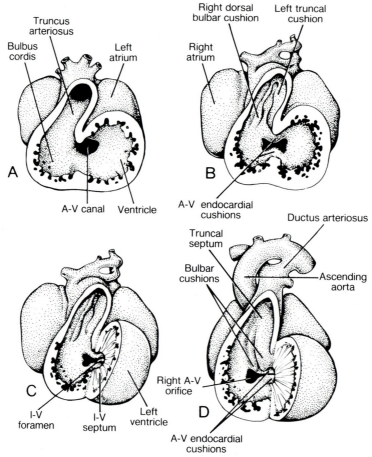

Figure 12.11. Initial stages in the separation of aortic and pulmonary cardiac outflow channels, shown in ventral views of the canine heart. Both left and right ventricles (i.e. the entire bulboventricle) have been removed in *A* (4 mm) and *B* (7 mm). *C* is the same stage as *B* but with the left ventricle and I-V septum included, and *D* is an older (10 mm) stage. (Redrawn after Langman, 1981, and von Moriep, Patterson and Schnarr, 1978.)

tricular (I-V) septum actually occur more as a result of caudal expansion and, especially, hypertrophy of the wall of the bulboventricle than from elongation of a median septum. The diameter of the midventral part of the bulboventricular loop remains relatively unchanged, while the ventricle, on the left, and bulbus, on the right, grow rapidly in a caudoventral direction.

Enlargement of these chambers occurs by a process called **trabeculation**. While mesenchymal and myocardial cells on the outer part of the cardiac wall are dividing and forming new tissues, those located beneath the endocardium degenerate. Local differences in the extent of cell death are the basis for the formation of the uneven luminal surface of the ventricles, and also for the retention of muscular and tendinous cords that cross the ventricular chambers, including the papillary muscles.

Since blood flowing through the bulboventricular loop is passing from the left to the right side, the median I-V septum appears to be perpendicular to the direction of fluid movement. In actuality, expansions of the ventricle and the bulbus, which forms most of the definitive **right ventricle**, coincide with the separation of the A-V canal and truncus into paired channels. This enables the embryonic heart to remain functional while separating blood flow into two systems. The original passageway between (left) ventricle and bulbus is now called the **interventricular foramen**.

The final separation of left ventricular from right ventricular (bulbar) channels is summarized schematically in Figure 12.12. First, the craniodorsal part of the I-V septum expands onto the A-V cushion. Simultaneously, the left ventral bulbar cushion elongates and fuses with this part of the I-V septum, and the right dorsal bulbar ridge expands onto the A-V cushion. The proximal ends of the bulbar cushions then fuse together, effectively separating pulmonary from systemic outflows.

Final closure of the I-V foramen is brought about by growth of the A-V cushion, which plugs the opening between left and right ventricles. This occurs at approximately 27 days of gestation in the pig (20-mm stage), 32 days in the dog (19-mm stage), 35 days in the horse (16-mm stage), and 45 days in humans (18-mm stage).

The A-V valves form by reshaping and selective tissue loss within the ventricular walls. As the chambers become dilated and the ventricular walls undergo hypertrophy and also trabeculation due to local cell death, strands of cardiac wall mesenchyme running from A-V endocardial cushions to the ventricular wall remain in their original locations. These form the cusps of the A-V valves and the chordae tendinae.

Following the formation and fusion of truncal ridges, three swellings appear within the walls of both the pulmonary and aortic trunks. The swellings expand into the lumen of each vessel. Originally quite broad, the bases of each of these primordia of **semilunar cusps** become thinned as a result of cell degeneration.

CONGENITAL HEART MALFORMATIONS

Congenital heart malformations, including patent ductus arteriosus and persistent right aortic arch, account for approximately 10% of the cardiovascular-related clinical presentations in domestic animals. A summary of the data on the incidence of specific cardiac anomalies in domestic animals is presented in Table 12.2. These data must be interpreted with caution, since the methods of collection and sample sizes vary considerably. Cardiac malformations are encountered less frequently in horses and cats than in cattle and dogs. For horses this is due to a higher incidence of early mortality in affected animals than occurs in other animals having comparable malformations. In cats both the relative lack of inbreeding and the lower frequency of presentation of kittens for postmortem examination are factors.

Patterson has assessed the frequency of congenital heart anomalies in various breeds of dogs presented at the University of Pennsylvania School of Veterinary Medicine. Based on screening of over 35,000 dogs, he

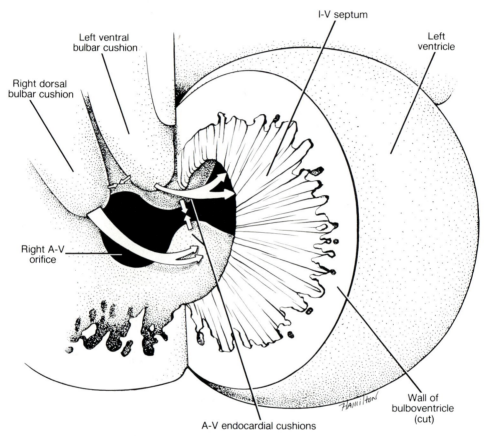

Figure 12.12. Schematic closure of the I-V foramen, shown in this enlarged aspect of Figure 12.11*D*. The heart is viewed from a ventral perspective with the ventral wall of the bulbus cordis removed to expose the interior of the right ventricle, the bulbar and A-V endocardial cushions, and the A-V orifices. All movements indicated by *arrows* occur simultaneously except the final fusion of the bulbar cushions, which is the last to occur.

found that 6.8/1000 dogs showed some form of congenital heart malformation. The incidence was appreciably higher in purebred strains (8.9/1000) than in mixed breeds (2.6/1000).

Some of the purebred strains showing a high incidence of one type of malformation were selected for breeding studies to learn whether there was a heritable pattern. Table 12.3 summarizes the results of Patterson's breeding experiments. In this study, both parents were of the same breed and both were diagnosed as having the same heart anomaly. Clearly, except for the persistent right aortic arch, these cardiac malformations show a definite pattern of heritability.

Table 12.2.
Incidence of cardiac malformations in domestic animals[a]

Species	Frequency (%)	Specific Malformations[b]	Reference
Horse	0.2	VSD (50%), aortic stenosis, pulmonary stenosis, persistent truncus arteriosus, A-V valve defects, interatrial septal defects, PDA, cor triloculare biatrium.	Mahaffey, 1958 Rooney and Franks, 1964
Cattle	0.17	VSD, aortic stenosis, tetralogy of Fallot, Eisenmenger complex, transposition of the aorta, PDA, ASD, duplicated cranial vena cava, coarctation of the aorta, ectopia cordis.	Van Nie, 1964 and 1966 Fisher and Pirie, 1965
Pig	0.16 to 4.1	VSD, aortic stenosis, tetralogy of Fallot, endocardial fibroelastosis, Eisenmenger complex, ASD, A-V valve defects, PDA.	Detweiler, 1960 Van Nie, 1963
Sheep	1.15	VSD (80%).	Dennis & Leipold, 1968
Dog	0.68	PDA, pulmonary stenosis, aortic stenosis, persistent right aortic arch, VSD, tetralogy of Fallot, ASD, persistent left cranial vena cava, A-V valve defects.	Das, et al., 1965 Patterson, 1968
Cat	1.85	Aortic stenosis, pulmonary stenosis, VSD, tetralogy of Fallot, persistent truncus arteriosus, persistent right aortic arch, PDA, endocardial fibroelastosis.	Das, et al., 1965 Tashjian, et al., 1965
Chicken	0.57	VSD, ASD, dextroposition of the aorta.	Siller and Hemsley, 1966

[a] Adapted from Whitney, 1975; and Okamoto, 1980.
[b] Listed in decreasing order of frequency.
[c] VSD, interventricular septal defect; PDA, patent ductus arteriosus; and ASD, interatrial septal defects.

Table 12.3.
Inheritance of congenital heart disease[a]

Breed	Parental defect	Number of progeny	Number (%) with same or similar malformation (%)
Poodle (10)[b]	Patent ductus arteriosus	35	29 (83)
Beagle (10)	Pulmonic stenosis	35	8 (26)
Newfoundland (5)	Subaortic stenosis	26	8 (31)
German Shepherd (3)	Right aortic arch	30	2 (6.7)
Keeshond (4)	Tetralogy of Fallot	11	10 (90)

[a] From Patterson DF and Pyle RL: Genetic aspects of congenital heart disease in the dog. 21st Gaines Veterinary Symposium, 1971, St. Louis, Mo.
[b] ( ) number of matings.

Cardiac malformations are usually classified as **acyanotic** or **cyanotic**. Acyanotic malformations permit the body to receive a sufficient amount of oxygenated blood to maintain life-sustaining levels of activity. In cyanotic malformations the body does not receive sufficient oxygenated hemoglobin in the peripheral capillary beds. This produces a blue color (kyano = blue) to most tissues, most easily seen upon examining the oral mucosa and gums. The above is at best an operational classification, and the same malformation might present differing degrees of oxygen insufficiency depending on the extent of secondary responses to the primary lesion.

Understanding and recognizing these secondary changes is a necessary aspect of diagnosing the condition. The two most prevalent changes that occur secondarily in the heart are **dilation** of a chamber and **hypertrophy** of the wall of a chamber. Dilation occurs if the volume of fluid in a chamber is chronically elevated, either as a result of restricted output or increased blood inflow. Hypertrophy of the muscular wall occurs if the contraction force needed to empty a chamber is chronically higher than normal.

ACYANOTIC HEART MALFORMATIONS

Acyanotic malformations are the most commonly encountered congenital heart anomalies. The frequencies obtained in the Patterson study are listed in Table 12.4.

Pulmonary Stenosis

Uncomplicated (i.e. without other heart anomalies) pulmonary stenosis is the most common cardiac defect in dogs, and is second only to persistent ductus arteriosus among congenital cardiovascular malformations. It is a narrowing of the pulmonary outflow tract (Fig. 12.14*A*) that can occur at one or more of several possible sites. **Infundibular pulmonary stenosis** is a narrowing of the pulmonary side of the partitioned bulbus cordis and truncus arteriosus. This condition

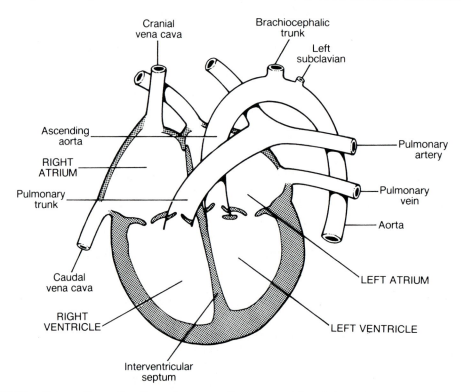

Figure 12.13. Schematic section through a normal heart cut obliquely in a plane passing from base to apex, viewed from a ventral perspective. Compare with Figures 12.14*A–D* and 12.15.

Table 12.4.
Occurrence of specific cardiovascular malformations in dogs[a,b]

Malformation	Percentage
Patent ductus arteriosus	28
Pulmonic stenosis	20
Aortic stenosis	14
Persistent right aortic arch	8
Interventricular septal defect	7
Tetralogy of Fallot	4 (cyanotic)
Interatrial septal defects	4
Persistent left cranial vena cava	4
Left A-V (mitral) valve defect	3
All other defects and anomalies	6

[a] From Patterson DF: Epidemiologic and genetic studies of congenital heart disease in the dog. *Circ. Res* 23:171–202, 1968.
[b] Based on 290 dogs having cardiovascular defects.

results from hypertrophy of the muscle in the wall of the right ventricle beneath the pulmonary valve. **Valvular pulmonary stenosis** is due to abnormal development of the cusps, with a resulting impediment to outflow from the right ventricle. **Subvalvular pulmonary stenosis** results from excessive fibrous tissue proliferation beneath the valve. Valvular stenosis is the most common form in dogs.

In animals with pulmonary stenosis the normally linear stream of blood flowing through the pulmonary valve during ventricular contraction is interrupted and blood is forced through a smaller orifice. This markedly increases the velocity of blood flow downstream from the site of narrowing. **Poststenotic turbulence** is produced, and causes a loud **systolic murmur**, which refers to an abnormal sound associated with ventricular contraction. In some cases the turbulence can be felt through the thoracic wall; this palpable tremor is called a cardiac thrill. After passing through the stenotic region, the high velocity stream of blood swirls in the pulmonary trunk. This puts increased pressure on the wall of the pulmonary trunk, causing it to dilate. Such chracteristic **poststenotic dilation** may be visible on radiographs. In addition, the increased resistence to pulmonary outflow caused by the stenosis

results in dilation of the right ventricle and hypertrophy of its wall.

Clinical signs may not occur in the puppy; however, onset of **right heart failure** usually occurs between 6 months and 3 yr of age. Typical signs of right heart failure include weakness, fatigue, dyspnea (difficult breathing) and venous congestion. The latter is characterized by systemic edema and ascites, which is an accumulation of fluid in the peritoneal cavity.

Pulmonary stenosis has been reported most frequently in the Beagle, in which strain it shows an inherited pattern of appearance. It is also found in above average frequency in the English Bulldog, Fox Terrier, Chihuahua, Samoyed, Old English Sheepdog and Miniature Schnauzer. It is much less common in the large domestic animals.

Aortic Stenosis

This narrowing of the systemic outflow (Fig. 12.14*B*) is usually caused by a proliferative thickening that forms a fibromuscular ring encircling the aortic outlet immediately below (proximal to) the aortic valve. Constriction in this location is called **subaortic** or **subvalvular aortic stenosis**. Less frequently, abnormal growth of the valves may result in **valvular aortic stenosis**.

Similar to pulmonic stenosis, a loud systolic murmur is produced on ventricular contraction. A poststenotic dilation eventually occurs in the ascending aorta distal to the valve. As a result of increased resistance to outflow, the left ventricle dilates and hypertrophies. Secondarily, the left atrium often becomes dilated. Clinical signs vary from none observed to chracteristic **left heart failure**, which includes pulmonary congestion and edema, panting, coughing and dyspnea. Insufficient aortic flow may produce syncope (fainting; loss of consciousness resulting from cerebral hypoxia) or, occasionally, convulsions. Sometimes dogs with this malformation appear normal and healthy, then die unexpectedly and suddenly. Surgery on this lesion has not been successful in dogs; most patients are managed medically.

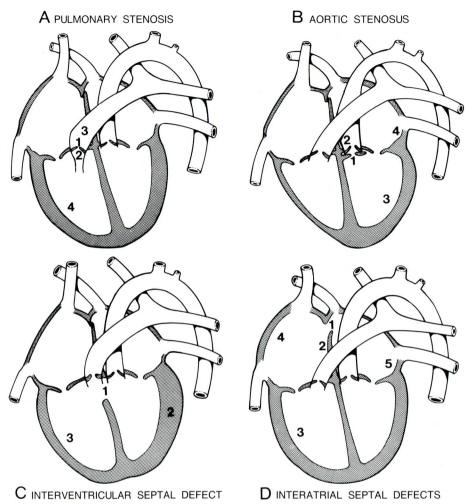

A PULMONARY STENOSIS B AORTIC STENOSUS

C INTERVENTRICULAR SEPTAL DEFECT D INTERATRIAL SEPTAL DEFECTS

Figure 12.14. Schematic representation of acyanotic cardiac malformations. *A*, Pulmonary stenosis, with the constrictions located at both valvular (*1*) and infundibular (*2*) levels. The characteristic poststenotic dilation of the pulmonary trunk (*3*) and right ventricular dilation and hypertrophy (*4*) are also indicated. *B*, aortic stenosis due to the formation of a fibrous subaortic ring (*1*). Poststenotic dilation of the ascending aorta (*2*), left ventricular dilation and hypertrophy (*3*) and left atrial dilation (*4*) often accompany this primary lesion. *C*, interventricular septal defect (*1*) with primary hypertrophy of the left ventricle (*2*) and secondary right ventricular dilation and hypertrophy (*3*). *D*, interatrial septal defects. As discussed in the text, there are many possible forms of this class of lesion. Shown here are an enlarged foramen secundum (*1*) and foramen ovale (*2*), with subsequent dilation and hypertrophy of the right ventricle (*3*), right atrium (*4*), and left atrium (*5*). Compare with Figure 12.13.

Aortic stenosis occurs in all domestic animals. In dogs, both Boxers and Newfoundlands may inherit the anomaly. It also occurs in unusually high frequency in German Shepherd, German Short-haired Pointer, Springer Spaniel, Fox Terrier and English Bulldog breeds. Note that some of these breeds also appear on the list of dogs susceptible to pulmonary stenosis. Among cats the Siamese have a higher incidence of aortic stenosis.

Interventricular Septal Defect

This malformation (Fig. 12.14*C*) is characterized by the presence of a small opening at the dorsal part of the I-V septum. The condition is caused by a deficient growth of one or more of the septa that normally close the interventricular foramen (I-V septum, left and right bulbar cushions, A-V endocardial cushions). At necropsy the defect is most commonly found under the septal cusp of the right A-V valve and, when viewed from the left side, in the left ventricular outlet; in this location it is referred to as a **subaortic I-V septal defect**.

When the defect is small the animal's physical condition may be normal. In fact, many bovine hearts are found to have small I-V septal defects at postmortem. In some instances there is a distinct systolic murmur caused by the turbulent forcing of blood through the defect from the left ventricle into the pulmonary trunk, and to a lesser extent the right ventricle, during ventricular contraction. Clinically, this condition usually presents features characteristic of left heart problems, often accompanied by pulmonary hypertension. Right ventricular dilation and hypertrophy also occur in severe cases. Often this septal defect is accompanied by other cardiac malformations, some of which probably arise secondarily. These produce cyanotic signs and will be discussed in the next section.

Interventricular septal defects are the most common cardiac malformation in the large domestic animals, and are especially frequent in cattle. Among dogs, it is most prevalent in the Siberian Husky. In the horse this condition is usually fatal prior to weaning; the same is true in cats.

Interatrial Septal Defects

As described earlier, animals with a patent foramen ovale in which the septum primum and septum secundum have not fused together but which are in all other respects normal, usually do not present any clinical abnormality. During atrial contraction the higher pressure on the left side forces the two septa together, thus preventing any left to right (or right to left) blood flow.

True interatrial septal defects (Fig. 12.14*D*) occur when the foramen ovale of the septum secundum overlies one (or more) openings in the septum primum. This can occur in any of several possible ways. If the foramen primum fails to close, the foramen ovale will overlap this opening. This condition, called **persistent foramen primum**, is often accompanied by abnormalities of the atrioventricular orifices resulting from de-

fective A-V endocardial cushion formation. More commonly the foramen secundum becomes greatly enlarged, which permits direct communication between the right and left atria. The condition is called **persistent foramen secundum**. It is common in these cases to find diminished growth of the septum secundum and subsequent enlargement of the foramen ovale.

Functionally the blood is shunted from left to right because of the higher left atrial pressure. The right heart is thus overloaded and overworked from the additional volume of blood it receives, and consequently dilation and hypertrophy of both right chambers results. The left heart often shows hypertrophic signs of overload in these animals. Thus, although right heart failure is the most acute result of an interatrial septal defect, all four chambers are effected.

Atrial septal defects have been reported in all domestic animals, but are extremely rare in horses. Among dog breeds it is more common in the Boxers and Samoyeds.

Left A-V Valve Defects

An abnormality in the development of the A-V endocardial cushions may lead to formation of valve cusps that are too short and do not fully close the left A-V orifice upon left ventricular contraction. Regurgitation of blood occurs upon systole, recognizable as a systolic murmur. This condition, called **left A-V valve insufficiency**, usually leads to left heart failure. It has been reported in all the domestic animals. In dogs it is most frequently found in the Keeshond, English Bulldog, Great Dane and Chihuahua.

Hypertophy of endocardial cushion tissues with subsequent closure of the left A-V orifice has also been reported. This leads to lack of left ventricular growth in utero, and is lethal at birth unless accompanied by other cardiac anomalies which permit some oxygenated blood to reach the systemic circulation. The term **left A-V (mitral) atresia** is used to describe this condition.

Ectopia Cordis

Ectopia of the heart is an anomaly of cardiac location rather than of internal organization. In this condition, which is most frequently reported in cattle, the heart is usually located in the neck region (**ectopia cordis cervicalis**). Normally the bovine fetal heart shifts into the thorax late in the 6th week of gestation, following which the thoracic inlet becomes surrounded by developing ribs. Delay in the onset of cardiac descent may result in it being trapped in a prethoracic location. In these calves the development of the great vessels may be anomalous but still compatible with normal growth.

Occasionally the paired sternal bars will not fuse to form a common sternum. In these cases the heart may be located ventrally outside the thorax, a condition called **ectopia cordis thoracis.**

Spiral Septal Defect

Incomplete development of the spiral septum can occur focally in the aortic sac (aorticopulmonary septum), truncus arteriosus or bulbus cordis, resulting in a small opening between the pulmonary trunk and the aorta. The clinical signs are similar to those of patent ductus arteriosis (PDA), with a left-to-right shunt of blood usually occurring. Complete failure of all these septal components to form results in the retention of a common truncus arteriosus; this cyanotic malformation will be discussed in the following section.

An aorticopulmonary septal defect can be experimentally caused in birds by surgically extirpating the primordium of the neural crest at the level of the first two somites. Normally it is this population of crest cells that forms the connective tissues in the walls of the 4th and 6th aortic arches.

Other Acyanotic Malformations

Aberrant pulmonary veins is a rare malformation in which the pulmonary veins grow out of the right rather than the left atrium. Usually both the left atrium and left ventricle are hypoplastic, and the period of survival after birth is very short. In order to survive postnatally a shunt must persist between the left and right sides in order that oxygenated blood can reach the systemic circulation.

Cor triloculare biatriatum and **cor triloculare biventriculare** are three-chambered heart conditions characterized by a single ventricle or single atrium, respectively. These are rare but have been reported in cattle and, in the second situation, in pigs. In both these anomalies there is considerable mixing of oxygenated and nonoxygenated blood, and both can produce cyanosis if the animal is stressed.

Dextrocardia is a "mirror image" heart that may occur as an isolated defect or with a complete **situs inversus** (all organ systems reversed). In this anomaly the left and right chambers are on opposite sides of the heart from normal, and the ductus arteriosus, aortic arch and pulmonary veins form on the right. This condition is compatible with normal health.

CYANOTIC HEART MALFORMATIONS

Most cyanotic cardiac malformations include the following two deviations from the normal intracardiac blood flow: (*a*) a venoatrial shunt, such that flow between right and left sides of the heart, can occur; and (*b*) an impediment to pulmonary trunk outflow.

Tetralogy of Fallot

This condition (Fig. 12.15*A*) is the most frequently encountered cyanotic malformation in domestic animals and humans. It is characterized by four lesions; three of these are primary, one is secondary. The primary defects consist of (*a*) an I-V septal defect, (*b*) pulmonary stenosis, and (*c*) **dextroaorta,** which means that the opening to the aortic outlet is shifted abnormally to the right. These all can be traced back to a single abnormality in the development of the proximal bulbar cushions. If these form so that the bulbar septum is displaced ventrally and to the right, the pulmonary outlet would be reduced in size. The aortic outlet would be larger than normal and partially override the plane in which the I-V septum was forming

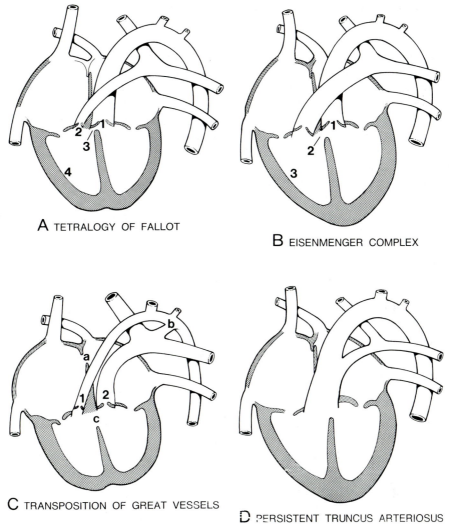

A TETRALOGY OF FALLOT

B EISENMENGER COMPLEX

C TRANSPOSITION OF GREAT VESSELS

D PERSISTENT TRUNCUS ARTERIOSUS

Figure 12.15. Schematic representation of cyanotic cardiac malformations. *A*, tetralogy of Fallot, which is characterized by dextroaorta (*1*), pulmonary stenosis (*2*), I-V septal defect (*3*) and dilation and hypertrophy of the right ventricle (*4*). *B*, Eisenmenger complex with dextroaorta (*1*), I-V septal defect (*2*) and right ventricular dilation with hypertrophy (*3*). *C*, transposition of the great vessels with the aorta (*1*) emanating from the right ventricle and the pulmonary trunk (*2*) from the left ventricle. In order for the animal to survive postnatally there must be one or more shunts allowing mixing of the left and right circulations. Possible shunts could occur as a result of an interatrial septal defect (*a*), a patent ductus arteriosus (*b*) and/or an I-V septal defect (*c*). *D*, persistent truncus arteriosus. In this situation both ventricles are of equal size.

(dextroaorta). This deviation would also prevent the normal closure of the I-V foramen.

Pulmonic stenosis causes resistance to flow from the right ventricle, which consequently dilates and hypertrophies. This is exaggerated by the left-to-right flow of left ventricular blood. The resulting right ven-

tricular hypertrophy is the fourth lesion characteristic of this tetralogy. Because of the dextroaorta, some unoxygenated blood in the right ventricle enters the aorta. When right ventricular hypertrophy is sufficient for the pressure generated in the right ventricle to equal or exceed left ventricular pressure, more of the unoxygenated blood will pass into the aorta, resulting in cyanosis. Many of these animals show such marked hypoplasia of the pulmonary arteries that enlargement of the bronchoesophageal artery is necessary to provide the lungs with blood.

Signs of this malformation usually occur in the young animal. Limited exercise will often elicit marked cyanosis. Poor growth, fatigue, dyspnea on exercise, and occasionally episodic syncope may accompany the cyanosis.

This malformation can be diagnosed using angiography. Dye injected into the right ventricle simultaneously fills the aorta and the pulmonary trunk. Surgical correction in humans has been performed by creating an artificial ductus arteriosus. This is done by anastomosing the aorta or the left subclavian artery to the pulmonary trunk.

Tetralogy of Fallot is found in most domestic animals, more commonly in ruminants and dogs, and has been proved to be inherited in the Keeshond. It is one of several cardiac anomalies found in this breed, although their appearance does not follow simple mendelian distribution.

Eisenmenger Complex

This anomaly (Fig. 12.15*B*) is similar to tetralogy of Fallot except that pulmonic stenosis does not occur. The primary defects include a slight dextroaorta and a large interventricular septal defect. Developmentally, this condition is thought to result from hypoplasia of the proximal bulbar ridges. The higher systemic pressure in the left ventricle causes blood to flow left to right through the I-V septal defect. This additional source of blood causes the right ventricle to dilate and hypertrophy, which constitutes the third and secondarily acquired lesion of this complex.

Without pulmonary stenosis there is no impediment to pulmonary outflow. In fact, the lung vessels become irritated from the large volume of high pressure circulation. In time this irritation results in obstructive lesions forming within the pulmonary vascular bed. The increased resistance to pulmo-

nary circulation is called **pulmonary hypertension.** Resistance often increases until the right ventricular pressure exceeds that of the left ventricle. When this occurs the flow of blood through the I-V septal defect will be reversed. Unoxygenated blood will then enter the aorta resulting in cyanosis.

Right Atrioventricular Stenosis or Atresia

Narrowing or obliteration of the right atrioventricular orifice is rare but has been reported in the dog, cat and horse. The right ventricle fails to expand normally, and the right atrium is enlarged. When atresia (total obstruction) occurs, both interatrial and I-V septal defects must be present for the animal to survive postnatally. The interatrial defect supplies the venoarterial shunt, while a persistent I-V foramen permits some left ventricular blood to enter the pulmonary trunk.

Transposition of Great Vessels

Reversal of pulmonary and systemic outflows (Fig. 12.15*C*) is rare, but has been observed in a Holstein calf and been reported in pigs. Failure of the aorticopulmonary and truncobulbar septa to develop in a spiral will cause the 4th aortic arches to connect with the right ventricle and the 6th aortic arches with the left ventricle. In this condition the ventricles are of the same size and generate comparable pressures. Since the systemic and pulmonary circulations are each separate and closed in this condition, the presence of a left-right shunt elsewhere in the heart is necessary for postnatal survival.

Persistent Truncus Arteriosus

In this malformation (Fig. 12.15*D*) the spiral septum completely fails to develop. The interventricular septum is developed, but, as would be predicted, an interventricular foramen persists. Both oxygenated and nonoxygenated blood mix upon leaving the heart through the common truncus. If pulmonary flow is adequate and no resistance is encountered, cyanosis will be minimal. Usually the pulmonary arteries are hypoplastic, restricting pulmonary flow and producing cyanosis. This condition has been reported in dogs and pigs, and is usually lethal within a few days or weeks of birth.

Persistent Atrioventricular Canal

This condition results from a failure of the A-V endocardial cushions to fuse together. Thus, the left and right A-V orifices do not become separated. Persistence of the foramen primum and the interventricular foramen also occurs.

Bibliography

NORMAL HEART DEVELOPMENT

Burlingame PL, Long JA: The development of the heart in the rat. Univ Calif *Publ Zool* 43:249–320, 1939.

Field EJ: The early development of the sheep heart. *J Anat* 80:75–88, 1946.

Girgis A: The development of the heart in the rabbit. *Proc Zool Soc* (London) 49:755–782, 1930.

Huntington GS: *The Anatomy and Development of the Systemic Lymphatic Vessels in the Domestic Cat.* Philadelphia, Lippincott, 1911.

Manasek FJ: Heart development: interactions involved in cardiac morphogenesis. In Poste G, Nicolson GL (eds): *The Cell Surface in Animal Embryogenesis and Development.* Amsterdam, Elsevier/North-Holland Biomedical Press, 1976.

McBride RE, Moore GW, Hutchins GM: Development of the outflow tract and closure of the interventricular septum in the normal human heart. *Am J Anat* 160:309–331, 1981.

Morrill CV: On the development of the atrial septum and the valvular apparatus in the right atrium of the pig embryo, with a note on the fenestration of the anterior cardinal veins. *Am J Anat* 20:351–373, 1916.

Oliveira P, et al: Observaciones anatomicas sobre el cierre del foramen oval en el perro (dog). *Anat Hist Embryol* 9:321–324, 1980.

Ottaway CW: The anatomical closure of the foramen ovale in the equine and bovine heart: a comparative study with observations on the foetal and adult states. *Br Vet J* 100:111–118 and 130–134, 1944.

Patten BM: *Embryology of the Pig*, ed 3. New York, Blakiston, 1948.

Rosenquist GC, Bergsma D: (eds): *Morphogenesis and Malformation of the Cardiovascular System.* New York, AR Liss, 1978.

Schulte HVonW: The fusion of the cardiac analagen and the formation of the cardiac loop in the cat (*Felis domestica*). *Am J Anat* 20:45–72, 1916.

Thompson RP, Fitzharris TP: Morphogenesis of the truncus arteriosus of the chick embryo heart: the formation and migration of mesenchymal tissue. *Am J Anat* 154:545–556, 1979.

van Mierop LHS, Patterson DF, Schnarr WR: Hereditary conotruncal septal defects in Keeshond dogs. *Am J Cardiol* 40:936–950, 1977. (Note: contains an excellent account of septation in the canine embryonic heart.)

Vitums A: The embryonic development of the equine heart. *Zbl Vet Med C Anat Histol Embryol* 10:193–211, 1981.

REVIEWS OF MALFORMATIONS

Bayly WM, Reed SM, Leathers CW, Brown CM, Traub JL, Paradis MR, Palmer GH: Multiple congenital heart anomalies in five Arabian foals. *JAVMA* 181:684–689, 1982.

Detweiler DK, Patterson DF: Congenital heart disease. In Kirk RW (ed): *Current Veterinary Therapy II.* Philadelphia, Saunders, 1966.

Hsu FS, Du SJ: Congenital heart diseases in swine. *Vet Pathol* 19:676–686, 1982.

Jackson BT: The pathogenesis of congenital cardiovascular anomalies. *N Engl J Med* 279:25–29, and 80–89, 1968.

Kemler AG, Martin JE: Incidence of congenital cardiac defects in bovine fetuses. *Am J Vet Res* 3:249–251, 1972.

Okamoto N: *Congenital Anomalies of the Heart.* Tokyo, Igaku-Shoin, 1980.

Patterson DF: Clinical and epidemiological studies of congenital heart disease in dogs. *JAVMA Proc* 100:128–135, 1963.

Patterson DF: Congenital heart disease in the dog. *Ann NY Acad Sci* 127:541–569, 1965.

Patterson DF: Canine congenital heart disease: epidemiology and etiological hypotheses. *J Small Anim Prac* 12:263–287, 1971.

Rooney JR, Franks WC: Congenital cardiac anomalies in horses. *Pathol Vet* 1:454–464, 1964.

Sandusky GE, Smith CW: Congenital cardiac anomalies in calves. *Vet Rec* 108:163–165, 1981.

Van de Linde-Sipman JS, et al: Congenital heart anomalies in the cat. A description of 16 cases. *Zbl Vet Med* A20:419–425, 1973.

PULMONARY AND AORTIC STENOSIS, VALVULAR DEFECTS

Carmichael JA, et al: A case of canine subaortic stenosis and aortic valvular insufficiency with particular reference to diagnostic technique. *J Small Anim Prac* 9:213–233, 1968.

Hamlin RL, Harris SG: Mitral incompetence in Great Dane pups. *JAVMA* 154:790–794, 1969.

Hamlin RL, Smetzer DL, Smith CR: Congenital mitral insufficiency in the dog. *JAVMA* 146:1088–1100, 1965.

Howe RS: Pulmonic stenosis in a cat. *J Am Anim Hosp Assoc* 17:777–782, 1981.

Krahwinkel DJ, Jr, Coogan PS: Endocardial fibroelastosis in a Great Dane pup. *JAVMA* 159:327–331, 1971.

Liu Si-K: Supravalvular aortic stenosis with deformity of the aortic valve in a cat. *JAVMA* 152:55–59, 1968.

Lord PF, Wood A, Liu S, Tilley LP: Left ventricular angiocardiography in congenital mitral valve insufficiency of the dog. *JAVMA* 166:1069–1073, 1975.

Ott BS, et al: Diagnosis and surgical repair of congenital pulmonary stenosis in the dog. *JAVMA* 144:851–856, 1964.

Ross JN, Jr: Diagnosis and surgical correction of patent ductus arteriosus and pulmonic stenosis in the dog. In Kirk RW (ed): *Current Veterinary Therapy III.* Philadelphia, Saunders, 1968.

Tashjian RJ, et al: Isolated pulmonic valvular stenosis in a dog. *JAVMA* 135:94–102, 1959.

Van der Linde-Sipman JS, Van der Luer RJT, Stokhof AA, Volvekamp WThC: Congenital subvalvular pulmonic stenosis in a cat. *Vet Pathol* 17:640–643, 1980.

Weirich WE, Blevins WE, Conrad CR, Ruth GR, Gallina AM: Congenital tricuspid insufficiency in a dog. *JAVMA* 164:1025, 1974.

Will JA: Subvalvular pulmonary stenosis and aorticopulmonary septal defect in the cat. *JAVMA* 154:913–916, 1969.

INTERVENTRICULAR AND INTERATRIAL SEPTAL
DEFECTS

Belling TH, Jr: Ventricular septal defect in the bovine heart—report of 3 cases. *JAVMA* 138:595–598, 1961.

Braden TD, et al: Correction of a ventricular septal defect in a dog. *JAVMA* 161:507–512, 1972.

Breznock EM: Spontaneous closure of ventricular septal defects in the dog. *JAVMA* 162:399–402, 1973.

Breznock EM, et al: Surgical correction of an interventricular septal defect in a dog. *JAVMA* 157:1343–1353, 1970.

Breznock EM, et al: Surgical correction using hypothermia of an interventricular septal defect in the dog. *JAVMA* 158:1391–1400, 1971.

Fisher EW, Pirie HM: Malformations of the ventricular septal complex in cattle. *Br Vet J* 120:253–272, 1964.

Hamlin RL, et al: Ostium secundum type interatrial septal defects in the dog. *JAVMA* 143:149–157, 1963.

Hamlin RL, et al: Interventricular septal defect in the dog. *JAVMA* 145:331–340, 1964.

Knauer KW, McMullan WC, Clark DR: Diagnosis of an interventricular septal defect in a horse. *Vet Med* 68:75–78, 1973.

Parry BW, Wrigley RH, Reuter RE: Ventricular septal defects in three familially-related female Saanen goats. *Aus Vet J* 59/3:72–77, 1982.

Scarrott, WK, et al: Ventricular septal defects in two goats. *Cornell Vet* 74:136–145, 1984.

OTHER ACYANOTIC MALFORMATIONS

Bowen JM, Adrian RW: Ectopia cordis in cattle. *JAVMA* 141:1162–1167, 1962.

Carrig CB, et al: Primary dextrocardia with situs inversus associated with sinusitis and bronchitis in a dog. *JAVMA* 154:1127–1133, 1974.

Milledge RD, et al: Physiologic and radiographic studies of cervical ectopia cordis in a calf. *JAVMA* 152:161–167, 1968.

Vacirca G, et al: Ectopia cordis cervicalis in a calf. Clinical and radiography study. *Clin Vet* 94:382–391, 1971.

Vitums A: Ectopic heart of a shorthorn bull. *Anat Anz*

114:48–61, 1964.

TETRALOGY OF FALLOT

Bolton GR, Ettinger SJ, Liu Si-K: Tetralogy of Fallot in three cats. *JAVMA* 160:1622–1631, 1972.

Bush M, et al: Tetralogy of Fallot in a cat. *JAVMA* 161:1679–1686, 1972.

Clark DR, et al: Tetralogy of Fallot in the dog. *JAVMA* 152:462–471, 1968.

Hamlin RL, et al: Antemortem diagnosis of tetralogy of Fallot in a dog. *JAVMA* 140:948–953, 1962.

Lacuata AQ, Yamada H, Hirose T, Yanagiua G: Tetralogy of Fallot in a heifer. *JAVMA* 178:830–836, 1981.

Lourens DC, van Heerden J: Tetralogy of Fallot in a two-and-one-half-year-old cat. *J Am Anim Hosp Assoc* 17:129–130, 1981.

Prickett ME, Reeves JJ, Zent WW: Tetralogy of Fallot in a thoroughbred foal. *JAVMA* 162:552–555, 1973.

Reef VB, Hattel AL: Echocardiographic detection of tetralogy of Fallot and myocardial abscess in a calf. *Cornell Vet* 74:81–95, 1984.

van Mierop LHS, Patterson DF: The pathogenesis of spontaneously occurring anomalies of the ventricular outflow tract in Keeshond dogs: embryologic studies. In Rosenquist GC, Bergsma D (eds): *Morphogenesis and Malformation of the Cardiovascular System.* New York, AR Liss, 1978, pp 361–375.

EISENMENGER'S COMPLEX, EISENMENGER'S
SYNDROME

Feldman EC, et al: Eisenmenger's syndrome in the dog: case reports. *J Am Anim Hosp Assoc* 17:477–483, 1981.

Fisher EW, et al: An Eisenmenger complex in an Ayrshire heifer. *Vet Rec* 74:447–452, 1962.

Sass B, Albert TF: A case of Eisenmenger complex in a calf. *Cornell Vet* 60:61–65, 1970.

OTHER CYANOTIC MALFORMATIONS

Liu Si-K: Persistent common atrioventricular canal in two cats. *JAVMA* 153:556–562, 1968.

Turk JR, et al: Double outlet right ventricle in a dog. *J Am Anim Hosp Assoc* 17:789–792, 1981.

Van Nie CJ: The ostium atrioventriculare commune persistens in animals. *Tijdschr Diergeneeskd* 88:205–211, 1963.

Vitums A, Grant BD, Stone EC, Spencer GR: Transposition of the aorta and atresia of the pulmonary trunk in a horse. *Cornell Vet* 63:41–57, 1973.

CHAPTER 13

Cardiovascular System III: Venous System and Lymphatics

The initial embryonic origin of venous endothelial cells has not been verified. Although the existence of angiogenic cords is often assumed, there is little direct evidence that the major intraembryonic veins develop from these precursors. Later, discrete venous channels form by the coalescing of isolated endothelial vesicles. Frequently, drainage from a particular region of the embryo will be accomplished by a plexus of small venous channels and only later, as muscles and skeletal and visceral tissues are forming, is a single channel selected. It is generally believed that selection of the definitive venous channel is the result of blood flow being increased along whichever pathway offers the least resistance.

Three pairs of venous channels drain into the sinus venosus in the early embryo: the **vitelline** (omphalomesenteric) and **umbilical veins**, and the **cardinal veins**. The latter set are intraembryonic, the others bring blood from the extraembryonic circulation into the heart. Initially these all are bilaterally symmetrical, but as a result of unequal patterns of vascular degeneration this symmetry is lost.

VITELLINE VENOUS SYSTEM

In the early embryo a pair of **vitelline veins** courses from the yolk sac into the **septum transversum** where they anastomose with those parts of the cardiac primordium that will later fuse and form the sinus venosus (Fig. 13.1). Intraembryonically the vitelline veins may be subdivided into proximal (cranial), middle and distal (caudal) parts, each of which subsequently develops differently.

The proximal part of each vitelline vein is located between the sinus venosus and the septum transversum after these two tissues separate. The LEFT proximal vitelline vein atrophies. On the RIGHT this segment is retained and forms the **hepatic** segment of the **caudal vena cava**.

The middle parts of the vitelline system become subdivided into numerous small channels within the liver. This transformation is brought about by the rapid proliferation of epithelial cords of hepatic tissue. The small vascular channels formed in this plexus are called **hepatic sinusoids;** they drain into **hepatocardiac channels** and then into the hepatic part of the **caudal vena cava**.

The distal part of the vitelline system, located in splanchnic mesoderm between the liver and the umbilical stalk, forms many branches. These establish a series of anastomosing channels passing around the developing duodenum both dorsally and, later, ventrally. Although some of these channels are transient, others are retained and form

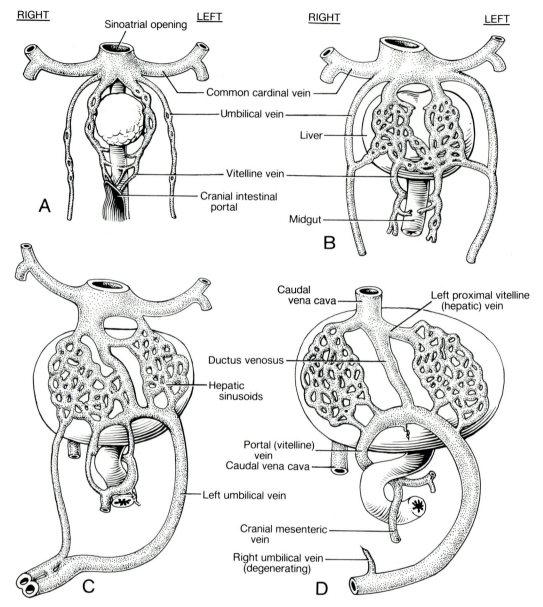

Figure 13.1. Development of intraembryonic vitelline and umbilical veins in the pig, shown in schematic ventral views of embryos at approximately *A*, 3- to 4-mm, *B*, 6-mm, *C*, 8- to 9-mm, and *D*, 20-mm stages. (Redrawn from Patten, 1948.)

most of the **portal venous system** and its branches.

UMBILICAL VENOUS SYSTEM

Early in development, paired **umbilical veins** pass from the allantois through the umbilical cord, then along the ventral body wall to the septum transversum. As the hepatic sinusoids are forming, anastomoses are established between the umbilical veins and hepatic sinusoids. Subsequently, the umbilical system cranial to these anastomoses degenerates, as shown in Figure 13.1 *B* and *C*. Increased flow of blood from the placenta to the liver results in the enlargement of these anastomoses on the LEFT side, while on the right the entire umbilical vein atrophies. The large vascular channel between the left umbilical vein and the hepatic part of the caudal vena cava is the **ductus venosus.**

Formation of the ductus venosus allows oxygenated blood from placental vessels to flow directly through the liver to the heart. This channel persists until birth in carnivores, ruminants, and primates. However, it disappears during gestation in the pig and horse, necessitating that the umbilical venous blood pass through the liver parenchyma in these species. Two umbilical veins pass through most of the length of the umbilical cord of carnivores and ruminants; these join to form the left umbilical vein before entering the body of the embryo.

The umbilical circulation ceases at birth. Concomitantly, spasmotic contractions of the wall of the umbilical vein cause constriction and subsequent occlusion of this vessel. This process is usually completed by the third postnatal week. In ruminants and the horse the umbilical cord and umbilicus are also ensheathed with smooth muscle, which contracts in response to stretching of the cord at parturition.

After birth that part of the umbilical vein which coursed through the ventral mesogastrium disappears, although vestiges of it may be found in the **falciform ligament** between the ventral midline of the body wall and the liver. In young puppies remnants of this vessel are often found in the **round ligament of the liver,** located in the free edge of the falciform ligament between the quadrate and left hepatic lobes. In carnivores and ruminants the ductus venosus becomes obliterated soon after birth; vestiges may remain in the form of the **ligamentum venosum.** Small parts of the original umbilical veins contribute to the intrahepatic part of the portal vein.

CARDINAL VENOUS SYSTEM

The large **cranial** and smaller **caudal cardinal veins**, which enter the sinus venosus via the **common cardinal veins,** arise early in development as an intraembryonic venous system. Transformations of these paired vessels, plus retention of parts of new cardinal vessels arising in conjunction with development of the intermediate mesoderm, establish the major venous channels.

Cranial Cardinal Veins

Cranial to the heart region the **cranial cardinal veins** are retained as the **internal jugular veins** and their branches. With growth of the first visceral arch and other components of the face, a branch of each cranial cardinal, the **external jugular vein,** appears. The **subclavian veins** arise as branches of the caudal cardinal veins near their junctions with the common cardinals. However, as shown in Figure 13.2, descent of the heart and elongation of the thorax result in the site of branching being shifted cranially, in the same manner as described for the subclavian arteries (Chapter 11).

Up until this stage the cranial cardinal venous system is bilaterally symmetrical. Following the formation of an anastomotic channel connecting the right and left cranial cardinal veins, the proximal part of the left cranial cardinal atrophies (Fig. 13.2 *B* and *C*). Both cranial cardinal veins now enter the **right common cardinal vein.** The anastomotic branch becomes the **left brachiocephalic vein.** In the neonate it is formed by the union of the external jugular vein and subclavian vein, and the internal jugular is considered a branch of this. The short **right brachiocephalic vein** is formed by the right cranial cardinal between the junction of the right external jugular and right subclavian veins and the attachment of the anastomotic branch (left brachiocephalic vein). The two brachiocephalic veins join to form the **cranial vena cava,** which is derived from the proximal part of the right cranial cardinal and the right comon cardinal veins.

Caudal Cardinal, Subcardinal and Supracardinal veins

Most of the venous drainage of the body wall, pelvic limbs axial muscles and viscera is formed from the cardinal venous network. During the course of embryonic development, three pairs of cardinal veins form in the trunk.

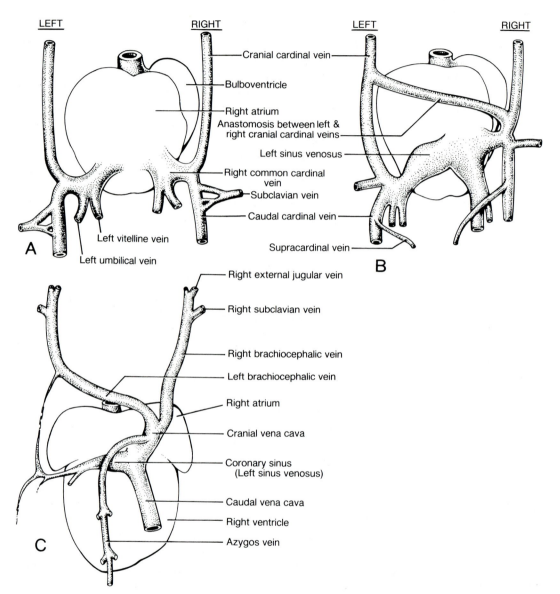

Figure 13.2. Schematic dorsal views of three stages in the development of the cranial cardinal veins and sinus venosus. The azygos vein is shown branching from the right caudal cardinal, as occurs in most domestic animals. In the pig and horse it branches from the left side, and is found branching from the coronary sinus in the adult. Note the cranial displacement of the subclavian veins.

The **caudal cardinal veins** (Fig. 13.3A) are the first to form and are evolutionarily the most primitive. They appear early in the intermediate mesoderm dorsal to the mesonephric duct (see Fig. 1.6). Subsequently the intermediate mesoderm on each side in the thoracolumbar region hypertrophies and forms the mesonephros, which functions as a kidney during part of fetal development in mammals and birds. Within this tissue are formed two bilateral sets of veins, the **subcardinals** and, later, the **supracardinals**. Their names indicate their original position relative to the caudal cardinal: the subcardinal veins are in the ventromedial part of the mesonephros, the supracardinal veins in the dorsal part of the organ. Both of these join the caudal cardinal veins near the heart. Caudally, the caudal cardinal vein shifts laterally and is found in the tissue of the body wall.

As the mesonephros develops and, later in gestation, regresses (when the definitive, metanephric kidney becomes functional), a major transformation of these three cardinal venous pathways of the trunk occurs. As a result of differential growth, fusion and degeneration, there is formed a **caudal vena cava** that incorporates portions of all these vessels. On the left side the cranial part of the caudal cardinal vein atrophies at its junction with the left common cardinal, which becomes the great cardiac vein and coronary sinus. However, the cranial part of the right caudal cardinal vein persists as the proximal part of the **azygos vein** (Fig. 13.2 *B* and *C*), joining the cranial vena cava in the horse, dog and cat. The remainder of the azygos vein is derived from the right supracardinal vein. In the ox and pig the azygos vein develops on the left side, as shown in Figure 13.3 *D* and *E*. It is derived from the left supracardinal vein, distally, and the left caudal cardinal vein proximally, plus the left common cardinal. This left azygos enters the right atrium via the coronary sinus.

Branches of the caudal part of the caudal cardinal veins include both the **iliac veins,** which drain the pelvic limbs and nearby tissues, and several anastomoses forming across the midline between them (Fig. 13.3 *C* and *D*). After the supracardinal veins join the caudal cardinals slightly cranial to the iliacs (Fig. 13.3*D*), the caudal cardinals degenerate except for the short segment between iliac and supracardinal veins.

Many anastomoses form between the right and left subcardinal veins (Fig. 13.3 *B* and *C*); these coalesce to form a large median **subcardinal sinus.** In addition a channel develops between the right subcardinal vein and the proximal part of the right vitelline vein (see Fig. 18.5). As a result blood from the embryonic kidneys (mesonephroi) enters the subcardinal veins, then is collected in a large subcardinal sinus and flows into the right vitelline vein, which is the proximal part of the caudal vena cava.

Initially there are many anastomoses in the mesonephros between subcardinal and caudal cardinal veins, seen best in a lateral view (Fig. 13.4). When the latter degenerate many of these channels are retained and are joined by branches from the supracardinals (Fig. 13.3*C*). Those branches which drain the adrenal and renal (metanephric kidney) tissues are retained in the adult.

The left subcardinal vein degenerates cranial to the subcardinal sinus, while the right subcardinal persists between the sinus and its anastomosis with the right vitelline vein. Caudally, part of the subcardinal veins are retained and form the **testicular** or **ovarian veins.** The definitive (metanephric) kidneys form caudal to the mesonephroi, and their drainage is facilitated by branches of the subcardinal-supracardinal anastomoses.

The **supracardinal veins** are paired veins that join with the remnants of the caudal cardinal veins both cranially near the common cardinal veins and caudally near the iliac veins. They form numerous intersegmental branches and also establish several anastomoses with the subcardinal veins and sinus.

Most of the **left supracardinal vein** degenerates soon after forming. Vestiges of it are represented only in those animals in which a left azygos vein is present. The **right supracardinal vein** degenerates cranial to its

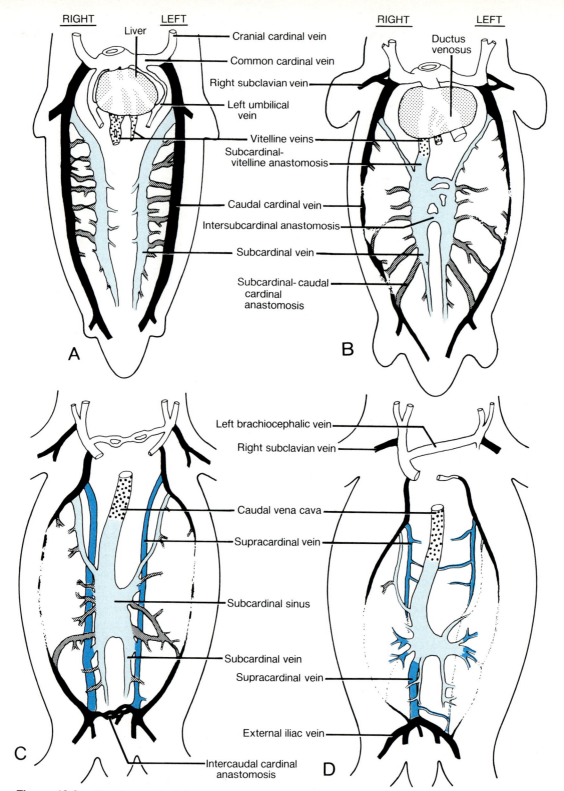

Figure 13.3. Development of the caudal vena cava and its branches in the pig, shown in ventral views. Note that the caudal cardinal (*black*), subcardinal (*light blue*), supracardinal (*dark blue*), vitelline (*stippled*), and various anastomoses between these all contribute to this major systemic vein. Since these anastomoses are difficult to trace in the embryonic mesonephros, there is considerable disagreement concerning the precise origins of veins draining the adrenal, kidney and gonads. *A*, 6-mm; *B*, 10-mm; *C*, 16- to 19-mm; *D*, 22- to 24-mm; and *E*, adult stages. (Redrawn with modifications from Patten, 1948.)

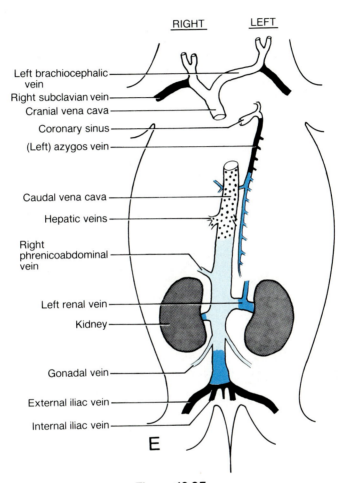

Figure 13.3*E*.

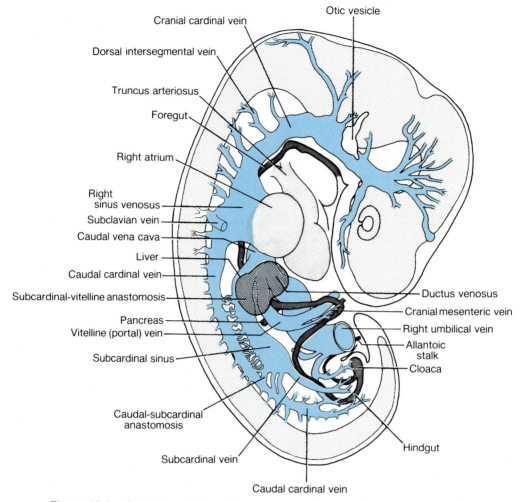

Figure 13.4. Right lateral view of the venous system of a 9.4-mm canine embryo.

anastomosis with the subcardinal sinus. The distal part of the azygos vein (right azygos if a pair are present) represents the only remains of the cranial part of the supracardinal vein. Caudally the right supracardinal is retained as the venous channel joining the iliac veins (caudal cardinal) to the rest of the caudal vena cava.

As a result of the events just described, blood flowing from the pelvic limbs would pass through the following vessels upon leaving the external iliac veins:

Adult vessel	*Embryonic components*
Common iliac vein	1. Interiliac anastomosis
	2. Caudal cardinal veins

Caudal vena cava

3. Right caudal cardinal veins
4. Right supracardinal vein
5. Right supracardinal-subcardinal anastomosis
6. Subcardinal sinus
7. Right subcardinal vein
8. Right subcardinal-right vitelline anastomosis
9. Right vitelline vein
10. Right sinus venosus

Right atrium

This circuitous route to arrive at a single major vein, the **caudal vena cava,** may appear to be unnecessarily complicated. However, it is in fact a quite conservative series of modifications on phylogenetically primitive patterns. The caudal cardinals and common cardinals are, both ontogenetically and phylogenetically, the earliest and most primitive veins of the trunk. This simple paired system is still present in the lamprey.

During the early evolution of some fishes, greater efficiency of kidney function was obtained by establishing separate venous channels flowing into the renal tissues. Such a venous system is called a **renal portal** network, and it permits greater contact between the nephric capsule and the circulatory system. The separate collecting veins that arose were the subcardinals. Gradually these assumed a greater role in carrying blood cranially, and the caudal cardinal veins became atretic cranially. Although it is not known why the vascular flow through certain vessels becomes diminished and augmented through others, it is clear that once a particular pathway has become evolutionarily reduced it cannot be "resurrected" in a later evolving species. The first two stages in caudal vena cava formation shown in Figure 13.3 are found in extant fishes. The supracardinal veins are the most recent to appear, and it is not known what (if any) their phylogenetic antecedents were.

The above scenario is teleological. Even less is known about the forces which affect the evolution of a complex set of structures than about their embryonic development. At issue is a fundamental problem in morphogenesis. Namely, what is the relationship between a gene or a set of genes or a class of gene products, and the elaboration of a pair of veins, of a limb from a limb field, or of a skull. The results of evolutionary pressures and selection are readily visible in the animal families; the mechanisms by which preferred changes in patterns of growth and morphogenesis are accomplished in development are matters of conjecture more than understanding.

MALFORMATIONS OF THE VENOUS SYSTEM

The precise patterns of branching of veins can vary considerably from one animal to another. In most cases these are of no clinical significance; however, this variability must be appreciated whenever surgery of internal organs is being performed. For example, in approximately 30% of the dogs presented with a right aortic vascular ring, a left cranial vena cava is also present (Fig. 13.5). Since it usually loops ventrally around the pulmonary trunk and directly across the ligamentum arteriosum, which must be transected to alleviate the esophageal constriction, its presence must be considered in these patients.

Many variations in the pattern of venous drainage of the kidneys, adrenals and gonads have been reported in man and the domestic animals. It is possible to have two caudal vena cavae between the iliac veins and the kidneys; presumably these result from retention of the left as well as the right caudal supracardinal veins. The hepatic portal veins are paired in avian species.

Portasystemic Anomalies

If an anastomosis persists between the caudal part of the vitelline veins, which form the portal system, and any of the cardinal

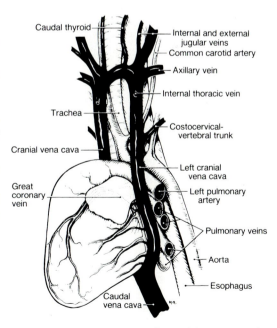

Figure 13.5. Persistent left cranial vena cava in a dog, left ventral view. (From Evans and Christensen, 1979.)

veins of the trunk, it can form a **portasystemic shunt**. In these cases one or several vessels connect the portal vein to the caudal vena cava or the azygos vein. Much of the blood which would normally enter the capillary plexus of the hepatic parenchyma, where potential toxic metabolic waste products are removed, goes instead directly to the heart.

Occasionally the ductus venosus persists and acts as a portacaval shunt within the liver parenchyma. Also, anastomoses between portal and systemic veins may arise in older animals in conjunction with chronic liver disease, such as cirrhosis or hepatitis.

Congenital portasystemic shunts are most frequently encountered in cats and dogs, but have been reported in calves and horses.

CASE STUDY

Signalment: A 3-month-old male English Springer Spaniel.

Chief complaint: Abnormal behavior.

History: A week before examination this puppy became depressed and walked aimlessly, often bumping into objects. He was disoriented and snapped at the owner. The next day he acted normal, but 2 days later he collapsed and seizures occurred. These signs continued episodically for several days.

Examination: Initial examination showed profound depression, visual impairment, recumbency and inability to walk. Several hours later he walked but acted blind, and a few hours after that his vision and gait were normal.

FACTS	INTERPRETATIONS
Depression, aimless walking, blindness, seizures, disorientation	These are all signs of abnormal cerebral function
Normal gait	Normal function of peripheral nerves, spinal cord and caudal brain stem
Recumbency, inability to walk	Disturbed function of peripheral nerves, spinal cord or caudal brain stem
Fluctuating clinical signs	Suggests a metabolic disturbance rather than a structural lesion in the nervous system

Hypothesis: This dog could have a primary disturbance of its prosencephalon that could be due to a metabolic disorder such as hypoglycemia, hypoxia from inadequate cardiac outflow, or hyperammonemia from liver dysfunction.

Laboratory tests:

Normal blood glucose and cerebrospinal fluid	Clinical signs probably not due to hypoglycemia or inflammatory brain disease
Elevated alkaline phosphatase, delayed bromosulphalein clearance, low total serum protein, low serum albumin, ammonium biurate crystals in urine	Suggest abnormal liver function

Hypothesis: Clinical signs may be due to **hepatic encephalopathy** resulting from excessive ammonia and other metabolites not being metabolized by the liver. These cause abnormal functioning of neurons in the central nervous system, especially the cerebrum.

Portal venogram:

Radiopaque dye in portal vein enters caudal vena cava with very little found in liver (Fig. 13.6A)	Confirms a **portasystemic shunt**

Puppies and kittens with portasystemic shunts grow poorly and are often chronically ill. They exhibit neurological signs such as episodic seizures, head pressing, circling, vis-

ual impairment, and sometimes even episodes of stupor or viciousness. Most of these are indicative of abnormal cerebral function. The chronic illness is characterized by pe-

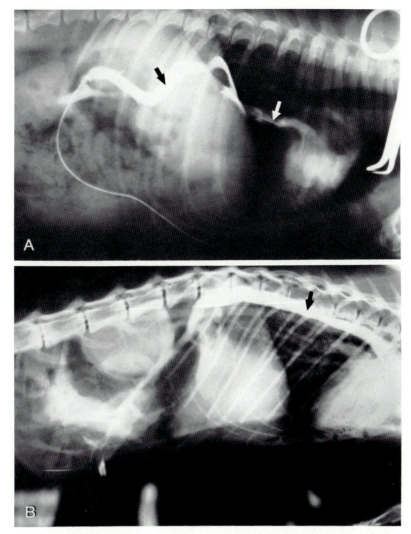

Figure 13.6.   Portasystemic shunts. *A*, shows a dog in which radiopaque dye was injected into the cranial mesenteric vein. Most of the contrast material passed through an abnormal shunt from the left gastric vein (*black arrow*) to the caudal vena cava (*white arrow*). *B*, is a cat in which dye injected into the cranial mesenteric vein passed into the azygos vein (*arrow*).

riods of anorexia (failure to eat), vomiting, diarrhea, intermittent fever, and occasionally polyuria (excessive urine output) and polydipsia (excessive thirst). Upon physical examination the liver may be difficult to palpate.

Although the exact cause of the neurological signs is not known, it is generally believed that they are related to high circulating levels of toxins, both from metabolic activity of the body's tissues and from intestinal flora. The best characterized of these is ammonia, which usually (but not always) is significantly elevated in the serum of affected animals.

Portal venography will confirm the clinical diagnosis of this disease. This may be performed by cannulation of an intestinal vein or the spleen, and injection of a radiopaque dye. If the dye directly enters either the caudal vena cava or the azygos vein (Fig. 13.6*B*) with only minimal opacification of the hepatic parenchyma, a portasystemic shunt is present.

Medical treatment consists of feeding a low protein diet and using an intestinal antibiotic to decrease enteric bacterial fermentation that produces ammonia. Surgical ligation of the shunt can be successful in those cases in which the normal hepatic portal vein and liver sinuses are present and patent.

A **persistent ductus venosus** has been reported in dogs. This also acts as a portasystemic shunt carrying portal venous blood directly to the caudal vena cava, bypassing the liver parenchyma. Portal venography will demonstrate this anomaly.

LYMPHATIC SYSTEM

The lymphatic system is derived from mesoderm and develops in parallel with many parts of the venous system. However, little is known about factors that control the assembly of these vessels or their pattern of branching. The branches of this system are closed; they collect fluids as well as macromolecules and discharge them into the venous circulation.

In the embryo, coalescence of the developing lymphatic channels forms six lymph sacs. The two large **jugular lymph sacs** at the thoracic inlet arise as outgrowths of the internal jugular vein. First visible in fetuses of about 10 mm in length, these connections persist in the adult animal. In addition there is one **retroperitoneal** lymph sac in the dorsal abdomen, the **cisterna chyli** in the dorsal abdomen and two **sciatic** lymph sacs for the pelvic limbs. Except for the cisterna chyli, these lymph sacs disappear in the late fetus.

Initially this is a bilateral system with lymph vessels from each pelvic limb and the abdomen entering the cisterna chyli. The cisterna is, in turn, drained by a pair of **thoracic ducts** that pass to the thoracic inlet, join with thoracic limb and head lymphatics, and connect to the venous system.

Lymph nodes develop along these lymphatic channels to filter the lymph. They are derived from the mesoderm adjacent to the lymphatics.

Congenital hereditary lymphedema has been reported in newborn puppies as an autosomal dominant inheritance of variable expression. Nonpainful pitting edema occurs in the limbs, and occasionally the trunk

and head. Lymphangiography has demonstrated malformed peripheral lymphatics consisting of an increase in the number, size and tortuosity of distal lymphatics associated with a failure of them to connect centrally. Lymph nodes may be absent. The condition may cause early death or slowly ameliorate by itself.

Fetal anasarca consists of diffuse subcutaneous edema at birth. Often the head and neck are most severely effected. It has been reported as due to an autosomal recessive gene in Ayshires and Swedish Lowland cattle. Also, it is a frequent result of teratological insult. Limited pathogenetic studies suggest that hypoplasia of lymph nodes and lymphatic endothelium may be one possible basis for this syndrome.

Bibliography

NORMAL DEVELOPMENT

Butler EG: The relative role played by the embryonic veins in the development of the mammalian vena cava posterior. *Am J Anat* 39:267–353, 1927.

Huntington GS, and McClure CFW: The development of the veins in the domestic cat. *Anat Rec* 20:1–30, 1920.

Lewis FT: The development of the lymphatic system in rabbits. *Am J Anat* 5:95–111, 1905.

Patten BM: *Embryology of the Pig.* Philadelphia, Blakiston, 1948.

Sabin FR: The origin and development of the lymphatic system. *Johns Hopkins Hospital Monographs, No. 5,* pp 1–94, 1913.

Sabin FR: On the fate of the posterior cardinal veins and their relation to the development of the vena cava and azygous in pig embryos. *Carnegie Inst Contrib Embryol* 3:5–32, 1915.

MALFORMATIONS

Barrett RE, de Lahunta A, Roenigk WJ, Hoffer RE, Coons FH: Five cases of congenital portacaval shunt in the dog. *J Small Anim Pract* 17:71, 1976.

Beech J, Dubielzig R, Bester R: Portal vein anomaly and hepatic encephalopathy in a horse. JAVMA 170:164–166, 1977.

Cornelius LM, Thrall DE, Halliwell WH, Frank GM, Kern AJ, Woods CB: Anomalous portosystemic anastomoses associated with chronic hepatic encephalopathy in six young dogs. JAVMA 167:220–228, 1975.

Ewing GO, Suter PF, Bailey CS: Hepatic insufficiency associated with congenital anomalies of the portal veins in dogs. *J Am Anim Hosp Ass* 10:463–476, 1974.

Keane D, Blackwell T: Hepatic encephalopathy associated with patent ductus venosus in a calf. JAVMA 182:1393–1394, 1983.

Levesque DC, Oliver JE, Cornelius LM, Mahaffey MB,

Rawlings CA, Wolata RJ: Congenital portacaval shunts in two cats: diagnosis and surgical correction. JAVMA 181:143–145, 1982.

Rothuizen J, Van den Ingh TS, Voorhout G, Van der Luer RJT, Wouda W: Congenital porto-systemic shunts in sixteen dogs and three cats. *J Sm Anim Pract* 23:67–81, 1982.

Sherdeng RG: Hepatic encephalopathy in the dog. *Compend Cont Ed* 1:53–63, 1979.

Strombeck DR, Weiser MG, Kaneko JJ: Hyperammonemia and hepatic encephalopathy in the dog. *JAVMA* 166:1105–1108, 1975.

Schmidt S, Suter PF: Angiography of the hepatic and portal venous system in the dog and cat: an investigative method. *Vet Radiol* 21:57–77, 1980.

Suter PF: Portal vein anomalies in the dog: their angiographic diagnoses. *J Am Vet Radiol Soc* 16:84–97, 1975.

Toombs JP, Hardy RM: Neurologic signs associated with congenital anomalies in a Yorkshire Terrier. *Vet Med Sm Anim Clin* 81:2072–214, 1981.

Vulgamott JC, Turnwald GH, King GK, et al: Congenital portacaval anomalies in the cat: two case reports. *J Am Anim Hosp Assoc* 16:915–919, 1980.

CHAPTER 14

Pharynx and Pharyngeal Pouches

ENDODERMAL TUBE

As the cranial and caudal intestinal portals move closer to each other, eventually meeting at the umbilicus, there is formed a tube of endoderm extending from the oral plate, cranially, to the cloacal membrane, caudally. Many diverticula will evaginate from this tube. Some, such as the middle ear cavity, liver, pancreas and lungs, will retain their connections with the original gut tube (via the auditory tube, bile duct, pancreatic duct(s), and trachea). In other cases, such as the thyroid and thymus, the original embryonic connections are normally lost.

The endodermal tube is divided into four regions, as shown in Figure 14.1: the pharynx, foregut, midgut and hindgut.

These are surrounded by mesoderm, which forms the stroma and supporting cells of all gut derivatives and the muscular wall of the digestive tract. The endoderm forms parenchymal cells, which are the tissue-specific functional cells of each organ. These include the mucosal epithelium of the stomach and intestine, the hepatocytes of the liver, and the bronchioles and alveoli of the lungs.

The pharynx is an endodermally lined, dorsoventrally flattened tube extending from the **oropharyngeal (oral) plate** (Fig. 14.2) to the esophagus, which begins at the level of the 1st and 2nd somites. Developmentally it differs from the rest of the endodermal tube in several essential ways. When first formed the rostral, ventral and lateral margins of the pharynx are closely approximated by the cephalic and lateral body folds, and the heart and aortic arches underlie it ventrally. Unlike the rest of the gut there is no coelom or cavity surrounding the pharynx and there is no separation of intraembryonic mesoderm into discernable somatic and splanchnic layers in the head.

Second, as described in Chapter 9, the pharynx becomes surrounded laterally and ventrally by mesenchyme derived from the neural crest, which forms the skeletal and connective tissues of the **visceral arches** (alternatively called pharyngeal or branchial arches). Finally, the pharyngeal region has undergone major changes during vertebrate evolution, concomitant with alterations in the visceral arches described in Chapter 9. The shift from filter-feeding to biting and chewing, and from gill to lung-mediated respiration allowed pharyngeal components to be modified for other functions.

The **pharyngeal pouches** are a series of 4–5 bilateral pairs of lateral evaginations of pharyngeal endoderm (refer to Fig. 11.2). These arise in a rostrocaudal sequence and, as shown in Figure 14.3, project laterally between the branchial arches. The distal (lateral) part of each pharyngeal pouch expands dorsally and ventrally (Fig. 14.4), and closely apposes medial indentations of the surface ectoderm called **visceral grooves**.

In mammals the 5th pharyngeal pouch is rudimentary and appears as a slight divertic-

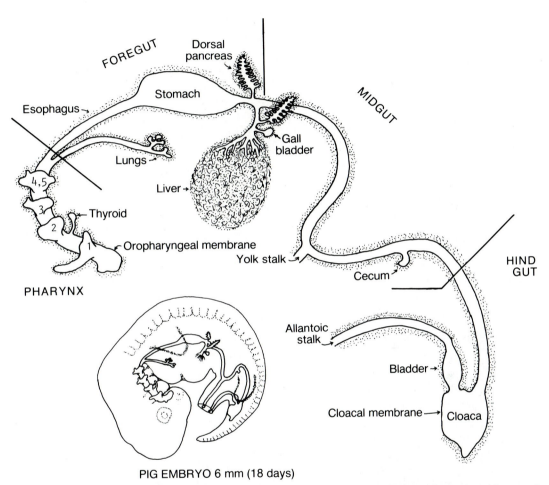

Figure 14.1.   Schematic lateral view of the endodermal tube, with pharynx, foregut, midgut and hindgut areas indicated. The *insert* illustrates the position of these structures with the body.

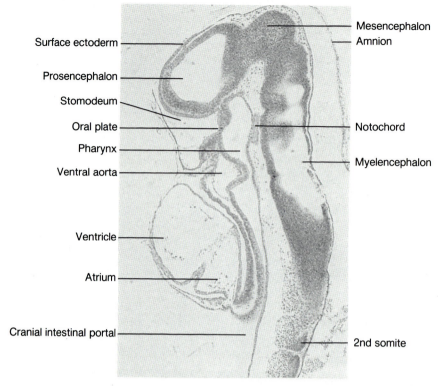

Figure 14.2. Median section of a 16-somite dog embryo showing the oral plate and pharynx.

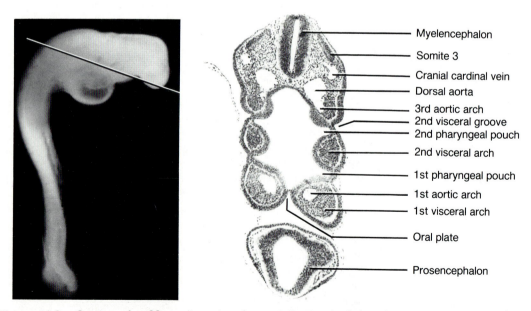

Figure 14.3. Section of a 22-somite cat embryo at the level of the pharynx and oral plate, as indicated on the *insert*. The embryo was cut in a dorsal plane.

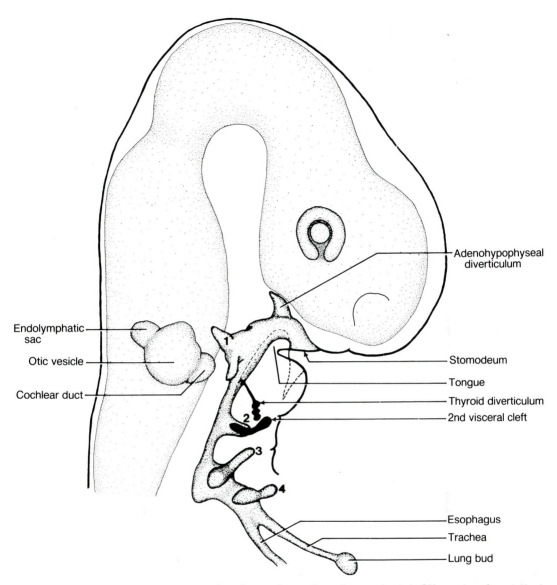

Endolymphatic sac

Otic vesicle

Cochlear duct

Adenohypophyseal diverticulum

Stomodeum

Tongue

Thyroid diverticulum

2nd visceral cleft

Esophagus

Trachea

Lung bud

Figure 14.4.   Schematic illustration of an 8-mm dog embryo (approximately 3½ weeks of gestation) showing the outpocketings of the pharynx. Only the second pharyngeal pouch fuses with the surface ectoderm to form a transient visceral cleft. *Dashed line* indicates the profile of the tongue. *1, 2, 3,* and *4* are pharyngeal pouches.

ulum off the 4th pouch. Only the first three pouches contact the surface ectoderm. In lower vertebrates the epithelia at these zones of endoderm-ectoderm apposition degenerate, creating openings between the pharynx and the extraembryonic environment. These openings, called **visceral clefts**, persist in fishes to form the gill slits. In contrast, the visceral clefts are transient and their number is reduced in all higher vertebrates, there

being only two (1st and 2nd pouches) in birds and, usually, one (2nd pouch) or none in mammals.

PHARYNGEAL POUCH 1

The ventral part of the first pair of pharyngeal pouches is obliterated by the developing tongue. The dorsal projection (Fig. 14.5) retains its close proximity to the otocyst and becomes the lining of the **auditory**

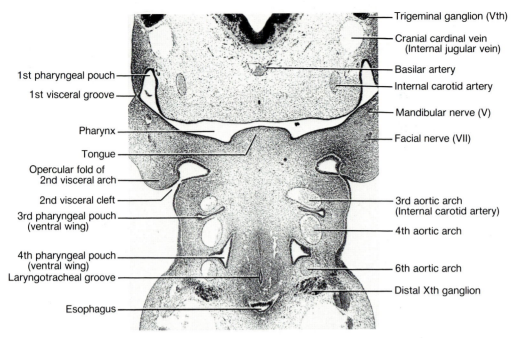

1st pharyngeal pouch

1st visceral groove

Pharynx

Tongue

Opercular fold of
2nd visceral arch

2nd visceral cleft

3rd pharyngeal pouch
(ventral wing)

4th pharyngeal pouch
(ventral wing)

Laryngotracheal groove

Esophagus

Trigeminal ganglion (Vth)

Cranial cardinal vein
(Internal jugular vein)

Basilar artery

Internal carotid artery

Mandibular nerve (V)

Facial nerve (VII)

3rd aortic arch
(Internal carotid artery)

4th aortic arch

6th aortic arch

Distal Xth ganglion

Figure 14.5. Section of an 11.5-mm calf embryo cut in the dorsal plane showing a transient visceral cleft between the 2nd pharyngeal pouch and 2nd visceral groove.

tube (Eustachian tube) and **middle ear cavity**, which is the cavity of the tympanic bulla. The auditory tube opens from the dorsal region of the pharynx designated the **nasopharynx**. In the middle ear the endoderm of this pouch forms the epithelial lining of the middle ear cavity and the **tympanum** (Fig. 14.6). In the horse a large diverticulum of each auditory tube becomes greatly enlarged to form the **guttural pouch**, illustrated in Figure 14.7.

The first visceral groove forms the **external ear canal**. At the base of the canal this ectodermal lining is closely apposed to the endoderm of the 1st pouch to complete the formation of the tympanum. The mesenchyme of visceral arches 1 and 2 adjacent to this groove will form the **pinna** of the external ear and the **ossicles** of the middle ear.

PHARYNGEAL POUCH 2

This pouch is greatly reduced by the proliferation of the tongue and adjacent tissues. Only part of the dorsal portion persists as the **fossa** for the **palatine tonsil**. The lymphatic tonsillar tissue is mesenchymal in origin, and the function served by endodermal epithelium is unknown. The epithelium covering the tonsil, called the **semilunar fold**, is also derived from second pouch endoderm.

PHARYNGEAL POUCH 3

The lumina of pharyngeal pouches 3 and 4 are obliterated, but the epithelial cells that form their lining proliferate and give rise to a number of endocrine glands. The endodermal epithelium of the dorsal wing of each 3rd pouch gives rise to the parenchymal cells of a **parathyroid gland**. These are called **parathyroid glands 3** or the **external parathyroids** because of their extracapsular relationship to the thyroid gland.

The ventral endoderm of each 3rd pouch (Fig. 14.6) gives rise to the epithelial reticular cells of the **thymus gland**. The thymic T cells, which are one class of lymphocytes, come from lymphopoietic stem cells initially derived from the mesoderm of the yolk sac, later from the liver, and postnatally from the bone marrow. These lymphocytes are activated in the thymus by an endocrine

mammals becomes intimately associated with the thyroid parenchyma. The crest cells within the ultimobranchial tissue form the **C cells (parafollicular cells)** of the thyroid gland. These produce **calcitonin** in response to hypercalcemia.

In sheep a small portion of the ventral 4th pouch epithelial cells also contributes to the developing thymus gland.

THYROID GLAND

The parenchymal cells of the thyroid gland are derived from endodermal epithelial cells. As shown in Figure 14.4 (see also Fig. 12.8), the primordium of the thyroid first appears as an evagination on the floor of the foregut between the first two pharyngeal pouches. This ventral outpocketing is called the **thyroid diverticulum**. A tube-like column of these epithelial cells grows ventrally and caudally into the adjacent mesenchyme. There it divides into two portions, each of which will give rise to a lobe of the thyroid. The tubular connection from the developing gland to the point of origin from the pharyngeal floor is the **thyroglossal duct**. In most mammals, including the dog, this duct is never patent. Unlike exocrine glands, which retain a connection with epithelium from which they arise (e.g. salivary glands, pancreas), the thyroid gland loses its original connection to the floor of the pharynx. The thyroid splits into two lateral lobes that in the large domestic animals usually remain connected ventral to the trachea by a **thyroid isthmus**. The exception is the pig, which has a single thyroid gland. In the dog the two lobes are completely separate.

As the primordial thyroid cells shift caudally, they contact tissues associated with the ventral portion of pharyngeal pouch 4. Some of these cells are presumptive calcitonin-secreting mesenchymal cells, which become incorporated into the thyroid during this period. The thyroid parenchymal cells organize in solid clusters, each of which subsequently forms a lumen and then becomes follicular. These follicles will be the source of thyroxine. The calcitonin-secreting cells disperse between follicles in the thyroid gland, thus the name parafollicular cells.

MALFORMATIONS OF PHARYNGEAL POUCHES

Given the complexity of pharyngeal pouch development, the system is remarkably low in the frequency with which malformations appear.

A **thyroglossal cyst** represents a developmental abnormality near the site of origin of the thyroid diverticulum. In this condition a cyst surrounded by thyroid follicular cells is found in the root of the tongue. These subepiglottic cysts may cause inspiratory dyspnea and exercise intolerance in athletic horses. Ectopic thyroid tissue in the vicinity of the basihyoid bone similarly is a remnant of the course taken by the thyroid diverticulum as it descends.

Branchial cyst, sinus, or **fistula**. A **cyst** is an epithelial lined cavity that does not communicate with an epithelial surface. A **sinus** is an epithelial lined cavity that communicates with one epithelial surface, and a **fistula** is an epithelial lined cavity that connects with two epithelial surfaces. When any of these abnormal structures are present congenitally, it usually is the result of an invaginating or evaginating epithelial vesicle failing to separate normally from its parent epithelium.

For example, improper closure of the **cervical sinus** (Fig. 14.6) by the caudal growth of the hyoid arch operculum may leave remnants of visceral grooves communicating with the skin of the neck. If a totally enclosed visceral groove persists, its epithelial lining secretes fluid into the lumen, resulting in formation of a **branchial cyst**. Visceral groove remnants such as these are more common in man than in domestic animals.

Noninflammatory cervical swellings are common in dogs, but only occasionally are they due to an abnormality of visceral groove development. More often these swellings contain a clear, slightly viscous salivary type of fluid and are **salivary mucoceles**, not branchial cysts. A mucocele is a cystic cavity that contains mucinous material but lacks an epithelial lining. A salivary mucocele is the result of a rupture or defect in a salivary duct or gland parenchyma. This involves the monostomatic sublingual gland or, occasionally, the mandibular salivary gland. As the saliva slowly leaks out of the duct or gland, it flows through the connective tissue spaces to a point in the neck where it begins to collect. The body responds by walling off this fluid collection with proliferated connective tissue.

Occasionally, salivary secretions collect in the oral cavity adjacent to the salivary duct alongside the tongue; this is called a **sublingual cyst** or **ranula**. Radiopaque dye injected into the orifice of the salivary duct will often demonstrate the site of the defect in the duct and show a communication with the mucocele. This technique is called **sialography** (sialon = saliva).

A branchial cyst is successfully treated by removal of the entire epithelial lining of the cyst. A salivary mucocele is successfully treated by removal of the involved salivary gland with or without removal of the mucocele. Simple aspiration of the fluid contents will not provide a permanent cure to either condition. It has been suggested that either injury or malformation may cause the salivary duct defect.

Ectopic derivatives of pharyngeal pouch epithelium, including thyroid, parathyroid, and thymus tissues, have been reported. In addition abnormal induction or migration of pouch tissues can result in finding several of these different tissue types in one organ. For example, it is possible while studying microscopic sections of the thymus gland to find a few thyroid follicles or parathyroid cells mixed in with the thymus gland parenchyma. These usually cause the animal no harm.

In the foal, abnormalities in the opening to a guttural pouch can lead to a gaseous distension of the pouch, which may be recognized by swelling caudal to the ramus of the mandible. This is referred to as **tympanites** or **guttural pouch emphysema**.

Bibliography

NORMAL DEVELOPMENT

Gerneke WH: The embryological development of the pharyngeal region of the sheep. *Onderstepoort J Vet Res* 30:191–250, 1963.

Godwin MC: Complex IV in the dog with special emphasis on the relation of the ultimobranchial body to interfollicular cells in the postnatal thyroid gland. *Am J Anat* 60:299–339, 1937.

Harrison BM, Mohn LA: Some stages in the development of the pharynx of the embryo horse. *Am J Anat* 50:233–249, 1932.

Hendrickx, AG: The pharyngeal pouches of the dog. *Anat Rec* 149:475–483, 1964.

Kingsbury BF: Ultimobranchial body and thyroid gland in the fetal calf. *Am J Anat* 56:445–479, 1935.

Kingsbury BF: On the mammalian thymus, particularly thymus IV. *Am J Anat* 60:149–183, 1936.

Ramsay AJ: The development of the palatine tonsil (cat). *Am J Anat* 57:171–203, 1935.

Sack, WO: The early development of the embryonic pharynx of the dog. *Anat Anz* 115:59–80, 1964.

CONGENITAL DEFECTS

Bergman, RT: Correction of branchial cysts. *JAVMA* 136:456–457, 1960.

Cook WR: The clinical features of guttural pouch mycosis in the horse. *Vet Rec* 83:336–345, 1968.

Glen JB: Salivary cysts in the dog: identification of sublingual duct defects by sialography. *Vet Rec* 78:488–492, 1966.

Glen JB: Canine salivary mucoceles: the results of sialographic examination and surgical treatment of fifty cases. *J Small Anim Pract* 13:515–526, 1972.

Hulland TJ, Archibald J: Salivary mucoceles in dogs. *Can Vet J* 5:107–117, 1964.

Karbe E: Lateral neck cysts in the dog. *Am J Vet Res* 26:717–772, 1965.

Karbe E, Nielsen SW: Canine ranulas, salivary mucoceles and branchial cysts. *J Small Anim Pract* 7:625–630, 1966.

Miskowiec JF, Hankes GH, Engel HN, Jr, Bartels JE: Internal branchial fistula in a kitten. *Vet Med Small Anim Clin* 69:259–269, 1974.

Stick, JA, Boles C: Subepiglottic cysts in three foals. *JAVMA* 177:62–64, 1980.

Wheat JD: Tympanites of the guttural pouch of the horse. *JAVMA* 140:453–454, 1962.

CHAPTER 15

Respiratory System and Partitioning of Body Cavities

TRACHEA AND LUNGS

Pulmonary Morphogenesis

Starting at the level of the 4th pharyngeal pouches a longitudinal diverticulum of endodermal epithelial cells grows ventrally from the foregut in the median plane. This solid cord of cells hollows out to form the **laryngotracheal groove** (Fig. 15.1*A*) which grows ventrally and caudally into the splanchnic mesoderm beneath the foregut. Initially this groove is open with the floor of the foregut over a considerable distance. Later, beginning from the caudal margin of the groove and progressing cranially, ridges of mesenchyme proliferate on both sides of the groove. Growth of these **tracheoesophageal ridges** causes the lateral endodermal epithelial surfaces to meet and fuse together, thus obliterating the communication between trachea and esophagus except at the level of the developing larynx. The partition formed by the ridges is called the **tracheoesophageal septum**.

The blind caudal end of the respiratory diverticulum continues to grow caudally in the mesoderm ventral to the esophagus. This diverticulum, shown in Figure 15.2, is the **lung bud**. It splits early to become bilobed. As it grows distally from its point of origin, the epithelium of the connecting stalk becomes the **laryngotracheal tube**. The mesoderm adjacent to this tube will ultimately form the connective tissues of the wall of the trachea and the tracheal cartilages.

As the lung bud extends caudally between the foregut and the developing heart, it is located in the embryonic mediastinum (see Separation of Pleural and Pericardial Cavities). Here the bilobed branches form the left and right **principal bronchi**. In the ruminant species and the pig a **tracheal bronchus** also develops on the right side.

Continued growth and subdivision of the principal bronchi will give rise to each lung as illustrated in Figure 15.3. The first bronchial branches formed will become the **lobar bronchi**; the future **segmental bronchi** form next, followed by smaller branches called **bronchioles**. The functional parenchymal unit on the end of this duct system is the **alveolus**. The distal bronchioles and alveoli continue to be formed postnatally. Histologically, there is a decrease in the amount of supporting connective tissue at more distal sites and an increase in the number of pulmonary blood vessels per unit area.

Repeated branching at the distal ends of the pulmonary epithelial diverticula is necessary to create a greatly increased surface area. Similar events occur in the other derivatives of the gut, but the pattern of branching is different for each.

In sheep the respiratory diverticulum appears on the 17th day of gestation, the lung

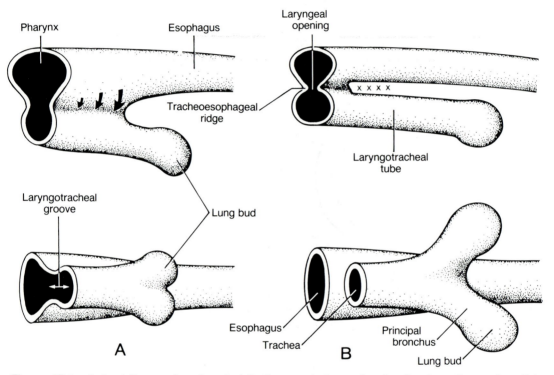

Figure 15.1. Lateral (*top row*) and ventral (*bottom row*) views showing the formation and partial separation of the laryngotracheal diverticulum from the floor of the caudal part of the pharynx. *A* and *B* represent successive stages of tracheoesophageal ridge apposition. *Arrows* in *A* indicate areas of the tracheoesophageal groove that will become occluded by ridge closure and will subsequently degenerate (X X X X).

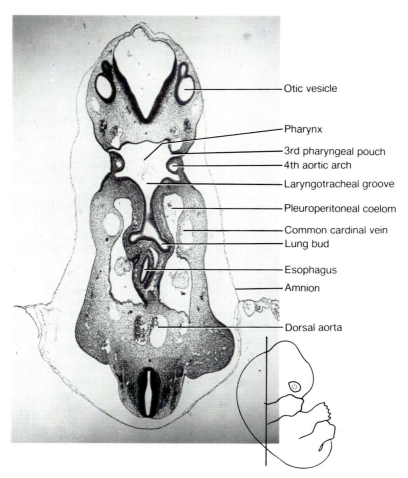

Figure 15.2.   Section cut in a dorsal plane through a 10-mm feline embryo to illustrate the early development of the lung buds and trachea. The location and plane of section are indicated on the *insert*.

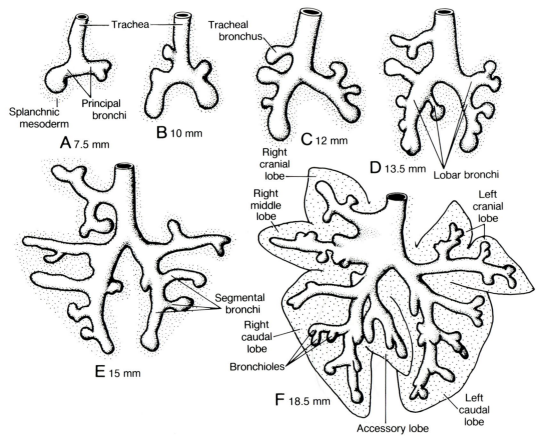

Figure 15.3. Sequential branching of the lung primordium in the pig embryo during the 4th week of gestation. Redrawn after Patten BM: *Embryology of the Pig. ed.* 3. Philadelphia, Blakiston, 1948.

bud is evident by the 19th day and is bilobed on the 20th day. The laryngotracheal tube is delineated on day 21 and the larynx develops over the next 10 days. Lobar bronchi surrounded by a dense mesoderm appear on day 22, and segmental bronchi by day 25. During this time the embryo grows from 4 to 12 mm in length.

Experimental analyses have shown that the endodermal epithelial component and the mesenchyme which surrounds it are both essential for normal lung morphogenesis. Lung bud epithelium stripped of its mesenchyme fails to continue growing and branching. If the mesenchyme is replaced, even with mesenchyme from a different organ (salivary gland or pancreas, for example), typical pulmonary-type growth and branching resumes. These heterologous mesenchymes will even elicit budding from the

trachea, as illustrated in Figure 15.4*A*. However, if distal (bronchial) mesenchyme is replaced with that normally surrounding the trachea, no branching occurs, as shown in Figure 15.4*B*. Thus, in early lung development the pattern of branching is largely an inherent property of the endodermal laryngotracheal diverticulum, but its expression is dependent upon mesenchymal cells with branching promoting properties.

Formation of Alveoli

When first formed the alveoli are solid cords of cuboidal cells. In time the lumen of the bronchioles expands into the alveoli and the alveolar epithelium becomes thin. Some of these epithelial cells produce a phospholipoprotein called **surfactant**, which reduces surface tension and aids in maintaining patency of the lumen of the alveolus.

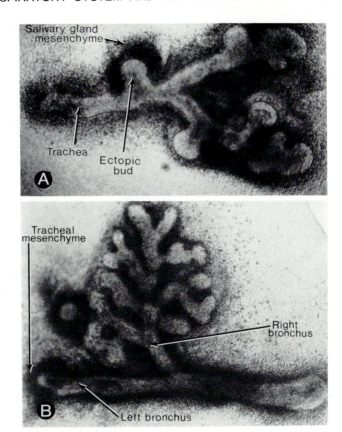

Figure 15.4. Interactions between pulmonary epithelia and mesenchyme demonstrated using organ culture of mouse lung primordia. In *A*, tracheal mesenchyme was removed and replaced with salivary gland mesenchyme; this resulted in the growth of an ectopic, tracheal bronchus. A tracheal bronchus is normally found in the pig and ruminants, but not in other domestic and laboratory animals. In *B*, tracheal mesenchyme grafted in place of bronchial mesenchyme was unable to elicit branching from the bronchial epithelium. (From Wessells NK: *Tissue Interactions and Development,* Menlo Park, W. A. Benjamin, Inc., 1977.)

In man alveoli become patent and the epithelial cells become narrow at 16 weeks of gestation, but surfactant is not produced until 30 weeks of gestation. In sheep the corresponding times are estimated to be 110 days and 125–130 days, respectively. Both patency of the alveolus and the presence of surfactant are necessary for survival. The administration of corticosteroids may accelerate surfactant production and permit respiratory function in animals born prematurely.

The fetal bronchial tree is filled with fluid, the origin of which is controversial. One theory is that it is derived from glandular secretions by the pulmonary mucosa and a small amount of vascular transudate. The other theory suggests it is predominantly ingested amniotic fluid that enters the bronchial tree via the opening of the glottis. While it is known that the fetal larynx has the capability to close the glottis and prevent the intake of amniotic fluid, and that fluid pressure within the fetal trachea generally exceeds that in the esophagus, the possibility that amniotic fluid enters the bronchial tree in utero cannot be excluded.

Recent experimental observations document the occurrence of shallow respiratory activity in the fetus. In the lamb these are first observed around 40 days of gestation and become deeper and more rapid towards term. This respiratory activity creates only a small change in thoracic volume, but is necessary to maintain functional articulations between ribs and vertebrae and tonus of respiratory muscles.

At birth an abrupt change must occur in the physiology of the fetus for it to survive in a gaseous environment. Cardiovascular and respiratory function are most immediately affected. The cessation of umbilical blood flow results in a rapid decrease of oxygen content of blood (hypoxemia) and an increase of CO_2 in the blood (hypercarbia). As a consequence of these events the blood pH decreases (acidosis). These chemical changes stimulate peripheral and central receptors that influence respiratory centers in the medulla. Additional stimuli include the body being released from immersion, cooling and external manipulation.

With the first few inspiratory gasps, the bronchial tree and alveoli expand and are maintained in this condition by the surfactant that lines the alveolar surface. Sudden expansion of the lungs produces a marked pulmonary vasodilation and decrease in the resistance to blood flow through the lungs. At the same time the ductus arteriosus be-

gins to constrict. Thus, blood from the pulmonary trunk that prenatally flowed through the ductus arteriosus now perfuses the lungs. Pulmonary blood flow increases 6–10 times over its flow in the fetus. A marked decrease in right heart pressure accompanies these pulmonary changes.

The fluid present in the fetal bronchial tree is removed from the newborn by a number of routes, which include direct flow to the pharynx and oral cavity, evaporation into the respired air, and absorption into the pulmonary lymphatics.

LARYNX

An elevation called the **epiglottal swelling** (Fig. 15.5) appears in the floor (ventral surface) of the pharynx immediately rostral to the laryngotracheal groove and caudal to the base of the tongue (see Chapter 9) at the level of the 4th visceral arches. This swelling elongates in the transverse plane as a result of local proliferation and dispersal of underlying mesenchyme. On either side of the laryngotracheal groove there appear longitudinal **laryngeal swellings**.

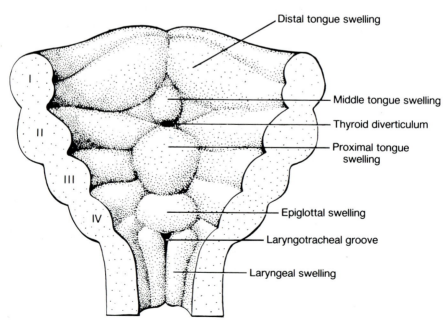

Figure 15.5.   Schematic representation of the floor of the pharynx to illustrate the location of the primordia of the epiglottis and laryngeal structures. Roman numerals identify visceral arches.

Growth of the epiglottal and laryngeal swellings causes the laryngeal opening (aditus) to become T-shaped. The lumen of the larynx becomes occluded by these swellings. Later, an epithelial-lined lumen is reformed and the paired **laryngeal ventricles** are formed.

It is generally stated that most (or all) the cartilages of the larynx are derived from visceral arch (neural crest) mesenchyme, and laryngeal muscles are correspondingly branchiomeric. This is based on the location of their formation, in close proximity to other known visceral arch structures, and their pattern of innervation.

However, recent experimental analyses in avian embryos negate these assumptions. Transplantation of labeled neural crest cells has shown that the arytenoid and cricoid laryngeal cartilages are formed from mesoderm, in much the same manner as the more caudally situated tracheal rings. Since the chick does not have a structure homologous to the mammalian thyroid cartilage, it is possible that this skeletal component is a neural crest derivative. Similarly, transplanted occipital somites 1 and 2 formed the muscle fibers within intrinsic laryngeal muscles, and grafts of somites 3-5 labeled extrinsic laryngeal and tongue muscles (see Fig. 9.13).

MALFORMATIONS OF THE RESPIRATORY SYSTEM
Laryngotracheal Defects

Choanal stenosis and **atresia** are discussed in Chapter 9.

Tracheal hypoplasia or **tracheal stenosis** refers to an abnormal narrowing of the trachea. This may be focal or, less commonly, involve the entire length of the trachea. Although the tracheal cartilages are usually abnormal in these animals, often being fused dorsally, it is not known whether this is a primary defect in cartilage morphogenesis or a secondary result of some abnormality in the tracheal epithelium. This condition occurs more commonly in the English bulldog.

A **collapsed trachea** occurs in toy and miniature breeds of dogs. The tracheal lu-

men is partly occluded and the tracheal cartilages are fusiform or flattened rather than circular. This may be due to a defect in the organic matrix of the tracheal cartilage. **Tracheal atresia**, which is a total lack of tracheal patency, is rare.

The signs evident in these situations vary according to the extent of occlusion. Chronic coughing and wheezing, attacks of dyspnea and poor endurance are common complaints. Usually palpation and radiography will identify the problem.

Malformations of the larynx, such as **subglottic stenosis**, have been reported in humans and domestic animals. It has been suggested that congenital anomalies of the larynx, which are thought to be rare, may be one of the causes of undiagnosed early postnatal mortality.

Tracheoesophageal fistulas (Fig. 15.6) result from improper separation of the caudal portion of the laryngotracheal groove from the foregut. They are often associated with stenosis or atresia of the esophagus. The inability to prevent ingesta from entering the trachea causes obstruction and infection.

Epiglottic entrapment is a condition in horses in which the mucosa beneath and beside the epiglottis extends over the entire margin of the epiglottis and may interfere with normal respiration. These have been referred to as ariepiglottic folds, but only the caudolateral aspect of these mucosal folds is equivalent to the laryngoepiglottic swellings. A malformed hypoplastic epiglottis is thought to predispose to this condition.

Pulmonary Abnormalities

Accessory lungs result from an extra lung bud developing in an abnormal site, such as the neck or abdomen. An abnormal outgrowth from the embryonic cervical trachea could develop into pulmonary tissue located in the cervical region. This condition is rare.

Pulmonary hypoplasia results in decreased lung development. Pulmonary **agenesis** or **aplasia** is the absence of lung development and is rare. Hypoplasia usually occurs if other organs in the thorax physically prevent normal lung growth. This often occurs con-

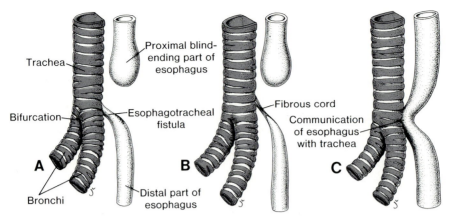

Figure 15.6. Tracheoesophageal anomalies. *A*, atresia of the esophagus and tracheoesophageal fistula. *B*, atresia of the esophagus with fibrous tracheoesophageal connection. *C*, persistent tracheoesophageal foramen, often accompanied by esophageal stenosis. From Langman J: *Medical Embryology*, ed. 4. Baltimore, Williams & Wilkins, 1981.

comitant with a congenital diaphragmatic hernia, in which abdominal organs enter the thorax.

Congenital pulmonary cysts can occur in the parenchyma of a lung. These result when one part of the bronchial tree loses its connection with the main branch. Continued secretion by the endodermal cells lining the bronchioles and alveoli results in fluid accumulation and enlargement of the cyst.

Endoderm has the capability of differentiating into many kinds of epithelial derivatives. For instance, in the digestive tract it can form a stratified squamous epithelium as in the esophagus, and a simple columnar epithelium with specialized glands as in the stomach. Liver and pancreatic parenchymal cells are endodermal. **Endodermal heteroplasia** describes the condition in which the epithelial cells differentiate inappropriately for their location. For example, the endoderm of bronchial cysts may form intestinal epithelium or pancreatic acinar cells. Usually such heteroplasias are small and focal, and produce no clinical signs.

The term **respiratory distress syndrome** includes many forms of neonatal breathing difficulties. One basis for this condition involves the inability of alveolar epithelial cells to produce enough surfactant to prevent collapse of the alveoli after their initial distension with air. In humans, this cause of the

syndrome is called hyaline membrane disease. There has been only limited investigation of this problem in domesticated mammals. Many premature and small full-term animals that do not survive the first few hours after birth are believed to be examples of this syndrome, but these are usually destroyed before a thorough examination can be made. An autosomal recessive genetic basis has been established for a neonatal respiratory distress (barker) syndrome in pigs.

In newborn foals with respiratory distress the signs manifested are neurologic, resulting from cerebral hypoxia caused by insufficient respiratory function. Seizures are commonly observed in these foals. Often during the onset of a seizure the foal may make barking sounds, which is the basis for calling this the barker foal syndrome.

Some cases rapidly progress to coma and death; others may slowly recover after passing through a period of visual deficit, stupor, and aimless wandering. At necropsy large portions of the lung are found to have extensive **atelectasis** (a = lack of; tel = end; ectasia = extension). This appears as collapsed or nonexpanded lung tissue that has failed to dilate or distend normally. Air injected into the atelectatic lung will expand the alveoli but they collapse after removal of the air. Physical studies on the contents of the partly aerated lung suggest decreased surfactant content. In some animals signs of this respiratory syndrome may not appear for 24–48 hr postnatally.

Another pathogenesis that has been proposed for this **neonatal maladjustment syndrome** in foals is that an insufficient volume of blood circulating in the newborn, which prevents normal full expansion of the lung and deprives the central nervous system of the oxygen it needs to function. It has been suggested that this vascular insufficiency results from there being a large volume of fetal blood left in the placenta at birth, which may occur if the umbilical cord is severed immediately after delivery. In an unattended delivery there is usually a long enough delay after delivery before the umbilical vessels are separated to allow blood to flow from the placenta back into the newborn. Up to 1.5 liters of blood may be involved in this placental loss.

Chronic bronchitis and rhinitis in young dogs can result from a congenital condition called the **immotile cilia syndrome**, in which some of the cilia projecting from epithelial cells lining the respiratory tract are structurally abnormal and appear to be randomly oriented. This reduces the ability of these animals to clear the lungs of mucous and particulate material. In some of these cases the cilia of spermatozoa have been found to be defective, also.

Approximately half of the animals (and humans) with immotile cilia syndrome have **situs inversus**, in which all internal organs show a reversed left-right asymmetry. The relation between ciliary function and the establishment of asymmetry during early cleavage and gastrula stages is not understood.

SEPARATION OF PLEURAL AND PERICARDIAL CAVITIES

Beginning immediately caudal to the level of the laryngotracheal groove, the gut is underlain and the heart surrounded by a splanchnic mesoderm-lined cavity, part of which originally formed in the cardiogenic plate prior to head fold formation. This cavity extends the length of the thoracic and abdominal regions, but does not reach the level of the pharynx, cranially. Formation of lateral body folds closes the cavity ventrally, except at the level of the umbilicus.

In the adult the parts of this intraembryonic coelom are identified by the tissues they surround (i.e. pleural, pericardial, peritoneal). However, in the embryo all regions of the intraembryonic coelom are continuous. The only partition present is the **septum transversum**, which lies in a transverse plane between the sinus venosus and the liver. Dorsal to this septum the common **pleuropericardial cavity** is continuous with the **peritoneal coelom**.

Caudoventral growth of the laryngotracheal diverticulum and associated mesoderm brings the lungs into the dorsal part of the body cavity near the level of the septum transversum (see Fig. 17.3) and into the **cranial mediastinum**, which in this region is derived from the dorsal mesocardium. The term mediastinum refers to any median partition, and is most commonly used in reference to that within the thoracic cavity. On either side of this tissue are the pleural cavities. The paired lung buds form and grow rapidly; as a result of their branching, the pulmonary tissue expands caudally and ventrolaterally, partially surrounding the heart. The pleural cavities expand dorsally and ventrally to accommodate this growth, as shown in Figure 15.7.

The formation of a pericardial cavity and its separation from the pleural cavity is initially related to the growth of the common cardinal veins. These vessels run along the lateral body wall dorsally then pass ventromedially to enter the sinus venosus near the level of the septum transversum. The mesenchymal tissue surrounding each common cardinal vein is the **pleuropericardial fold**. These folds grow medially and fuse with the mediastinum ventral to the esophagus, forming a **pleuropericardial septum**, as shown in Figure 15.7. As the lungs grow laterally into the body wall, this horizontal septum expands laterally. Similarly, as the

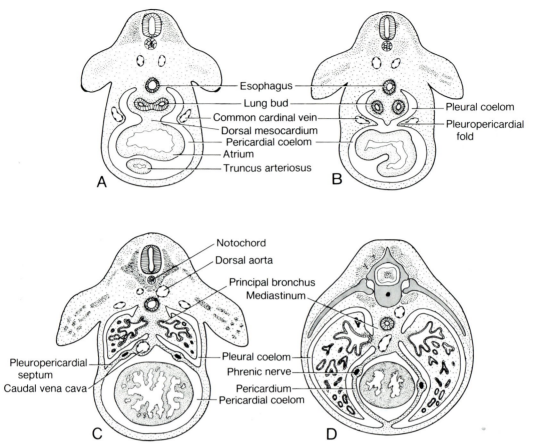

Figure 15.7. Schematic transverse sections to show the separation of pleural and pericardial cavities by the formation of the pleuropericardial septum, and shaping of the pleural cavity by growth of the lungs. Note in *C* and *D* how the pleuropericardial septum envelopes the heart to form the pericardium. Redrawn after Patten BM: *Embryology of the Pig*, ed. 3. Philadelphia, Blakiston, 1948.

heart descends, the pleuropericardial septum becomes elongated craniocaudally.

With continued lateral and ventral expansion of the lungs, the sites of attachment of the pleuropericardial septum from the lateral body wall shift progressively towards the ventral midline. This results in the heart being completely surrounded by a heavy sheath, the **pericardium**, which is continuous dorsally with the mediastinum and ventrally is attached to the thoracic wall. The cavity between the pericardium and the epicardium, which is the outermost serous lining of the heart, is the **pericardial cavity**. These growth changes completely isolate the pericardial cavity from the common pleuroperitoneal cavity.

FORMATION OF THE DIAPHRAGM

The tissues that participate in the formation of the diaphragm (Fig. 15.8) are diverse in their origins, and include paraxial mesoderm, somatic and splanchnic mesodermal layers, and the dorsal mesentery of the caudal part of the esophagus. The ventral component, the **septum transversum**, develops early during cardiogenesis, and later forms the central tendon of the diaphragm. The second component is the **caudal mediastinum**, through which the esophagus and (right) caudal vena cava pass. This septum, sometimes called the dorsal mesentery of the esophagus (mesoesophagus), becomes elon-

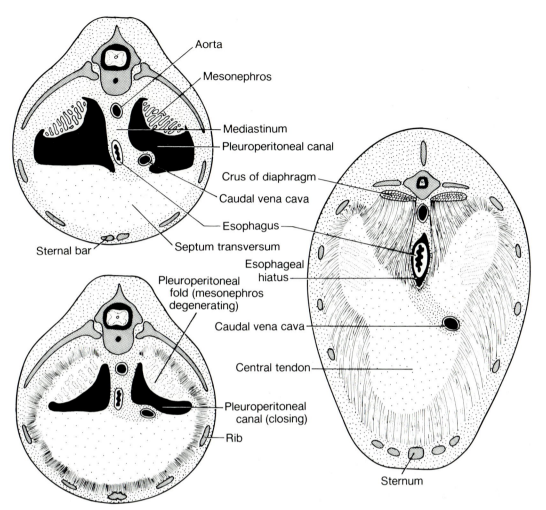

Aorta

Mesonephros

Mediastinum

Pleuroperitoneal canal

Crus of diaphragm

Caudal vena cava

Esophagus

Septum transversum

Sternal bar

Pleuroperitoneal fold (mesonephros degenerating)

Esophageal hiatus

Caudal vena cava

Central tendon

Pleuroperitoneal canal (closing)

Rib

Sternum

Figure 15.8. Formation of the diaphragm from septum transversum, mesoesophagus (caudal mediastinum), pleuroperitoneal folds and body wall mesenchyme. The exact contributions of pleuroperitoneal folds to the central tendon are not known. Schematic transverse sections viewed from a caudal perspective.

gated dorsoventrally as a result of caudodorsal growth of the lungs. Because of this expansion, which causes the roof of the pleural cavities to elevate on either side of the midline, the left and right **pleuroperitoneal canals** enlarge dorsally.

Final closure of the pleuroperitoneal canals is accomplished by formation of a pair of **pleuroperitoneal membranes**. These arise as folds of tissue that project into the peritoneal cavity from its dorsolateral margin. They are continuous caudally with the mesonephroi. Simultaneous with ventrolateral expansion of the lungs and enlargement of

the mesenephroi, these pleuroperitoneal folds expand and fuse with the septum transversum, ventrally, and the caudal mediastinum, medially, to close the pleuroperitoneal canals.

As the thoracic cavity enlarges during later stages of fetal growth, tissues of the body wall become incorporated into the diaphragm circumferentially. It has been suggested that most of the lateral and dorsal muscular components (pars costalis and lumbaris) are derived from this body wall tissue. However, the exact contribution of body wall to the diaphragm is not known.

MALFORMATIONS OF THE DIAPHRAGM

Pleuroperitoneal hiatus defects are clefts in the dorsal tendinous part of the diaphragm near the esophagus that are thought to represent defective closure of the pleuroperitoneal canals. These are rare but would permit herniation of abdominal organs into the pleural cavity.

A **pericardioperitoneal communication** is an abnormal opening between these two cavities. It may be associated with a defective closure of the midline of the abdominal wall near the diaphragm. In dogs and cats there is often an abnormal swirling of the hair in this region.

The origin of this congenital diaphragmatic hernia has often been explained erroneously as a direct, persistent connection between the peritoneal and pericardial cavities. However, there is never a natural communication here to be closed. Therefore, this condition has to arise as a secondary phenomenon in the development of the diaphragm.

After the liver grows out of the septum transversum, the peritoneal cavity extends between the liver and septum transversum. If this separation is faulty, a gap may occur ventrally within the septum, or the remaining tissue may be so thin that it ruptures, allowing the peritoneal and pericardial cavities to communicate through an opening in the ventral part of the diaphragm. This allows abdominal organs to pass through the defect in the diaphragm directly into the pericardial cavity, where they may interfere with cardiac function, produce signs of digestive system abnormality or produce no clinical signs except muffled heart sounds. Radiography following a barium meal will confirm the diagnosis. These defects can be surgically repaired.

Bibliography

NORMAL DEVELOPMENT

Boyden EA, Thompsett DH: The postnatal growth of the lung in the dog. *Acta Anat* 47:185–215, 1961.
Bryden MM, Evans HE, Binns W: Embryology of the Sheep. III. The respiratory system, mesenteries, and colon in the fourteen to thirty-four day embryo. *Anat Rec* 175:725–736, 1973.
Dameron F: An experimental study of the organogenesis of the lung. *J Embryol Exp Morphol* 20:151–167, 1968.
de Reuck AVS, Porter R (eds): *Ciba Foundation Symposium on the Development of the Lung.* Boston, Little, Brown, 1967.
Engel S: *The Prenatal Lung.* Oxford, Pergamon Press, 1966.
Hashimoto Y: Histologic studies on the lung of the cattle foetus. *Bulletin of the Naniwe University, Series B,* vol 3, 1953.
Lenkscheidt W: Uber das Wachstum von Herz und Lunge wahrend der Entwicklung beim Schwein. Berlin, Diss, 1925.
Spooner BS, Wessels NK: Mammalian lung development: interactions in primordium formation and bronchial morphogenesis. *J Exp Zool* 175:445–454, 1970.
Willsman NJ, Farnum CE, Reed DK: Variability of ciliary ultrastructure in normal dogs. *Am J Anat* 164:343–352, 1982.

MALFORMATIONS OF THE RESPIRATORY SYSTEM

August JR, Teer PA, Bartels JE: Kartagener's syndrome in a dog. *J Am Anim Hosp Assoc* 18:822–826, 1982. (Note: Kartagener's = immotile cilia syndrome.)
Azelius BA: The immotile-cilia syndrome and other ciliary diseases. *Int Rev Exp Pathol* 19:1–43, 1979.
Boles CL, Raker CW, Wheat JD: Epiglottic entrapment by arytenoepiglottic folds in the horse. *JAVMA* 172:338–342, 1978.
Bradley R, Wrathall AE: Barker (neonatal respiratory distress) syndrome in the pig: the ultrastructural pathology of the lung. *J Pathol* 122:145–151, 1977.
Carrig CB, Suter PF, Ewing GO: Primary dextrocardia with situs inversus, associated with sinusitis and bronchitis in a dog. *JAVMA* 164:1127–1134, 1974.
Done SH, Drew RA: Observations on the pathology of tracheal collapse in dogs. *J Small Anim Pract* 17:783–791, 1976.
Edwards DF, Patton CS, Benis DA, Kennedy JR, Selcer BA: Immotile cilia syndrome in three dogs from a litter. *JAVMA* 183:667–672, 1983.
Eigenmann UJE, Schoon HA, Tahn D, Grunert E: Neonatal respiratory distress syndrome in the calf. *Vet Rec* 114:141–144, 1984.
Haynes PF, Qualls CW Jr: Cleft soft palate, nasal septal deviation, and epiglottic entrapment in a thoroughbred filly. *JAVMA* 179:910–913, 1981.
Martens RJ: Neonatal respiratory distress: a review with emphasis on the horse. *Compend Cont Ed* 4:523–533, 1982.
O'Brien JA, Buchanan JW, Kelly DG: Tracheal collapse in the dog. *J Am Vet Radiol Soc* 7:12–20, 1966.
Rossdale PD: Modern concepts of neonatal disease in foals. *Equine Vet J* 4:1–12, 1972.
Suter PF, Colgrove DJ, Ewing GO: Congenital hypoplasia of the canine trachea. *J Am Anim Hosp Assoc* 8:120–127, 1972.
Venker-van Haagen AJ, Engelse EJJ, van den Ingh T: Congenital subglottic stenosis in a dog. *J Am Anim Hosp Assoc* 17:223–225, 1981.
Wrathall AE, Bailey J, Wells DE, Hebert CN: Studies on the barker (neonatal respiratory distress) syndrome in the pig. *Cornell Vet* 67:543–598, 1971.

Malformations of the Diaphragm

Atkins CF: Suspect congential peritoneopericardial diaphragmatic hernia in an adult cat. *JAVMA* 165:175–176, 1974.

Barrett RB, Kittrell JE: Congenital peritoneal-pericardial diaphragmatic hernia in a cat. *J Am Vet Radiol Soc* 7:21–26, 1960.

Bjorck GR, Tigerschiold A: Peritoneopericardial diaphragmatic hernia in a dog. *J Small Anim Pract* 11:585–590, 1970.

Bolton GR, Ettinger S, Roush JC: Congenital peritoneopericardial diaphragmatic hernia in a dog. *JAVMA* 155:723–730, 1969.

Clinton JM: A case of congenital periocardio-peritoneal communication in a dog. *J Am Vet Radiol Soc* 8:57–60, 1967.

Detweiler DK, etal: Diagnosis and surgical correction of peritoneal-pericardial diaphragmatic hernia in a dog. *JAVMA* 137:247–250, 1960.

Frye FL, Taylor D: Pericardial and diaphragmatic defects in a cat. *JAVMA* 146:481–482, 1968.

CHAPTER **16**

Digestive System

Table 16.1.
Gut components and derivatives

Region	Components	Derivatives
Foregut	Esophagus	
	Stomach	
	Cranial (descending)	Liver
	duodenum	Pancreas
Midgut	Caudal duodenum	
	Jejunum	
	Ileum	(Yolk stalk)
	Cecum	
	Colon (ascending,	
	one-half trans-	
	verse)	
Hindgut	Colon (one-half trans-	
	verse, descending)	
	Cloaca	Rectum
		Bladder
Attlantoic		Urachus
stalk		

GUT TUBE

Concomitant with the formation of body folds that provide the embryo with lateral and ventral body walls, a ventrally located tube of endoderm surrounded by splanchnic mesoderm is established. In addition to the pharynx, this simple tubular structure consists of the **foregut**, **hindgut** and, later, the **midgut**, which remains connected with the original extraembryonic yolk sac via the **yolk stalk**. (Table 16.1) These regions of the gut approximate the areas supplied by the celiac, cranial and caudal mesenteric arteries.

Histologically the tubular digestive tract consists of three tunics. The inner layer is the **tunica mucosa**, which consists of an epithelium derived from the endoderm and a mesodermal connective tissue component. The epithelium is the parenchyma of the organ. The middle layer is the **tunica muscularis** consisting of various layers of muscle, most of which are smooth and are derived from the splanchnic mesoderm. The outer layer is the mesodermal **tunica serosa**, which is formed from the visceral peritoneum.

Although the gut is initially a hollow tube, many regions will close during development and then re-open. The reason for this transient loss of patency is not known, and has been suggested as one possible basis for congenital intestinal atresia.

DEVELOPMENT OF THE FOREGUT

Esophagus

The primordium of the esophagus is established during the neurula stage, at which time it is located ventral to the first two or three somites. This short segment of foregut elongates extensively during growth of the cervical and thoracic regions of the body. Like the pharynx, the cranial part of the esophagus is not enveloped by a coelom, but is incorporated in the dorsal wall of the pleuroperitoneal cavity. Following growth of the lungs, the mediastinum becomes its non-muscular supporting tissue, and only at the diaphragm is there a short mesoesophagus.

In domestic animals the esophageal tunica muscularis largely differentiates into striated muscle. However, in the pig there is a short segment near the junction with the stomach in which smooth muscle is present. In the horse and cat this zone extends along the caudal one-third, and in birds the entire length is ensheathed with smooth muscle.

Stomach

The primordium of the stomach is first recognized as an enlargement of the foregut cranial to the level of the septum transversum. Subsequently, the stomach shifts caudally and undergoes changes in orientation. First, the ends of the stomach arch ventrally, due largely to differential increase in growth of the dorsal wall. As a result, the dorsal surface becomes convex and the ventral margin concave; these are referred to as the **greater** and **lesser curvatures**, respectively. Later, an expansion of the cranial aspect of the greater curvature forms the fundus.

In animals with a simple stomach two rotations occur that bring the stomach to its definitive location in the abdomen. The first begins shortly after the foregut is delineated. It is an approximately 90° rotation during which the greater curvature shifts to the *left* of the animal, as illustrated in Figure 16.1.

The second 90° rotation occurs around a *dorsoventral* axis; when viewed from a dorsal perspective, this shift is in a counterclockwise direction. The caudal end of the stomach shifts to the right side and cranially; this second rotation occurs gradually during the fetal and early postnatal period.

The morphogenesis of the ruminant stomach is initially similar to that of other mammals. By the 10- to 12-mm (5th week) stage, the bovine stomach has rotated approximately 90°, bringing the zone of attachment of the dorsal mesentery (**dorsal mesogastrium, greater omentum**) to the left side, as shown in Figure 16.2*A*. Early in the 6th week

of gestation, the fundus undergoes a marked craniodorsal, leftwards enlargement, forming the primordium of the **rumen**. A smaller, caudoventral outpocketing of the fundus establishes the **recticulum**. By the 28-mm stage (Fig. 16.2*B*), the **omasum** is recognizable externally as a swelling of the lesser curvature, which is located on the right ventral surface of the stomach. Internally, the lumen of the stomach is subdivided into a large fundic canal on the left and gastric canal on the right by the formation of ventral and dorsal furrows.

During the 7th week of development (28- to 40-mm stages), the bovine stomach exhibits a change in orientation and differential growth of each chamber. The rumen shifts caudodorsally, as indicated by the *upper arrow* in Figure 16.2*B*. This inverts the original dorsal and ventral parts of the rumen. Thus the definitive ventral sac of the rumen arises from what was originally the (right) dorsal aspect of the fundic outgrowth. The blind sacs arise later as caudal outgrowths of the rumen.

The pyloric region of the **abomasum** also changes in relative position during this period. It shifts first ventrally (*lower arrow*, Fig. 16.2*B*), then to the right and, finally, loops caudally. The cardiac region of the abomasum expands greatly during the second half of gestation, and is the largest gastric chamber in the neonate.

The external morphogenesis of the reticulum and omasum are less complicated. The former expands to the left and shifts cranially relative to the rest of the stomach. The omasum remains on the right ventral side of the stomach. By the 10th week of gestation, most morphological features of the adult bovine stomach are present, although the relative sizes of the chambers are not established until after birth.

Liver and Gall Bladder

The liver is a derivative of the embryonic gut. It arises as a large ventral outgrowth from the region of foregut endoderm that will differentiate into the cranial portion of

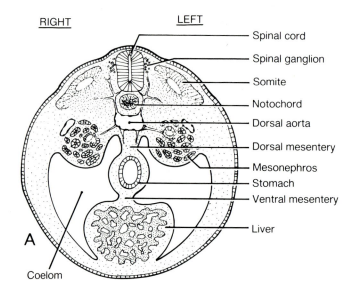

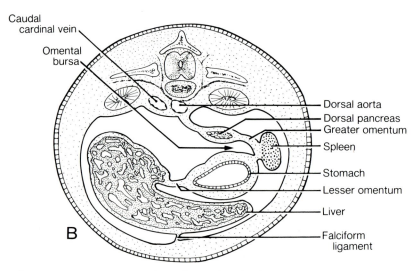

Figure 16.1. Schematic transverse sections illustrating the foregut and mesenteries *A*, before and *B*, after rotation of the stomach. Compare with Figure 16.5.

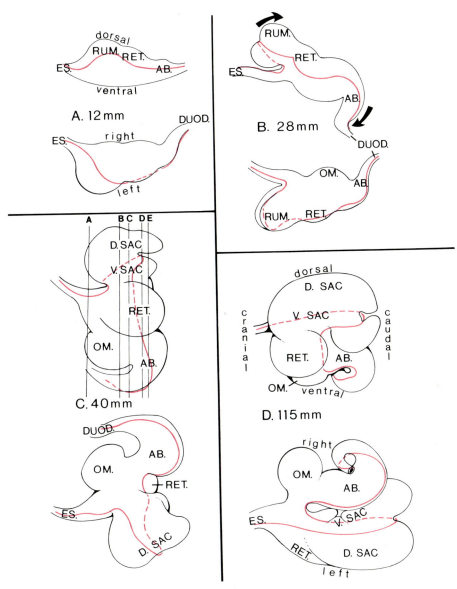

Figure 16.2. *A–D*, Development of the bovine stomach. For each of the four stages illustrated both a left lateral (*upper drawing*) and dorsal (*lower drawing*) are shown. The *red line* indicates the site of attachment of the dorsal mesogastrium. In the dorsal views of *C* and *D* the dorsal sac of the rumen has been pulled to the left. *ES*., esophagus; *RUM*., rumen; *RET*., reticulum; *AB*., abomasum; *DUOD*., duodenum; *OM*., omasum; *D. SAC* and *V. SAC*, dorsal and ventral sacs of the rumen. The lines in *C* indicate the levels of sections shown in Figure 16.6. In *B*, the rumen shifts caudodorsally (*upper arrow*); and the abomasum shifts ventrally (*lower arrow*).

the duodenum. This **hepatic diverticulum** (Figs. 16.3 and 16.4) grows cranioventrally through the mesenchyme of the primitive ventral mesentery (ventral mesogastrium) and into the adjacent mesoderm of the septum transversum. The diverticulum develops two outgrowths, a **pars hepatica** that will form the liver parenchyma and a **pars cystica** that will form the gall bladder. The latter is absent in those species lacking a gall bladder, including the horse and some lab rodents.

The endodermal epithelial cells of the pars hepatica proliferate extensively, forming plates or sheets of cells that differentiate into the functional parenchymal cells of the liver, the hepatocytes. Other pars hepatica-derived cells give rise to the biliary duct system. These include the interlobular ductules most closely associated with the parenchymal cells, the biliary ductules, and the hepatic ducts that leave the liver lobes. The common stem of the ventral hepatic diverticulum for the pars hepatica and pars cystica becomes the **bile duct** (choledochal duct) that enters the cranial duodenum at the site of origin of the diverticulum.

The initial site of origin of the hepatic diverticulum is from the ventral side of the foregut. As the duodenum differentiates, unequal growth in the wall adjacent to where the hepatic diverticulum was located brings the origin of the diverticulum, now the entrance of the bile duct (the **major duodenal**

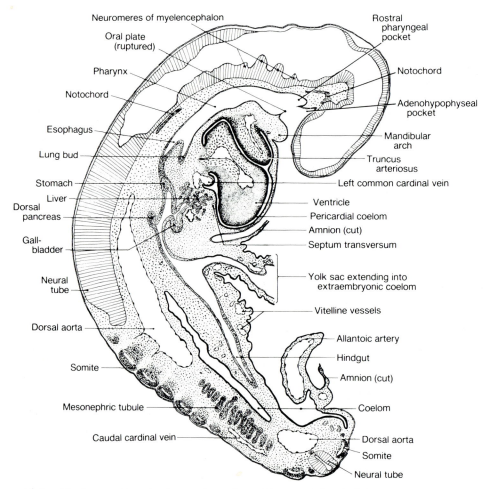

Figure 16.3. Median section of a 5-mm pig embryo. The caudal end of the embryo is twisted to the left and thus does not appear in this plane of section. (From Patten and Carlson, 1974.)

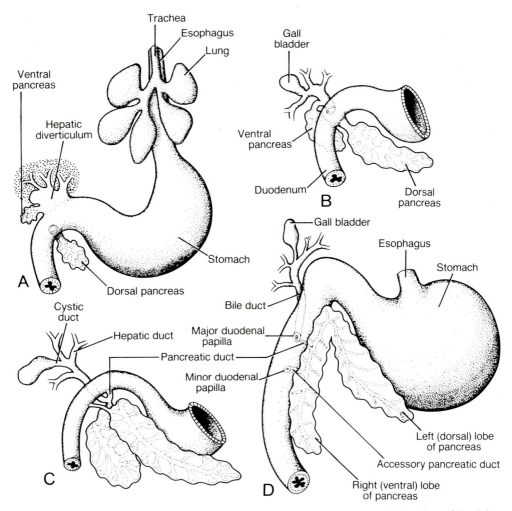

Figure 16.4. Ventral views of the canine foregut illustrating the changes in location of the lobes of the pancreas and associated ducts. *A* was drawn from a 9-mm embryo, *D* from an adult; *B* and *C* are intermediate stages.

papilla), to the dorsal surface of the duodenum. The bile duct courses in the free edge of the lesser omentum to this site.

The liver is extensively vascularized with venous sinusoids adjacent to the plates of hepatocytes. These blood vessels arise from the mesoderm of the septum transversum and from embryonic vitelline and umbilical venous channels that coursed through the septum to enter the sinus venosus of the heart.

Pancreas

The pancreas forms from two separate endodermal outpocketings. The **dorsal pan-**creatic diverticulum arises dorsally from the cranial duodenum, distal to the hepatic diverticulum (Fig. 16.3). It grows into the primitive dorsal mesentery (mesoduodenum) and the adjacent dorsal mesogastrium that will become the deep portion of the greater omentum. Thus it is growing from right to left across the dorsal aspect of the abdomen. This forms the **left lobe** of the pancreas.

The endodermal epithelium of this pancreatic diverticulum proliferates and branches. At the ends of the smaller branches, clumps of cells form the secretory pancreatic **acini**. The acini and branches remain patent, forming an exocrine duct system. This duct, which enters the duodenum at the site of the origin of the dorsal pancreatic diverticulum, is the **accessory pancreatic duct**. It opens into the descending duodenum on the minor duodenal papilla. Scattered between acini are groups of cells derived from the same pancreatic diverticulum but isolated from the duct system. These form the **pancreatic islets** (Langerhans islets), which secrete insulin and glucagon.

The **ventral pancreatic diverticulum** arises from the main stem of the hepatic diverticulum near its origin, as shown in Figure 16.4. Thus, it is a derivative of the ventral surface of the foregut. However, when the hepatic diverticulum becomes repositioned onto the dorsal aspect of the duodenum, the ventral pancreatic diverticulum goes along with it. In that position it grows caudally in the mesentery of the duodenum, crossing and fusing with the origin of the dorsal pancreatic diverticulum. This forms the **right lobe** of the pancreas, and the duct of the ventral pancreatic derivative is the **pancreatic duct**. It opens into the cranial duodenum on the major duodenal papilla, together with or adjacent to the bile duct.

When these two pancreatic derivatives cross, they partially fuse, forming a common body at the site of crossing. Their duct systems anastomose so that pancreatic secretions can pass by either the pancreatic or accessory pancreatic duct into the duodenum. Species differences occur with respect to which one of the pancreatic ducts is present or is the largest, as summarized in Table 16.2. In domestic animals the major papilla and associated ducts are located cranial to the minor papilla; this situation is reversed in humans.

MESENTERIES AND THE GREATER OMENTUM

The embryonic stomach is suspended dorsally and ventrally by mesenteries, the **dorsal** and **ventral mesogastriums**. As the stomach changes in shape and position, these mesenteries maintain their original connection with the greater curvature (original dorsal border) and lesser curvature.

Following the leftward rotation of the stomach, the dorsal mesogastrium extends caudally and to the left, as shown in Figures 16.1 and 16.5. Subsequently, this mesentery expands and becomes folded. The cavity formed between its dorsal and ventral sheets is the primordium of the **omental bursa**.

Beginning in the fetal period and continuing postnatally, the dorsal mesogastrium expands tremendously. It extends caudally between the ventral abdominal wall and the intestinal mass to the level of the bladder. This extended dorsal mesogastrium is the **greater omentum**. In the adult it appears as a thin structure, lacelike in appearance because of the fat that is found in it associated with its many small blood vessels.

The spleen develops in the superficial portion of the greater omentum near to the stomach, as shown in Figures 16-1, 16.5 and 16.6. In the dog the left lobe of the pancreas expands into the deep portion of the greater omentum near the dorsal body wall cranial to the transverse colon.

Initially, the ventral mesogastrium is attached to the lesser curvature of the stomach and extends to the ventral body wall. The liver primordium grows caudally between the left and right sheaves of this ventral mesogastrium, which then becomes the hepatic serosa. The short ventral mesogastrium

Table 16.2.
Species variation in pancreatic duct retention

Species	Pancreatic duct	Accessory pancreatic duct
Dog	Small (absent 8%)	Large
Pig-cow	Absent	Present
Goat-sheep	Present	Absent
Cat	Present	Absent (80%)
Horse	Large	Small

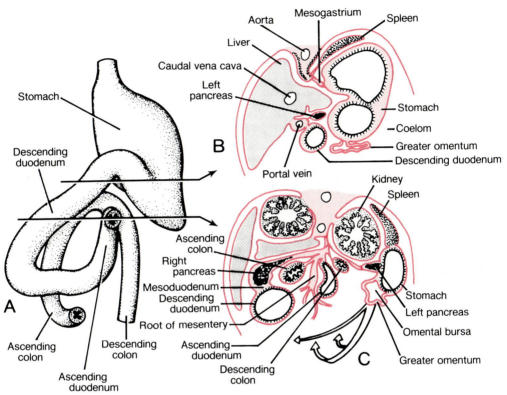

Figure 16.5. The spatial relationships of the foregut and colon in the neonatal ferret. *A* is a ventral view in which the jejunum, ileum and other internal organs have been removed. *B* and *C* are transverse views at the levels indicated on *A*. *C*, which is comparable to Figure 16.6*E*, shows the root of the mesentery and early expansion of the greater omentum; the *arrows* illustrate the later directions of growth of this dorsal mesentery.

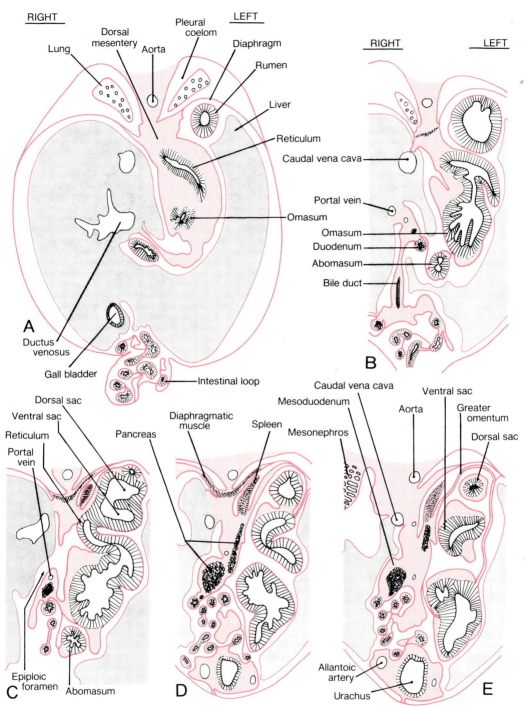

Figure 16.6. Transverse sections of a 40-mm bovine fetus, illustrating the development of the stomach and mesenteries. *A–E* represent cranial to caudal sections, as indicated in Figure 16.2C.

between the stomach and liver is retained as the **lesser omentum**.

The ventral mesentery located between the liver and ventral body wall persists as the falciform ligament. The rest of the ventral mesentery degenerates except for a short segment between the urachus and ventral body wall, part of which persists after birth as the median ligament of the bladder.

DEVELOPMENT OF THE INTESTINE

Intestinal Loop

After the primordium of the gut tube has closed, the intestine is suspended by a dorsal mesentery and is relatively straight. The exception to this occurs at the site of yolk sac attachment, where the gut loops ventrally towards and, later, through the umbilicus (Fig. 16.7A). At this site the dorsal mesentery is expanded and a large blood vessel courses through it. This is the right vitelline artery that supplies the yolk sac during its period of function and becomes the cranial mesenteric artery in the fetus and adult.

The yolk stalk attachment to the yolk sac is lost soon after the development of the intestinal loop, permitting the loop a considerable degree of movement within the abdomen. Shortly after the loss of the yolk stalk, an evagination occurs in the wall of the caudal limb of the loop. This is the primordium of the **cecum**, which demarcates the small intestinal portion of the loop from the large intestinal portion.

The segment of foregut immediately caudal to the stomach forms the descending duodenum. During the subsequent changes in position of the intestinal loop, this portion of the gut tube is held in place on the right dorsal aspect of the peritoneal cavity by the mesoduodenum.

Rapid elongation of the small intestine causes most of the cranial limb of the loop to pass out of the body cavity into the umbilical stalk. This normal embryonic herniation of the intestine is illustrated in Figure 16.8. While the intestinal loop is externalized, the cranial limb continues to elongate.

This asymmetric expansion of one part of the gut causes the loop to rotate around the cranial mesenteric artery, with the cranial limb of the loop passing caudally and to the right of the caudal limb, as shown in Figure 16.7B. The process continues as the (original) cranial limb expands cranially and to the left of the rest of the midgut (Figs 16.7 C and D). Orienting on the cranial mesenteric artery as the axis of rotation, the intestinal loop undergoes an approximately 270° clockwise rotation, when viewed dorsoventrally.

The sequence of withdrawal of the loop determines the final placement of the intestines. The cranial limb, which gives rise to the ascending duodenum and most of the jejunum, returns into the abdomen first. During internalization this gut segment passes to the left of the median plane and pushes the descending colon to the left side. The mass of coiled jejunum fills much of the ventral abdomen and the distal jejunum passes cranially on the right side of the abdomen.

When the caudal limb withdraws, the cecum and ileum pass directly to the right side, in front of the cranial mesenteric artery. This extends the transverse colon from the descending colon at the left colic flexure to the right side. After reaching this position, the cecum passes caudally a short distance on the right of the cranial mesenteric artery. This forms the ascending colon and right colic flexure.

During the process of rotation and final placement, some parts of the dorsal mesentery are brought into apposition. When this occurs the two apposed layers usually fuse. The twisted mesentery that attached the intestine to the dorsal body wall around the cranial mesenteric artery is called the root of the mesentery (Figs 16.5 and 16.7).

In man, the smooth muscle of the intestinal tunica muscularis is well enough developed to produce peristaltic contractions when the fetus is 6-cm long (11 weeks of gestation). The material which accumulates in the colon and rectum prior to birth is called **meconium**. It consists of gastrointes-

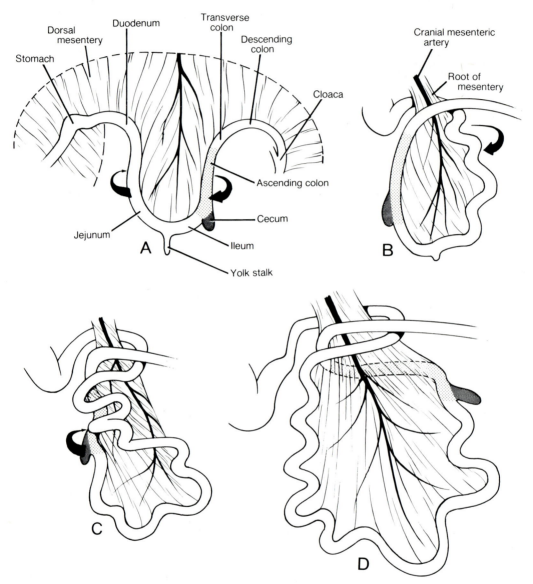

Figure 16.7. *A–D*, four stages in the development of the intestinal loop of the dog, illustrated schematically from a left perspective. *Arrows* show rotation. The cranial mesenteric artery acts as the axis for looping of the gut. Note that the small intestine elongates much more than the large. (Redrawn after Horowitz.)

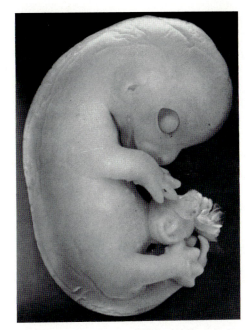

Figure 16.8. A 16-mm (25 day) feline embryo. Note the presence of the intestinal loop in the umbilical stalk.

tinal glandular secretions, bile, epithelial debris, and hair that was swallowed.

Comparative Development of the Colon

The colon, which is shaped like an inverted J in dogs and cats (Fig. 16.9*A*), has a more complicated configuration in the larger domestic animals. The comparative morphology of this structure can be readily appreciated if considered from a developmental standpoint. In all of these larger domestic animals the locations of the transverse and descending colons are not significantly different from that seen in the dog. The most extensive changes occur in the **ascending colon** and **cecum**.

In the dog and cat the ascending colon is a short straight tube between the ileum and transverse colon on the right side of the dorsal abdomen (Fig. 16.9*A*). Attached to the beginning of the ascending colon is a small, coiled cecum. The ascending colon is

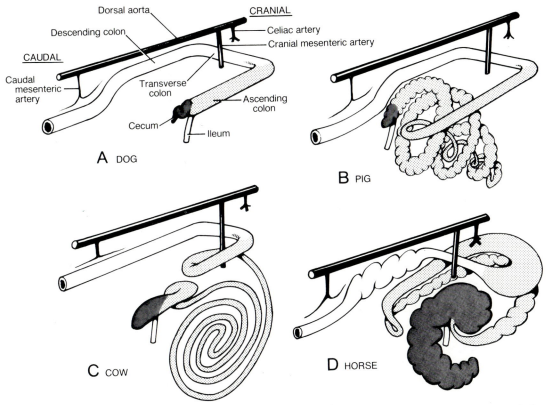

Figure 16.9. *A–D*, Schematic representation of the position and morphology of the cecum (dark stipple) and ascending colon, (light stipple) in domesticated animals. (Redrawn after Preuss.)

suspended by a short, straight portion of the mesocolon.

If one were to imagine grasping the center of the ascending colon, pulling it cranially then to the left around the root of the mesentery and, finally, stretching it caudally on the left side to the level of the pelvic inlet, the general morphology of the equine ascending colon would be obtained (Figs. 16.9D and 10 A and B). The point where the colon was grasped becomes the pelvic flexure. The two limbs that were stretched out become the **dorsal** and **ventral colons**, which are continuous at the pelvic flexure.

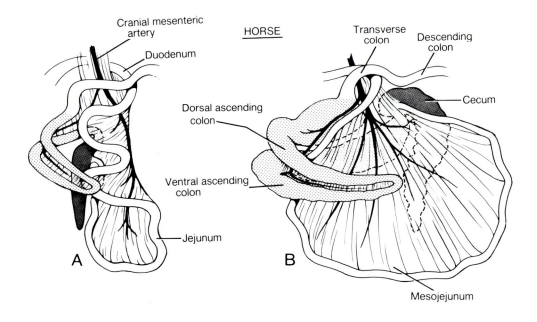

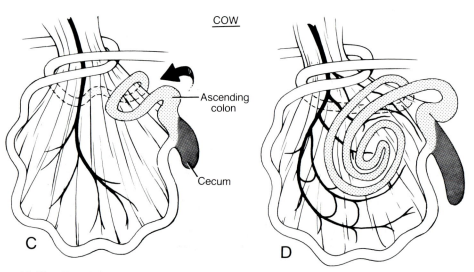

Figure 16.10.   Development of the intestinal loop and colon in *A* and *B*, the horse; and *C* and *D*, the cow. Schematic left lateral views. (Redrawn after Horowitz.)

The **mesocolon** remains between the dorsal and ventral colons. As a result, this portion of bowel, especially near the pelvic flexure, is subject to volvulus that compresses the local blood supply and may cause colic. The cecum remains on the right side, enlarges tremendously, and its apex extends cranioventrally on the abdominal wall.

In ruminant species the center of the ascending colon expands caudally around the root of the mesentery (Fig. 16.10C), then cranially on the left side and, finally, coils like a rope on the left side of the mesentery to produce the adult arrangement (Fig. 16.10D). The cecum is straight and dilated. It is located on the right side of the dorsal abdomen with its blind end caudally.

The same process establishes the morphology of the ascending colon of the pig, except that the coiled portion is shaped like a pyramid with its base on the left side of the mesentery, as shown in Figure 16.11. The cecum is straight and dilated, but has been pulled with the ascending colon to the left side of the dorsal abdomen.

SUBDIVISION OF THE CLOACA

The caudal portion of the embryonic hindgut is called the **cloaca**, and it serves as a common terminus for the urinary and digestive systems. The allantoic stalk, a ventral diverticulum of the hindgut, extends cranially and passes through the umbilicus and into the extraembryonic coelom where it participates in fetal membrane formation.

The cloaca is bounded caudally by the **cloacal membrane**, which is a septum formed by the apposition and fusion of hindgut endoderm and surface ectoderm. The mesenchyme surrounding the cloacal membrane expands, so that the membrane comes to lie in a shallow depression called the **proctodeum**, shown in Figure 16.12A. Mesonephric (urinary) ducts enter the cloaca laterally.

The hindgut and allantois are surrounded by splanchnic mesoderm. The hindgut is suspended dorsally by a dorsal mesentery, and the allantois is attached ventrally to the abdominal wall by a fold of splanchnic mesoderm. There is no mesenteric attachment between the hindgut and allantois.

Beginning at the junction of hindgut and allantois, the endoderm and surrounding mesenchyme thicken, forming the **urorectal septum**. This septum grows caudally, separating the cloaca into two chambers (Fig. 16.12 B and C). The dorsal chamber, which is continuous with the rest of the gut, is the

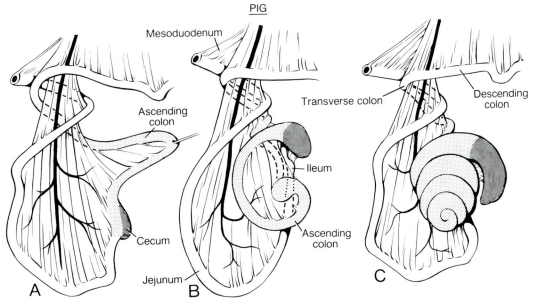

Figure 16.11. *A–C*, development of the intestinal loop and colon in the pig. Schematic left lateral views. (Redrawn after Horowitz.)

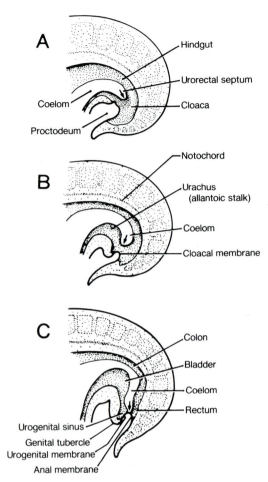

Figure 16.12. *A–C*, formation of the hindgut, and separation of the cloaca into urogenital sinus and rectum. *Arrow* indicates movement of the urorectal septum.

primordium of the **rectum** and part of the **anal canal**. The ventral chamber, continuous with the allantois and mesonephric ducts, is the **urogenital sinus**.

This separation continues until the urorectal septum contacts the cloacal membrane, dividing it into a dorsal **anal membrane** and a ventral **urogenital membrane**. The tissue between these two thin plates is the **perineal body**, the external surface of which will become the **perineum**. The anal membrane lies in a depression (anal pit). When this membrane degenerates, a patent **anal canal** is formed. It is lined with endoderm cranially and ectoderm caudally.

The proximal part of the allantois, to-

gether with the adjacent cranial portion of the urogenital sinus, enlarge to form the bladder. The remainder of the allantois extending from the apex of the bladder to the umbilicus is called the **urachus**. It is patent in the embryo, allowing urinary excretions to pass into the lumen of the allantois. The fold of peritoneum that attaches the bladder and urachus to the ventral body wall is the **median ligament of the bladder**. In the embryo and fetus it also contains the two umbilical arteries. After birth the urachus and umbilical arteries collapse and slowly degenerate in the free edge of the median ligament of the bladder.

MALFORMATIONS OF THE INTESTINAL TRACT

Stenosis and Atresia

The most common congenital malformations of the gut are local narrowing (stenosis) or closure (atresia) of the lumen of the gut. These can occur at any part of the gut, and while usually singular, are occasionally found in several locations in the same animal.

As was shown in Figure 15.4, **esophageal stenosis** or **atresia** can occur singly or associated with a tracheoesophageal fistula. Occasionally hydrops of the amnion accompanies this malformation. Hypoplasia of the esophageal wall may cause a focal weakness; also, an abnormal evagination of the wall, an **esophageal diverticulum**, may occur.

The various forms of intestinal stenosis and atresia are illustrated in Figure 16.13. There is considerable debate concerning the cause(s) of these conditions. Failure of the gut to initially form a continuous tube is an unlikely explanation, since the closure of each segment of the gut is dependent upon the preceding closure of the adjacent segment. Thus, a failure at this initial stage would create a large visceral schisis.

The most frequently given explanation is that small regions of the gut either fail to become vascularized or the vessels degenerate early in development. The avascular segments of gut become hypoplastic or completely degenerate, depending upon the severity of the vascular deficit. Support for this hypothesis comes from studies in which intestinal atresia can be produced by experimentally disrupting the mesenteric arteries.

Similar conditions would result if the intestine failed to reestablish patency after the transient stage of luminal occlusion. Alternatively, local abnormalities in the proliferation or cytodifferentiation of the muscular tunic could create a stenotic situation. This would be especially deleterious if the situation arose during the period of maximal gut tube elongation.

Intestinal atresia occurs with greater frequency at particular locations in different domestic animals, as summarized in Table 16.3. Intestinal atresia is found only in the colon in kittens and foals, and in the small intestine and rectum in puppies. Among the domestic animals, it is most prevalent in

calves and can occur either in the jejunum, the colon or the rectum.

An atresia of the coiled portion of the ascending colon has been reported in calves and unfortunately has been erroneously termed "duocecum." This is because the proximal stump of the ascending colon, up to the level of the atresia, is dilated from the obstructed contents and it appears the same shape as the normal cecum. These animals die 2–5 days after birth.

An hereditary-recessive cause of intestinal atresia has been reported in the jejunum of Jersey cattle and the ileum of Swedish Highland cattle. An hereditary-recessive cause of atresia of the ascending colon at the pelvic flexure has been reported in Percheron horses.

Atresia Ani

Atresia ani, more commonly called **imperforate anus**, is the failure of the anal membrane to break down and remain patent. In these animals the rectum is intact and attached to the membrane. Atresia ani is most frequently encountered in calves and pigs. If the rectum ends blindly as a cul-de-sac a short distance cranial to the anal membrane, the condition is called **rectal atresia**.

Urorectal Fistual

Often associated with the above defects is an abnormality in the development of the urorectal septum that permits communication between the rectum (or descending colon) and a derivative of the urogential sinus. These are collectively called **urorectal fistu-**

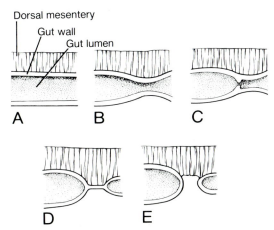

Figure 16.13. Schematic median views of *A*, normal; *B* and *C*, stenotic; and *D* and *E*, atretic sections of the gut.

Table 16.3.
Intestinal atresia and stenosis in domestic animals[a,b]

Region	Dog	Cow	Lamb	Pig	Cat	Foal
Duodenum	a					
Jejunum	s	A,s	a	a		
Ileum	a		a	a		
Colon		A	a,s	a	A,s	A
Rectum	a	A	a	A	a	a

[a] Data from Van der Gaag and Tibboel, 1980.
[b] A, atresia, frequent; a, atresia, uncommon; and s, stenosis, uncommon.

las, but more specifically may be named for the exact site of the communication, such as:

Rectovesicular fistula—connection to the bladder
Rectovestibular fistula—connection to the vestibule
Rectourethral fistula—connection to the urethra

If the fistula is large, fecal excretions may pass through the urogenital system. The urachus frequently remains patent in these animals. While individuals, especially females, with a urorectal fistula may survive for long periods, secondary infections due to the presence of fecal material in the vestibule or urethra are common. However, these animals often have atresia ani, in which case the situation becomes critical within a few days of birth.

Situs Inversus

Situs inversus is a malformation in which all the body organs develop opposite to their normal position, forming a "mirror-image" of normal. This usually involves both thoracic and abdominal organs. For example, the pylorus would be on the left, the descending duodenum on the left, the cecum and ascending colon on the left, and the descending colon on the right. This malformation is completely compatible with normal function. Occasionally these animals will also have a condition called the immotile cilia syndrome, in which cilia on epithelial cells lining the respiratory and upper digestive tracts do not move normally. This often leads to respiratory infection.

Umbilical Anomalies

The yolk stalk may persist from the distal jejunum to the umbilicus as a fibrous cord (Fig. 16.14A) or as a patent vitellointestinal duct. The latter is called an **umbilical fistula**, and it allows direct communication from the intestine to the surface of the body.

Remnants of the yolk stalk at its normal attachment to the intestine are common.

Occasionally the bowel is evaginated at this site, producing a **diverticulum** (Meckel's diverticulum). In horses, parts of the distal left vitelline artery and associated mesenteric folds may persist, in addition to those normally found on the right side (cranial mesenteric artery). These **mesodiverticular bands** (Fig. 16.14B) surround the small intestine at the former site of yolk stalk attachment. Usually their presence is an incidental finding at necropsy. Occasionally, part of the small intestine will pass through a tear or fold in this mesentery, which may produce sufficient constriction or twisting of the gut to obstruct the passage of digesta.

Normally the urachus closes and degenerates along the border of the median ligament of the bladder. If it remains open, this is a **patent urachus** or **urachal fistula** and urine will be excreted from this tube at the umbilicus. This is a source of infection for the bladder. Persistence of only the distal end of the intraembryonic allantoic stalk at the umbilicus creates a **urachal umbilical sinus**. Persistence of the proximal urachus at its union with the bladder creates a diverticulum that may be a site of chronic cystitis.

An **umbilical hernia** is a defect in the muscular wall around the umbilicus that allows abdominal organs to protrude through the umbilicus under the skin. In dogs and cats it is usually the small intestine that herniates; in calves it is the abomasum. This common abnormality may in some instances be inherited.

An **omphalocele** (Fig. 16.15) is a hernia that occurs in the embryo in which the abdominal contents protrude through the umbilicus, and remain within the umbilical stalk, and are therefore covered by the amnion. This probably results from a failure of normal withdrawal of the developing intestinal loop. A complete absence of the ventral abdominal wall results in externalization of the viscera, a condition inappropriately called **gastroschisis**. This is most prevalent in cats.

Nonrotation of the intestine occurs if, during the process of being brought back into the abdominal cavity, the intestinal loop

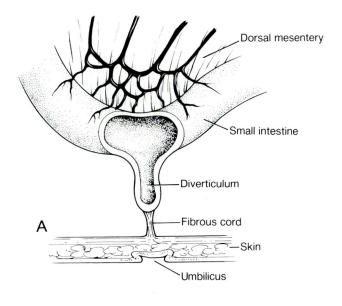

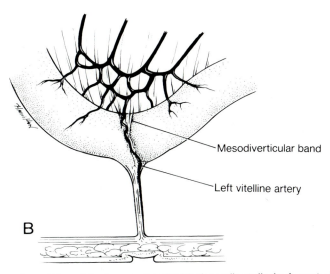

Figure 16.14. Anomalies of the midgut associated with the yolk stalk. In *A*, part of the stalk remains patent as a diverticulum; in some cases this remains attached to the umbilical site by a fibrous cord, as shown. Cysts may be present in this cord. *B* shows a persistent left distal vitelline artery and associated left sheet of the mesentery, which has formed a mesodiverticular band.

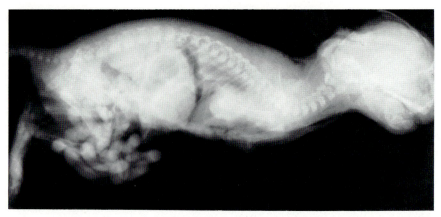

Figure 16.15. An omphalocele in a newborn kitten, shown radiographically. This animal also had bilateral thoracic ectromelia.

fails to undergo its 270° rotation. Often this will result in a **volvulus**, which is an acute twisting of a segment of gut around its mesentery.

Neuromuscular Disorders of the Gut

Neuromuscular disorders of the esophagus and intestine may present many of the same clinical signs as stenosis. Most of these are called achalasia, which means a lack of relaxation of the gut wall.

Colonic achalasia is a failure of a segment of the descending colon to relax and dilate. As discussed in Chapter 7, this is caused by a congenital lack of enteric neurons in the myenteric plexus of that segment of bowel. Feces accumulate cranial to the constricted area, and cause the colon to dilate (**megacolon**).

A **neuromuscular esophageal disorder** occurs occasionally in dogs and less often in cats. The defect probably involves the esophageal neuromuscular plexus that controls the normal sequence of peristaltic contraction during swallowing. The lack of normal esophageal peristalsis results in a failure of the functional sphincter at the gastroesophageal junction to relax (esophageal achalasia). As a consequence, food fails to pass into the stomach and accumulates cranial to this junction in the caudal esophagus. This causes stretching of the esophageal wall and a dilation of the lumen termed **megaesophagus.**

Megaesophagus may also be a manifestation of defects in the preganglionic vagal parasympathetic neurons. This has been suggested because experimental bilateral vagotomy causes signs similar to this condition. Studies of brain stem nuclei in one affected dog revealed a decreased number of neuronal cell bodies in the motor nucleus (nucleus ambiguus) whose axons innervate the striated esophageal muscle via branches of the vagus nerve.

There is a breed predilection for this disease, which, in some instances, has occurred in an hereditary pattern. The breeds most commonly affected include German Shepherds, Wirehaired Fox Terriers, Miniature Schnauzers, German Short-Haired Pointers, and Dachshunds. The disease is usually congenital, with signs occurring in the puppy. However, a similar but acquired disease can occur in older dogs. As a rule, while the puppy is on a liquid diet no signs of the problem occur because the liquid can pass through the gastroesophageal junction. When solid food is consumed at weaning, regurgitation commonly occurs, associated with eating or shortly thereafter. The vomitus is undigested, having failed to reach the stomach.

Radiographs following consumption of barium sulfate reveal a dilated esophagus cranial to the diaphgram and a narrow terminal segment. Functional studies may further reveal the neuromuscular deficiency.

Many treatments have been tried with variable success. These include surgical procedures to cause relaxation of the gastroesophageal junction and feeding of these dogs in an upright position.

Heterotopic Tissues

Heterotopic pancreatic tissue develops from endodermal epithelial cells that differentiate inappropriately for the organ in which they are located. These are most often associated with the area of origin of the pancreatic diverticulae. Pancreatic acini most commonly are found in the duodenal submucosa in the area of the pancreatic ducts, or are mixed in with the duodenal glands in the duodenal mucosa. Occasionally they occur in the gall bladder mucosa. They do not cause clinical signs.

Bibliography

NORMAL DEVELOPMENT

Kano Y, Kufkaya K, Asari M, Eguchi Y: Studies on the development of the fetal and neonatal bovine stomach. *Anat Histol Embryol* 10:267–274, 1981.

Lambert PS: The development of the stomach in the ruminant. *Vet J* 104:302–310, 1948.

Warner ED: The organogenesis and early histogenesis of the bovine stomach. *Am J Anat* 102:33–59, 1958.

ATRESIA, STENOSIS, HYPOPLASIA

Clark WT, Cox JE, Birtles MJ: Atresia of the small intestine in lambs and calves. *NZ Vet J* 26:120–122, 1978.

Dennis SM, Leipold HW: Atresia ani in sheep. *Vet Rec* 91:219–222, 1972.

Freeman DE, Koch DB, Boles CL: Mesodiverticular bands as a cause of small intestinal strangulation and volvulus in the horse. *JAVMA* 175:1089–1094, 1979.

Johnson R, Ames NK, Coy C: Congenital intestinal atresia in calves. *JAVMA* 182:1387–1389, 1983.

Liepold HW, Sapperstein G, Johnson DD: Intestinal atresia in calves. *Vet Med Small Anim Clin* 74:1037–1040, 1979.

McGeady TA, Murphy EC, Twomey T: Atresia coli in a calf. A note on its pathogenesis. *Ir Vet J* 21:148–150, 1967.

Norrish JG, Rennie JC: Observations on the inheritance of atresia ani in pigs. *J Hered* 59:186–187, 1968.

Osborne JC, Legates JE: Six cases of bovine intestinal anomaly. *JAVMA* 142:1104, 1963.

Rawlings CA, Capps WF, Jr: Rectovaginal fistula and imperforate anus in a dog. *JAVMA* 159:320–326, 1971.

Van der Gaag I, Tibboel D: Intestinal atresia and stenosis in animals: a report of 34 cases. *Vet Pathol* 17:565–574, 1980.

NEUROMUSCULAR DEFECTS OF THE ESOPHAGUS

Clifford D: Diseases of the canine esophagus due to prenatal influence. *Am J Dig Dis* 14:578–602, 1969.

Clifford DH, Gyorkey F: Myenteric ganglial cells in dogs with and without achalasia of the esophagus. *JAVMA* 150:205–211, 1967.

Clifford DH, et al: Congenital achalasia of the esophagus in four cats of common ancestry. *JAVMA* 158:1554–1560, 1971.

Gray GW: Acute experiments in neuroeffector function in canine esophageal achalasia. *Am J Vet Res* 35:1075–1082, 1974.

Harvey CW, et al: Megaesophagus in the dog: a clinical study of 79 cases. *JAVMA* 165:443–446, 1974.

Hoffer RE, Valdes-Dapena A, Baue AE: A comparative study of naturally occurring canine achalasia. *Arch Surg* 95:83–88, 1967.

Osborne CA, et al: Hereditary esophageal achalasia in dogs. *JAVMA* 151:572–581, 1967.

Sokolovsky V: Achalasia and paralysis of the canine esophagus. *JAVMA* 160:943–955, 1972.

CHAPTER 17

Derivatives of the Intermediate Mesoderm: Urinary System, Adrenal Gland

The urogenital system is derived from the nonsegmented intermediate mesoderm (nephrogenic plate) and the adjacent mesodermal coelomic epithelium. The early proliferation and development of this mesoderm produces a longitudinal swelling along the dorsolateral aspect of the abdomen. This is referred to as the urogenital ridge.

URINARY SYSTEM

The classical, evolutionary approach to the development of the urinary system is to consider the formation of three "kidneys," the **pronephros**, **mesonephros**, and **metanephros**, which develop in sequence from cranial to caudal along this urogenital ridge. Another approach is to consider the developing nephric system as one kidney, a **holonephros**, of which the cranial portions form first and degenerate during fetal development. To relate better to published literature, the classical approach will be considered.

The **pronephros** is rudimentary in mammals. Seven or eight pairs of pronephric tubules form briefly at the level of somites 7–14 (Fig. 17.1). In the intermediate mesoderm of this same region a duct develops

and grows caudally to the cloaca. Because of its time of origin and relationship to these tubules this is called the **pronephric duct**.

In most domestic animals the pronephric tubules are nonfunctional and do not establish patent connections with the duct. The exception occurs in sheep, in which the tubules are well developed and connect to the longitudinal duct. Caudal to this, at approximately the level of somites 9 through 26, 70–80 pairs of **mesonephric tubules** develop (Fig. 17.2; see also Figs. 18.3–5). These are apposed on one end to a blood vessel and on the other they connect into a caudal extension of the pronephric duct, which is now called the **mesonephric duct**. The formation of mesonephric tubules, most of which are functional in the fetus, is initiated by the presence of the pronephric duct.

A rich vascular plexus forms within the mesonephros. This is composed of numerous lateral branches from the dorsal aorta as well as anastomotic branches of the caudal, supra- and subcardinal veins.

The size of the mesonephros is correlated with the type of placenta. It is smallest in carnivores (Fig. 17.3) and man, (endothelio- and hemochorial), largest in pigs (epithelio-chorial), and intermediate in sheep. In many of these domestic animals the mesonephros takes up so much room in the abdomen that it is partly responsible for the normal herniation of the growing intestinal loop.

Soon after their formation, most of the mesonephric tubules degenerate. This atrophy occurs craniocaudally, leaving only the

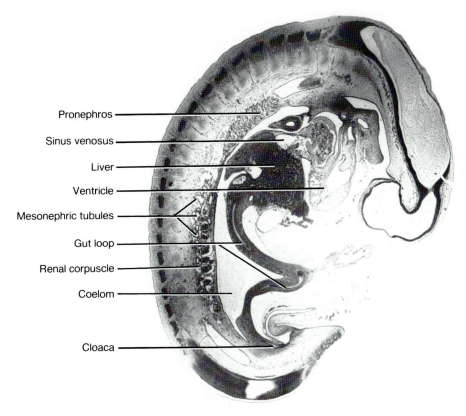

Pronephros

Sinus venosus

Liver

Ventricle

Mesonephric tubules

Gut loop

Renal corpuscle

Coelom

Cloaca

Figure 17.1. Paramedian section of a 9.5-mm calf embryo illustrating the locations of the pronephros and mesonephros. Note the vascular plexus associated with the mesonephric tubules.

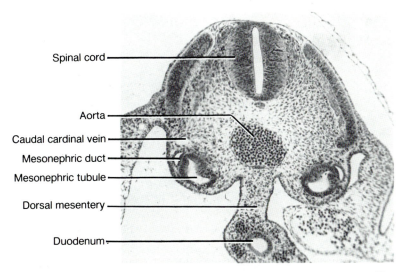

Spinal cord

Aorta

Caudal cardinal vein

Mesonephric duct

Mesonephric tubule

Dorsal mesentery

Duodenum

Figure 17.2. Transverse section at the cranial thoracic level of a 6-mm cat embryo. The mesonephric tubules at this level are transient and do not develop as fully as their more caudal counterparts.

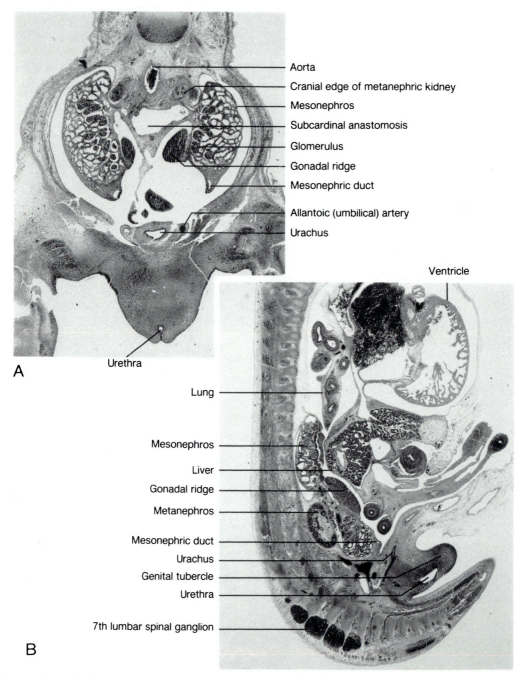

Aorta
Cranial edge of metanephric kidney
Mesonephros
Subcardinal anastomosis
Glomerulus
Gonadal ridge
Mesonephric duct

Allantoic (umbilical) artery
Urachus

Ventricle

Urethra

A

Lung

Mesonephros
Liver
Gonadal ridge
Metanephros

Mesonephric duct
Urachus
Genital tubercle
Urethra

7th lumbar spinal ganglion

B

Figure 17.3.   The urogenital organs in a 16-mm canine embryo. *A*, cross section through the cranial pole of the metanephric kidney and the genital tubercle. *B*, paramedian section through the right mesonephric and metanephric kidneys and the gonadal ridge.

caudal ⅙ to function for awhile. Degeneration of the cranial part of the mesonephros occurs between 4 and 8 weeks in man, around 8–9 weeks in the horse, and 10 weeks in cattle.

Development of the **metanephros** begins at the level of somites 26 through 28 when the embryo is 6–7 mm in length. It appears as an evagination from the caudal end of the mesonephric duct (Fig. 17.4); this is called the **metanephric diverticulum (ureteric bud)**. The diverticulum grows craniodorsally into the overlying caudal intermediate mesoderm which is proliferating and aggregating to

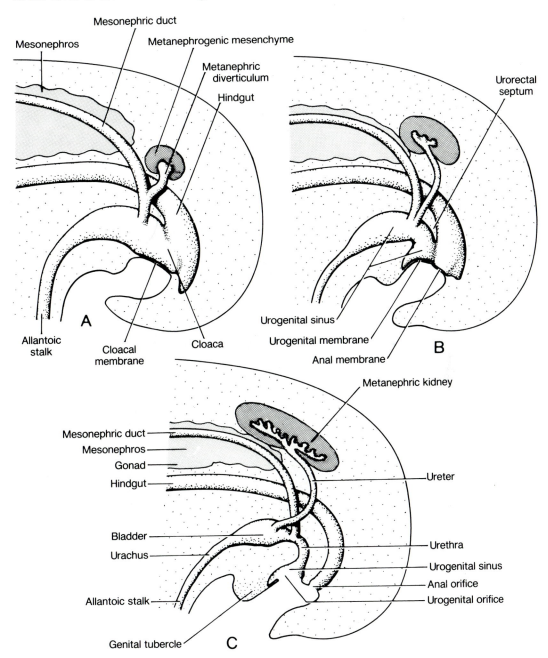

Figure 17.4. Schematic lateral views showing the formation of the metanephric diverticulum and subsequent partial incorporation of the mesonephric and metanephric ducts into the urogenital sinus.

form the **metanephrogenic mass**. As the diverticulum grows towards this mass, its distal end dilates to form the **pelvis**.

The subsequent morphogenesis of the metanephric diverticulum varies depending upon the species (Fig. 17.5). However, in all species the smallest, terminal branches are **collecting tubules**. Urine passes from nephrons into these tubules, and from there into larger **papillary ducts**.

As the collecting tubules form, each causes the adjacent metanephric mesoderm to coalesce into a solid cluster which then hollows to form a **renal vesicle**. The vesicle elongates into a tube that progressively grows in length

and forms **metanephric tubules** (Fig. 17.6). The aggregation of these metanephrogenic mesenchymal cells to form epithelial tubules is dependent upon their producing a specific glycoprotein component in the basement membrane. This material may be responsible for the increased cellular adhesiveness critical to tubule formation.

The morphogenesis of the metanephric kidney requires reciprocal inductive interactions between both components. The ureteric bud will not undergo branching in the absence of metanephric mesenchyme, similar to situations described earlier for lung and pancreas (Chapters 15 and 16)

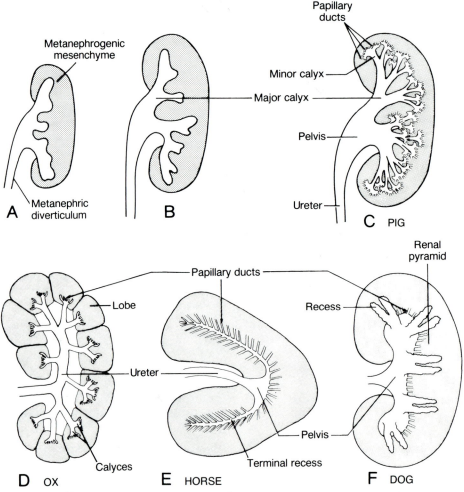

Figure 17.5. *A–C,* branching of the distal part of the metanephric diverticulum in the developing pig. *D–F,* schematic representation of the branching patterns in bovine, equine and carnivore kidneys. The papillary ducts have been drawn disproportionately larger than they actually are.

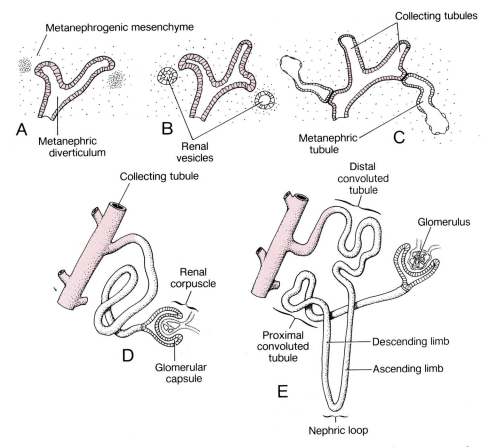

Figure 17.6. Schematic representation of the formation of the nephron from metanephrogenic mesenchyme and its fusion with the collecting duct, which is derived from the metanephric diverticulum. The epithelia will degenerate at the site where metanephric and collecting tubules are in contact. *D* and *E* illustrate early stages in the formation of the convoluted tubules and glomeruli. Redrawn after Langman J: *Medical Embryology*, ed. 4. Baltimore, Williams & Wilkins, 1981.

primordia. In addition, the transformation of metanephric mesenchymal cells into epithelial tubules is dependent upon the presence of the ureteric bud.

After attaining a certain length, one end of each metanephric tubule attaches to a collecting tubule. The other end of the metanephric tubule widens and invaginates to form a cup-shaped structure, the **glomerular capsule**. This cup is invaded by a proliferating plexus of blood vessels. The capillary plexus is called a **glomerulus**, and the entire structure is the **renal corpuscle**. Continued growth of the tubule will form the definitive segments of the secretory tubule between the glomerulus and the collecting duct (Fig. 17.6 *D* and *E*).

The mature **nephron** includes the glomerular capsule and the secretory tubule. Nephrons are organized so that the renal corpuscles are located in the outer, **cortical** portion of the kidney, and the elongated loops of the nephron extend centrally to form the inner, **medullary** portion of the kidney.

The first renal corpuscles to form are located at the corticomedullary junction, and many of these early formed nephrons degenerate during later fetal stages. Collecting tubules elongate and new nephrons are induced to form at progressively more superficial levels throughout fetal development. Nephrogenesis ceases by birth or shortly thereafter depending on the species. New nephrons continue to arise in the first few weeks after birth in the dog. It is estimated that about 200,000 nephrons form in the feline kidney, 300,000–500,000 in the dog, and 1.5–4 million in the pig and ox.

The lack of ability to regenerate new nephrons is an important consideration in kidney disease. Following destruction of a population of nephrons, none of these can be replaced. The remaining nephrons attempt to compensate for the increased load by physiological adjustments as well as by increasing their size. The number of existing nephrons does not change.

The variations in macroscopic anatomy seen in kidneys of different mammals (Fig. 17.5) result from differences in the branching of the metanephric diverticulum and arrangement of nephrons associated with these branches. The bovine kidney has 12–25 separate lobes; the papillary ducts within each lobe drain into a **calyx**, which opens into a branch of the ureter.

The cortical region of the porcine kidney is not lobated, but the medulla is subdivided into **renal papillae**. Each of these papillae consists of nephric loops and the collecting tubules and ducts that empty into terminal branches of a minor (secondary) calyx (Fig. 17.5C). In horses, small ruminants and carnivores there are no calyces, and the papillary ducts drain directly into a common chamber. In the horse the renal pelvis is elongated, with two long, thin-walled processes called **terminal recesses** in which urine is collected.

In the dog, all of the collecting ducts enter the renal pelvis along a ridge in the roof of the pelvis called the **renal crest**. The recesses present in the canine kidney (Fig. 17.5F) do not serve to collect urine, but do segregate the medullary region into wedge-shaped regions called **renal pyramids**.

The metanephric kidney forms initially in the pelvic region of the embryo. It ascends a short distance relative to the extensive growth and elongation of the caudal aspect of the fetus, becoming situated ventral to the cranial lumbar vertebrae in most species. The ureter elongates commensurate with this growth of the fetus.

The metanephric kidneys are functional in the fetus. One evidence for this is that if a ureter is stenotic or atretic, the kidney it drains becomes swollen and **hydronephrotic**. This is due to the distention of the collecting system by execreted urine. However, this function is not critical to the fetus, as indicated by the birth of animals lacking kidneys (renal aplasia). Apparently the placenta can adequately function for the exchange of waste products normally eliminated from the body by the kidney. Without kidney function, the animal cannot survive after birth.

UROGENITAL SINUS

Subdivision of the cloaca by the urorectal fold and septum into the rectum and the urogenital sinus was described with the digestive system (Chapter 16). Following the degeneration of the urogenital membrane, the urogenital sinus opens caudally into the amniotic cavity via the **urogenital orifice** and cranially into the allantoic cavity via the **urachus** and **allantoic stalk**. For developmental considerations the urogenital sinus is divided into **pelvic** (cranial) and **phallic** (caudal) regions.

The bladder develops from the proximal urachus and the cranial part of the pelvic region of the urogenital sinus. The mesonephric duct enters the pelvic part of the urogenital sinus, and the metanephric diverticulum develops as a branch of the duct close to its junction with the wall of the sinus. With growth and expansion of the sinus, the caudal segment of the mesonephric duct and part of the metanephric diverticulum are incorporated into the dorsal wall of the developing neck of the bladder. As shown in Figure 17.4, this results in the establishment of separate openings for the mesonephric duct and ureter on each side. Subsequently these orifices shift position so that the ureter opens cranially in the neck of the developing bladder and the entrance of the mesonephric duct is located caudally in the pelvic part of the urogenital sinus, which will form the cranial **urethra**. In the male the mesonephric duct becomes the **ductus deferens**.

The dorsal wall of the neck of the bladder and the cranial urethra form the **trigone**, which represents the region of mesonephric and metanephric duct incorporation. The base of the trigone is delineated cranially by the entrance of the ureters. The apex is located at the site of the entrance of the ductus deferens on either side of a small swelling, the urethral crest.

In the female the **urethra** is derived from the cranial part of the pelvic urogenital sinus and the remainder of the sinus becomes the **vestibule**. The vagina and uterus develop from a separate set of ducts discussed in Chapter 18. In the male the entire urogenital sinus contributes to the formation of the urethra. The **pelvic urethra** is derived from the pelvic part of the sinus, and the **spongy urethra** found in the penis is from the phallic part of the sinus.

MALFORMATIONS OF THE URINARY SYSTEM

Agenesis of the kidneys can be bilateral or unilateral. Bilateral agenesis is lethal. In unilateral agenesis the opposite kidney undergoes **compensatory hypertrophy**. It is common for genital system anomalies to be associated with renal agenesis. In the female there is often an ipsilateral uterine aplasia (see Chapter 18).

Renal dysplasia includes a wide range of abnormal development of nephrons and collecting ducts, and is often associated with the formation of cysts. The reduced kidney function may be initially manifest as a skeletal defect directly caused by an endocrine imbalance. The kidney lesion causes retention of phosphorus in the blood, and the body adjusts by eliminating calcium through the intestine. The hypocalcemia stimulates parathyroid hormone secretion which acts by mobilizing calcium from bone. The latter causes bones to become soft. This condition, which is called **osteodystrophy fibrosa** secondary to **renal hyperparathyroidism** is usually most apparent in the mandible.

Renal cortical hypoplasia has been reported as a possible hereditary condition in Cocker Spaniels. The congenital kidney abnormality induces secondary renal hyperparathyroidism which in turn induces a fibrosis of the kidney further compromising its already insufficient function. Renal dysplasia is probably familial in Norwegian Elkhounds and there is a high incidence in the Samoyed, Keeshond, and Bedlington Terrier.

Hypoplasia of a portion of the ureteric bud or abnormal differentiation of its lumen causes stenosis of the ureter and secondary hydronephrosis.

The cause of **polycystic kidneys** is not clearly understood. One suggestion is that it represents failure of nephrons to join the collecting ducts. Urine is formed and retained in the nephron, which dilates and becomes cystic.

Ectopic kidneys consist of either a **pelvic kidney** that fails to ascend normally or a **horseshoe kidney**, which represents two kidneys that fused at their origin in the pelvic region and fail to ascend due to the presence of the caudal mesenteric artery and, possibly, the mesonephric ducts. **Supernumerary kidneys** result from an extra or branched (bifid) metanephric diverticulum in the embryo. The kidney tissue that develops in association with the extra ureteric bud may be fused with or separate from the normal kidney.

Ectopic ureters occur in all domestic animals but are most common in dogs. This condition most commonly presents a clinical problem in the female whenever a ureter enters the urethra distal to the sphincter located in the neck of the bladder and proximal urethra. There is nothing to prevent the continual slow dripping of urine from the vulva.

This is a common cause of congenital **incontinence**, which is the loss of voluntary control of micturition. In some cases the ectopic ureter can be located using endoscopy of the genital tract. Frequently this condition is confirmed by radiographic urography following injection via either the intravenous route or into the suspected ectopic ureter. Phenol red dye injected intravenously will be excreted in the urine and may help visualize the ectopic ureter. In many cases the ectopic ureters can be surgically corrected.

Other malformations of the urinary or genital system may accompany this defect. Hydroureter and hydronephrosis are the most common. A high risk for ectopic ureters exists in the Siberian Husky, West Highland White Terrier, Fox Terrier and Miniature and Toy Poodles.

A **common cloaca** results from failure of the urorectal septum to develop. This has been seen in the Manx cat in conjunction with absence of caudal vertebrae (Fig. 17.7).

An inherited malformation called **rectovaginal constriction** occurs in Jersey cattle. This autosomal recessive condition is due to the presence of fibrous bands that circumscribe the anorectal junction and the vestibule. The resulting anovestibular stenosis makes rectal examination difficult and causes dystocia.

A **vesicourachal diverticulum** occurs most commonly in dogs and often leads to chronic bladder infection. The diverticulum results from failure of the urachus to close and separate from the apex of the bladder. Other congenital malformations involving the urachus or the urorectal septum are presented in Chapter 16.

ADRENAL GLAND

The adrenal gland develops in the intermediate mesoderm at the cranial pole of the mesonephric kidney. The **adrenal medulla** is ectodermal in origin, being formed by cells derived from the neural crest (see Chapter 7). The **adrenal cortex** is derived from the surrounding intermediate mesoderm. The initial proliferation of intermediate mesoderm causes a bulge medially into the abdominal cavity. This is the transient **fetal adrenal cortex** that surrounds the neuroectodermal cells of the medulla. A second mantle of intermediate mesoderm proliferates and surrounds the first. This is the permanent cortex, which replaces the fetal cortex postnatally. The function of the provisional fetal cortex is unknown. In the dog the fetal cortex is absent at birth.

At birth the weight of the adrenal gland is $\frac{1}{3}$ that of the kidney, but in the adult it is only $\frac{1}{28}$ the weight of the kidney.

Malformations consist mostly of **ectopias** or **accessory adrenal cortices**. These are usually found near the adrenal, kidney, or gonad. Because the male gonad is derived from intermediate mesoderm medial to the mesonephros near the developing adrenal and descends into the scrotum, it may pull ectopic or accessory adrenal cortical tissue

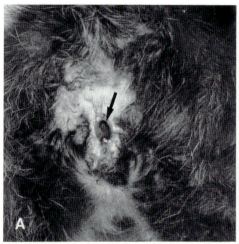
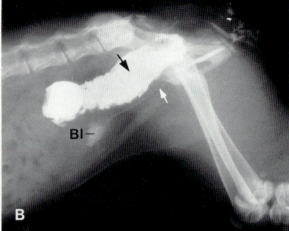

Figure 17.7. Persistent cloaca in a Manx cat. *A* is a caudal view illustrating the appearance of a single cloacal orifice (*arrow*) and absence of a tail. *B* is a radiograph of same animal following injection of contrast medium into the cloaca. Radiopaque material is visible in the colon (*black arrow*), urethra (*white arrow*) and bladder (*Bl*).

with it. This accounts for the presence of adrenal cortical tissue in the spermatic cord of horses.

Bibliography

NORMAL DEVELOPMENT

Berton JP: Anatomie vasculaire du mesonephros chez certain mammiferes. I. Le mesonephros de l'embryon de porc. *Comput Rendu Assoc Anat* 124:272–290, 1965.

Bryden MM, Evans H, Binns W: Development of the urogenital system in the sheep embryo. *Ciencias Morfologicas en America* 2:21–29, 1980.

Canfield P: Development of the bovine metanephros. *Anat Histol Embryol* 9:97–107, 1980.

Chandra, H: The correlation of growth and function in the developing mesonephros and metanephros in goat embryos. *J Anat Soc India* 13:18–23, 1964.

Du Bois AM: The embryonic kidney. In Rouiller C, Muller AF (eds): *The Kidney*, vol 1. New York, Academic Press, pp 1–60, 1969.

Eisenbrandt DL, Phemister RD: Postnatal development of the canine kidney: quantitative and qualitative morphology. *Am J Anat* 154:179–194, 1979.

Ekblom P, Alitalo K, Baheri A, Timpl R, Saxen L: Induction of a basement membrane glycoprotein in embryonic kidney. Possible role of laminen in morphogenesis. *Proc Natl Acad Sci USA* 77:485–489, 1980.

Fine H: The development of lobes of the metanephros and fetal kidney (human). *Acta Anat* 113:93–107, 1982.

Grobstein C: Inductive interaction in the development of the mouse metanephros. *J Exp Zool* 130:319–340, 1955.

Hay DA, Evan AP: Maturation of the glomerular visceral epithelium and capillary endothelium in the puppy kidney. *Anat Rec* 193:1–22, 1979.

Latimer HB: The growth of the kidneys and the bladder in the fetal dog. *Anat Rec* 109:1–12, 1951.

Leeson TS, Baxter JS: The correlation of structure and function in the mesonephros and metanephros of the rabbit. *J Anat* 91:383–390, 1957.

Torrey TS: The development of the urogenital system of the albino rat. I. The kidney and its ducts. *Am J Anat* 72:113–144, 1943.

CONGENITAL DEFECTS

Bardley WP: Unilateral ureteral ectopia in a Holstein-Friesian heifer. *JAVMA* 173:485–486, 1978.

Bebko RL, Prier JE, Biery DN: Ectopic ureters in a male cat. *JAVMA* 171:738–740, 1977.

Carrig CB, et al: Ectopic ureter, ureteral stricture, and hemivertebra in a hiefer. *JAVMA* 155:143–148, 1969.

Cordes DO, Dodd DC: Bilateral renal hypoplasia of the pig. *Pathol Vet* 2:37–48, 1965.

Crowell WA, Hubbell JJ, Riley JC: Polycystic renal disease in related cats. *JAVMA* 175:286–288, 1979.

Finco DR, Kurtz HR, Low DG, Perman V: Familial renal disease in Norwegian elkhound dogs. *JAVMA* 156:747–760, 1970.

Goulden B, Bergman MM, Wyburn RS: Canine urethro-rectal fistulae. *J Small Anim Pract* 14:143–150, 1973.

Hayes HM: Ectopic ureter in dogs: Epidemiologic features. *Teratol* 10:129–132, 1974.

Johnson CA: Renal ectopia in a cat: a case report and literature review. *J Am Anim Hosp Assoc* 15:599–602, 1979.

Johnson ME, Denhart, JD, Graber ER: Renal cortical hypoplasia in a litter of cocker spaniels. *J Am Anim Hosp Assoc* 8:268–274, 1972.

Johnston GR, Osborne CA, Wilson JW, Yano BL: Familial ureteral ectopia in the dog. *J Am Anim Hosp Assoc* 13:168–170, 1977.

Kaufman CF, Soirez RF, Tasker JB: Renal cortical hypoplasia with secondary hyperparathyroidism in the dog. *JAVMA* 155:1679–1685, 1969.

Krook L: The pathology of renal cortical hypoplasia in the dog. *Nord Vet Med* 9:161–176, 1957.

Leipold HW, Watt B, Vestweber JGE, Dennis SM: Clinical observations in rectovaginal constriction in Jersey cattle. *Bovine Pract* 16:76–79, 1981.

Lennox JS: A case report of unilateral ectopic ureter in a male Siberian Husky. *J Am Anim Hosp Assoc* 14:331–336, 1978.

Lucke VM, Kelly DF, Darke PGG, Gaskell CJ: Chronic renal failure in young dogs—possible renal dysplasia. *J Small Anim Pract* 21:169–181, 1980.

Maizels M, Simpson, SB, Jr: Primitive ducts of renal dysplasia induced by culturing ureteral buds denuded of condensed renal mesenchyme. *Science* 219:509–510, 1983.

Marshall LS, Oehlert ML, Haskins ME, Selden, JR., Patterson DF: Persistent Mullerian duct syndrome in Miniature Schnauzers. *JAVMA* 181:798–802, 1982.

Mawdesley-Thomas LE, Birtley RDN: Unilateral hypoplasia of the urogenital system in a beagle. *Vet Rec* 82:89–90, 1968.

McGhee CC, Leipold HW: Morphologic studies of rectovaginal constriction in Jersey cattle. *Cornell Vet* 72:427–436, 1982.

O'Handley P, Carrig CB, Walshaw, R: Renal and ureteral duplication in a dog. *JAVMA* 174:484–487, 1979.

Olsson, SE: Ectopic ureteral orifice causing urinary incontinence in a dog. *J Small Anim Pract* 3:75, 1962.

Osborne CA, Perman V: Ectopic ureter in a male dog. *JAVMA* 154:273–278, 1969.

Owen RR: Canine ureteral ectopia—a review. I. Embryology and etiology. *J Sm Anim Pract* 14:407–417, 1973.

Owen RR: Canine ureteral ectopia—a review. II. Incidence, diagnosis and treatment. *J Sm Anim Pract* 14:419–428, 1973.

Pearson H, Gibbs C: Urinary tract abnormalities in the dog. *J Sm Anim Pract* 12:67–84, 1971.

Smith CW, Stowater JL, Kneller SK: Ectopic ureter in the dog—a review of cases. *J Am Anim Hosp Assoc* 17:245–248, 1981.

Wilson JW, Klausner JS, Stevens JB, Osborne CA: Canine vesico-urachal diverticulum. *Vet Surg* 8:63–67, 1979.

CHAPTER **18**

Derivatives of the Intermediate Mesoderm: Reproductive Organs

The internal organs of reproduction, including the gonads, arise together with excretory structures from **intermediate mesoderm**. The primordia of both male and female reproductive structures develop in all embryos. The time when both sets of primordia are present is called the **indifferent stage** of organogenesis; this occurs during the 4th week of gestation in the dog, the 6th in cattle (Table 18.1). Shortly thereafter gender-specific characteristics develop, usually accompanied by degeneration of the inappropriate structures. This chapter describes the morphogenesis of internal and external organs of reproduction; the following chapter will discuss the hormonal control of this process.

GERM CELLS

Primary germ cells do not arise within the gonadal precursors, but rather are formed elsewhere and secondarily invade the presumptive gonads. In birds these cells are first seen at about 18 hr of incubation in the **germinal crescent**, which is located in front of the rostral tip of the embryo (Fig. 18.1). These large, glycogen-rich cells are formed from the epiblast during gastrulation and then accumulate between the endoderm and ectoderm. As blood vessels develop in the area vasculosa, primordial germ cells enter the extraembryonic circulation. During the 3rd day of incubation they leave the vascular

Table 18.1.
Formation of reproductive organs

Feature	Stage
Formation of gonadal ridge	9–10 mm
Dog, sheep	(24 day)
Horse	(27 day)
Ox	(28 day)
Genital tubercle externally visible	10–12 mm
Appearance of paramesonephric ducts	14–18 mm
Initial appearance of tunica albuginea[a] (denotes onset of testicular development)	16–20 mm
Formation of anogenital raphe in males[b]	
Dog	20 mm (31 day)
Ox	27 mm (42 day)
Anogenital distance greater in male	
Dog	25 mm (32 day)
Ox	36 mm (45 day)

[a] It requires several days for tunica albuginea to fully encapsulate testis; the process is completed by 30 days (boar), 35 days (ram), or 45 days (bull).
[b] Raphe appears 1 day later in females.

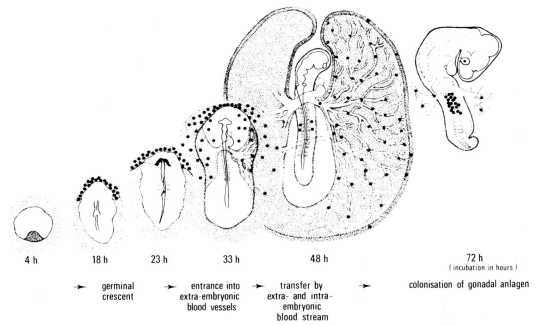

4 h	18 h	23 h	33 h	48 h	72 h
					(incubation in hours)

germinal crescent → entrance into extra-embryonic blood vessels → transfer by extra- and intra-embryonic blood stream → colonisation of gonadal anlagen

Figure 18.1.   The development of germ cells in birds. Primordial germ cells (*black spots*) first appear in the germinal crescent, then travel via the circulatory system to the gonadal ridge. (From Nieuwkoop PD, Sutasurya LA: *Primordial Germ Cells in the Chordates*, Cambridge, Cambridge University Press, 1979.)

network in the mesonephros and colonize the gonadal primordia.

Evidence for this vascular route comes from experiments in which the germinal crescent was removed from a neurula-stage chick embryo and replaced with the crescent from a different strain of bird. The host's gonads were later found to contain germ cells from the graft. How the circulating germ cells selectively colonize only the gonadal ridges is not well understood. Circumstantial evidence indicates that there is an attractant which the circulating cells recognize and respond to chemotactically.

In mammals the germ cells can first be recognized in the caudal yolk sac endoderm and adjacent splanchnic mesoderm (Fig. 18.2) at about the time that somitogenesis begins. They contain large amounts of both alkaline phosphatase and glycogen. The germ cells shift dorsally to the dorsal mesentery of the hindgut and then to the mesonephros, which is the site of gonad formation. While some germ cells enter the circulatory system in mammals, there is no evidence that these circulating germ cells colonize the gonads.

GONADOGENESIS
Indifferent Stage

The first sign of gonad development is a swelling called the **gonadal ridge** (genital or urogenital ridge) on the medial side of the middle part of each mesonephros. This ridge initially forms in embryos of approximately 9–10 mm and quickly enlarges (Fig. 18.3) due to local hypertrophy of the coelomic epithelium and arrival of approximately 100–300 primary germ cells.

The development of the gonadal primordium is closely linked with the partial degeneration of the mesonephros, especially the mesonephric tubules. Cords of epithelial cells from mesonephric tubules and degenerating glomerular capsules invade the area of the gonadal ridge (Fig. 18.4) then coalesce to form clusters and small vesicles that incorporate primary germ cells. These epithelial components form the **gonadal cords**

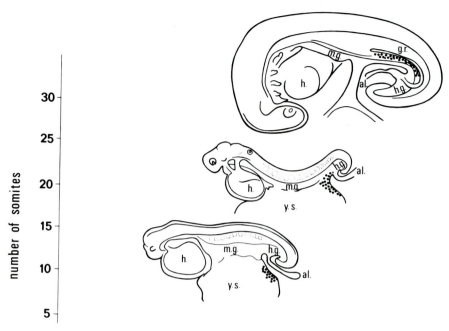

Figure 18.2. The development of germ cells in mammals. Primordial germ cells first appear in the endoderm of the yolk sac (*y.s.*) They shift dorsally to occupy the dorsal mesentery, and finally move into the medial margin of the mesonephros at the time of gonadal ridge formation (*al.*, allantois; *g.r.*, gonadal ridge; *h.*, heart; *h.g.*, hindgut; and *m.g.*, midgut). (From Nieuwkoop PD, Satasurya LA, 1979.)

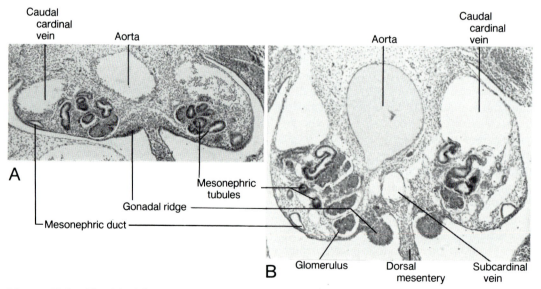

Figure 18.3. The initial formation of the gonadal ridge is illustrated in these transverse sections from *A*, an 8mm, and *B*, an 11-mm bovine embryo.

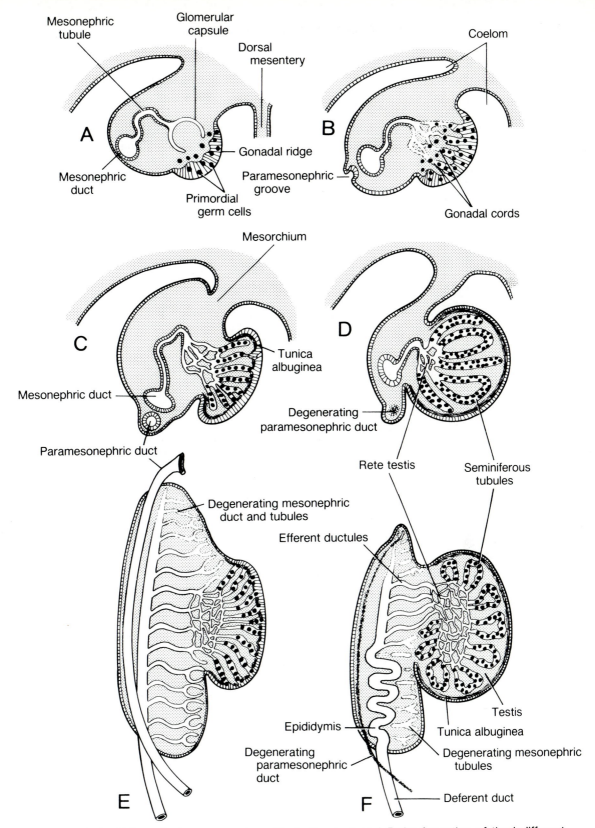

Figure 18.4. Schematic transverse views illustrating in *A* and *B* the formation of the indifferent gonad and in *C* through *F* the subsequent development of the testis. *E* and *F* are ventral views at the same stages as *C* and *D*.

(primitive sex cords). They establish an epithelial network between the gonadal ridge epithelium and the remnants of the mesonephric tubules.

The best evidence regarding the precise origins of gonadal cords comes from analyses of sheep and cattle gonadogenesis. These species have a giant nephron (Fig. 18.5) that is located in the cranial part of the mesonephros and has a large, multisegmental glomerular capsule connected to many tubules. As this nephron breaks down, the capsular epithelial cells colonize the gonadal ridge and form the primary sex cords. This is referred to as the indifferent stage of gonadogenesis.

Testis

The subsequent development of the male gonad (Fig. 18.4) takes place in the medullary region of the gonadal ridge. The gonadal cords form solid tubes that postnatally become patent and form the **seminiferous tubules**. These tubules are arranged in loops that connect via a network of ductules, the **rete testis**, to the **efferent ductules**. Both of these duct systems are derived from mesonephric tubules.

The gonadal cords become separated from the coelomic epithelium by a distinct mesenchymal sheet, the primordial **tunica albuginea**. The appearance of this tunic, which serves as the pathway of blood supply to the gonad, is the first histological evidence that the gonad is a testis, as shown in Figure 18.4. In the definitive testis the germ cells become the **spermatogonia**. They line the seminiferous tubule in association with **sustentacular cells** (Sertoli cells), which are derived from mesonephric tubule epithelial cells. The origin of **interstitial cells** (Leydig cells), which are located between seminiferous tubules, is uncertain; descriptive data suggest they are formed by mesodermal mesenchyme cells that originally occupied the gonadal ridge. These interstitial and sustentacular cell populations produce androgens and other secretions of the male gonad (discussed in Chapter 19).

Ovary

In the female the epithelial gonadal cords break up into many small clusters called **follicles** (Fig. 18.6), each of which has one or more germ cells in the center. Most of the cell clusters are situated peripherally, close to the hypertrophied epithelium that will form the mesothelial surface of the gonad. Those clusters located deep in the medullary region degenerate. No tunica albuginea develops in the ovary, and the medullary

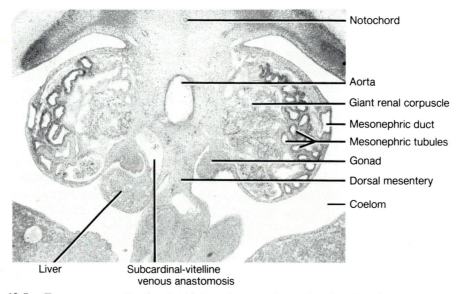

Notochord

Aorta

Giant renal corpuscle

Mesonephric duct

Mesonephric tubules

Gonad

Dorsal mesentery

Coelom

Liver

Subcardinal-vitelline venous anastomosis

Figure 18.5. Transverse section from a 10-mm sheep embryo showing the appearance of the giant renal corpuscle in each mesonephros, and its close relation to the gonadal ridge.

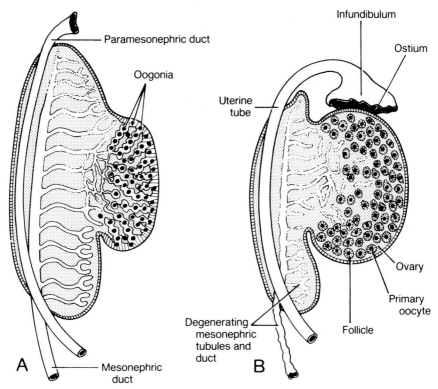

Figure 18.6.   Schematic ventral views of the development of the ovary. Compare with sections *E* and *F* of Figure 18.4.

region remains as a loosely arranged stroma through which blood vessels to the developing ovary grow. The ovary of the mare is an exception in that the cell clusters are distributed throughout the ovary, not just in the cortical region, and it has a peripheral vascular supply.

Although a few oogonia enter meiotic prophase shortly after entering the gonadal ridge, most continue to divide mitotically throughout fetal stages and shortly after birth. When they stop dividing they form **primary oocytes** (see Chapter 2).

The precise origin(s) of follicular cells has not been defined. By analogy with the male, it is usually stated that estrogen-producing follicular cells are of gonadal ridge mesenchymal origin. However, descriptive evidence indicates that gonadal cord epithelial cells, which are the predominant cell type during early stages of ovarian development, contribute to fetal follicles and probably persist in the adult. Possibly both cell types contribute to the follicular population,

which may explain the functional heterogeniety of mature follicular cells. During development many more oogonia are produced than will survive. In the pig there are approximately 5,000 germ cells in the fully formed indifferent gonad (24 days of gestation), 1,100,000 oogonia at 50 days and 500,000 at term.

INTERNAL DUCTS

The mesonephros degenerates from cranial to caudal. In the male, some of the mesonephric tubules that fused with gonadal cords persist and form the **efferent ductules** (ductuli efferentes; Fig. 18.4). That portion of the mesonephric duct originally located within the mesonephros remains closely associated with the testis and forms the **epididymis**. As shown in Figure 18.7, the caudal part of each mesonephric duct forms a **deferent duct** (ductus deferens).

In contrast, the entire mesonephric duct and tubules degenerate in the female fetus (Fig. 18.8). Vestigial traces of mesonephric

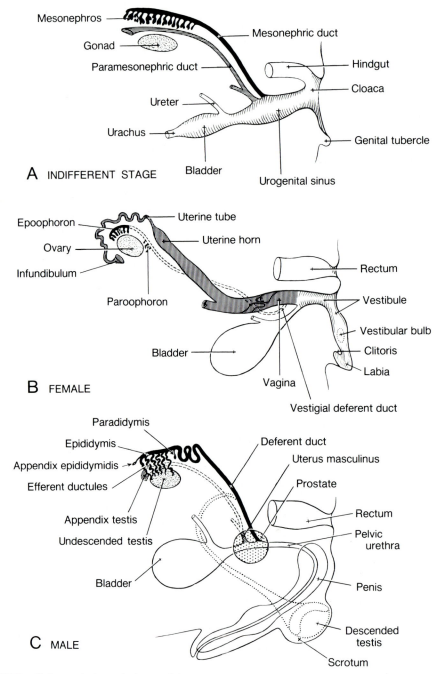

Figure 18.7. Schematic lateral views of the canine urogenital system at *A*, the indifferent stage, at which time primordia of both male and female ducts are present; in *B*, the female; and *C*, the male. (Modified from HE Evans and GC Christensen, 1979.)

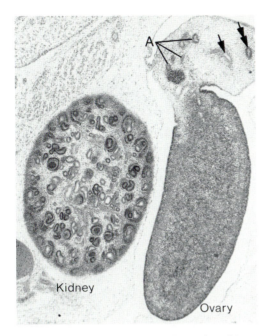

tubule and duct tissues can occasionally be found in mesenteries surrounding the ovary (epoophoron, paroophoron) or near the wall of the vagina (Gartner's duct) or urethra.

A second duct, the **paramesonephric duct** (müllerian duct), forms in both male and female embryos on the lateral side of the mesonephros, close to the mesonephric duct (Figs. 18.9, 10). Initially, a longitudinal **paramesonephric groove** develops in the mesothelium. This deepens then separates from the peritoneal lining, forming a solid cord of cells that grows caudally along the lateral then ventral wall of the mesonephros. Subsequently a lumen forms in the cord. In the caudal region of the abdomen this growing tube curves medially and meets the paramesonephric duct from the opposite side (Fig. 18.10). The two tubes fuse and extend caudally as one tube to enter the urogenital sinus caudal to the mesonephric and metanephric ducts.

In the female the **uterine tubes** (Fallopian tubes, oviducts), **the horns**, **body** and **cervix**, and part of the **vagina** are derived from these fused paramesonephric ducts. The urogenital sinus and, to a lesser extent, mesonephric

Figure 18.8. Transverse section of a 41-mm feline fetus showing the metanephric kidney and ovary. The ovary is occupied by proliferating oogonia surrounded by follicular cells. Note that most of the mesonephric tubules have degenerated (*A*), and only a remnant of the mesonephric duct (*single arrow*) is still present. The *double arrow* indicates the paramesonephric duct.

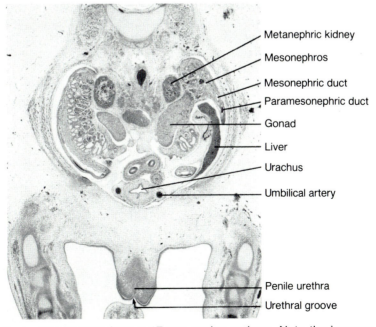

Metanephric kidney

Mesonephros

Mesonephric duct

Paramesonephric duct

Gonad

Liver

Urachus

Umbilical artery

Penile urethra

Urethral groove

Figure 18.9. Transverse section from a 17-mm canine embryo. Note the increase in size of the indifferent gonad (compare with Figs. 18.3 and 18.5), and the presence of both male (mesonephric) and female (paramesonephric) ducts. If this animal was genetically a male, the tunica albuginea would begin to form near the base of the gonad at about this stage.

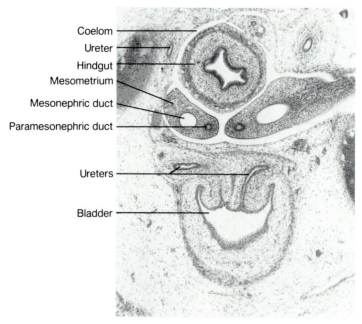

Coelom

Ureter

Hindgut

Mesometrium

Mesonephric duct

Paramesonephric duct

Ureters

Bladder

Figure 18.10. Transverse section through the cranial aspect of the urogenital sinus (bladder) and hindgut of a 41-mm female canine fetus. The paramesonephric ducts are shown immediately cranial to their fusion to form the body of the uterus. Note that the mesonephric ducts have not yet degenerate.

ducts also contribute to the vagina. The caudal part of the urogenital sinus is retained as the **vestibule.**

The paramesonephric ducts initially form identically in the male embryo, but largely degenerate following the onset of gonadal function. In male bovine embryos these ducts form during the beginning of the 6th week of gestation (17–18 mm) and degenerate within 3 weeks. Remnants of the paramesonephric ducts in the male include the appendix testis and, caudally, the uterus masculinus (Fig. 18.7*C*). Table 18.2 summarizes the fate of the mesonephric and paramesonephric duct systems in each sex.

The morphology of the uterus varies considerably among mammals, reflecting differences in the extent of fusion between the two paramesonephric ducts (Fig. 18.11). In monotremes and most marsupials the paramesonephric ducts do not fuse, but enter separately into the urogenital sinus. Most rodents and lagomorphs (rabbits) have a duplex uterus, which means that both cervices of the uterus open separately into a common

vagina. Domestic animals have a bicornuate uterus in which the uterine horns join to form a uterine body that opens into the vagina at the cervix. The openings of the two horns into the body may be largely (cow) or partially (sow) separated internally.

ACCESSORY SEX GLANDS

Accessory sex glands (Figs. 18.7 and 18.16; Table 18.3) develop as evaginations from the epithelium of the urogenital sinus or associated ducts. Their basic formation is typical of exocrine glands as described elsewhere for the salivary glands and pancreas.

The bull, ram, boar, stallion and most small laboratory animals have prostate, bulbourethral, and seminal vesicle glands. The cat lacks seminal vesicles, and the dog has only a prostate gland.

EXTERNAL GENITALS
Indifferent Stage

The development of the external genitals is related to the development of the phallic

Table 18.2.
Derivatives of the mesonephric and paramesonephric ducts[a]

Indifferent	Male	Female
Mesonephric tubules	Efferent ductules [Paradidymis]	[Epoophoron] [Aberrant ductules] [Paroophoron]
Mesonephric duct	Epididymis Ductus deferens [Epididymal appendage]	[Vesicular appendage] [Epoophoron] [Vestigial deferent (Gartner's) duct]
Paramesonephric duct	[Appendix testis] [Prostatic utricle] [Uterus masculinus]	[Vesicular appendage] Uterine tube Uterus—horn, body and cervix Vagina (in part: completed by mesonephric ducts and urogenital sinus)

[a] Brackets indicate vestigial structures.

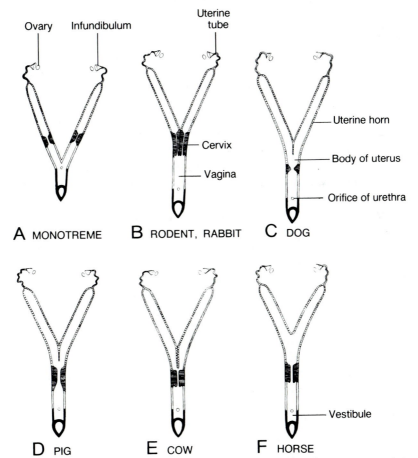

Figure 18.11. Schematic representation of the different degrees of paramesonephric duct fusion found in mammals. *A*, both ducts enter separately into the urogenital sinus; *B*, the ducts of most rodents and rabbits fuse but remain separated internally; *C*, dog; *D*, pig; *E*, cow; and *F*, horse. From Schummer A, Nickel R, Sack WO: *The Viscera of Domestic Mammals*, Berlin, Verlag Paul Parey, 1979.

Table 18.3.
Origin of accessory sex glands

Origin	Male	Female
Urogenital sinus	Prostate gland (from pelvic urethra)	Urethral glands (microscopic in wall of urethra)
	Bulbourethral glands (from caudal part of pelvic urethra)	Major vestibular glands (dorsolateral in vestibule)
	Lateral urethral glands, (microscopic in pelvic urethra)	Minor vestibular glands (ventral in vestibule)
Mesonephric duct	Seminal vesicle	No homolog

portion of the urogenital sinus and surrounding mesenchyme. Simultaneous with body and tail folding, lateral mesoderm derived from the primitive streak passes lateral and ventral to the cloaca. This lateral mesoderm forms the mesenchymal components of the ventral abdominal wall at the level of the pubovesicle pouch, and the ventral wall of the bladder.

Proliferation of mesoderm adjacent to the cloacal membrane creates a series of swellings. At the cranioventral end of the cloacal membrane the **genital tubercle** is formed (Figs. 17.3, 18.12 and 18.13). Lateral to the membrane and extending most of its length are the **cloacal folds**. Peripheral to these, caudolateral to the cloacal membrane, are the **genital** or **labioscrotal swellings** that overlie the site of inguinal canal development. These are all present and similar in both sexes prior to sex differentiation.

After the caudally growing urorectal septum separates the rectum from the urogenital sinus, the urogenital and anal membranes rupture. This establishes the anal orifice caudodorsally and urogenital orifice cranioventrally. The cloacal folds fuse in the midline between these two orifices; the site of fusion is demarcated by the **genital** (perineal) **raphe** (Fig. 18.12). The dorsal portion of the cloacal folds forms the **anal folds**, while the elongated ventral portion enlarges to form the **urogenital folds**.

Shortly after the appearance of the genital tubercle and prior to completion of urorectal septal development, the epithelial lining of the floor of the urogenital sinus expands

cranioventrally along the ventral margin of the elongating genital tubercle. These endodermal cells initially form a solid cord called the **urethral plate** extending inward from the ventral surface of the tubercle (Fig. 18.13). Concomitant with the breakdown of the urogenital membrane, the urethral plate hollows to form a canal. Proliferation of mesenchyme on both sides of the urethral plate enlarges the urogenital folds and establishes a median **urethral groove** (Fig. 18.9) on the ventral surface of the genital tubercle. The urethral groove and urethral plate are directly apposed along the base of the tubercle. As always occurs when surface ectoderm and endoderm are in direct contact, the zone of apposition degenerates. This creates a deep trough, still called the urethral groove, along the ventral surface of the genital tubercle.

Female

In the female domestic animal the urogenital folds that bound the sides of the urogenital orifice remain separate and form the **labia** or lips of the **vulva**. They overgrow the genital tubercle, which becomes internalized in the floor of the vestibule. The tubercle forms the **clitoris**, which is vestigial in most species. With elongation of the body, the genital swellings shift cranial to the genital tubercle; in most species these disappear during fetal development.

Male

The first external indication that the embryo is developing as a male is an elongation of the genital raphe. This results from both

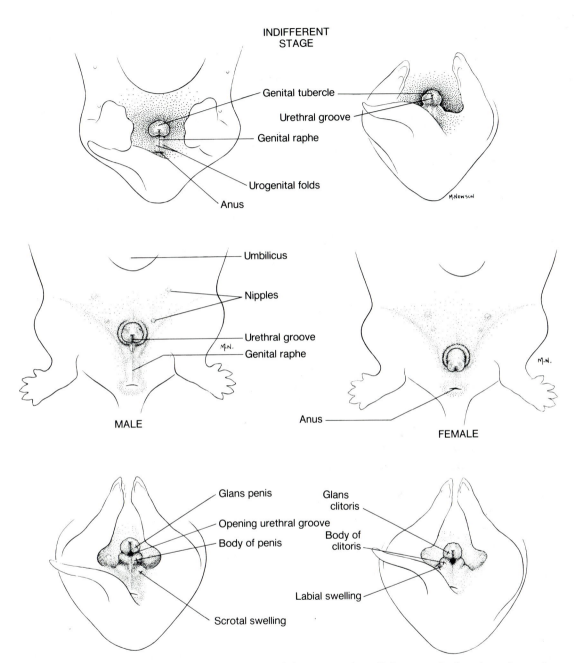

Figure 18.12.   Schematic early development of the external genital organs in the dog, shown in ventral and caudal views of (*top row*) 19-mm (30-day) and (*below*) 35-mm (35-day) embryos. (From HE Evans and GC Christensen, 1979.)

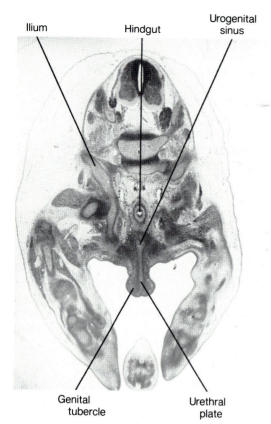

Figure 18.13. Transverse section at the level of the pelvic limbs in a 13-mm feline embryo showing the urethral plate extending from the urogenital sinus onto the genital tubercle.

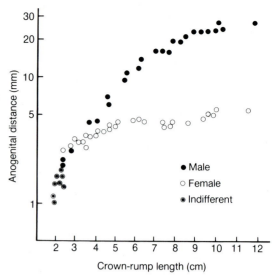

Figure 18.14. Changes in the anogenital distance of developing bovine embryos. (After Inomata T, et al: *Japanese Journal of Veterinary Science* 44:489, 1982.)

a cranial shift in the genital tubercle and fusion of the urogenital folds over the urogenital orifice. This closure extends in a caudal-to-cranial (distal) direction along the urethral groove, leaving the urethra opened only on the ventral surface of the genital tubercle. Later, the urogenital folds fuse ventrally along the entire length of the genital tubercle, establishing the **penile urethra**. The site of fusion is indicated by the genital raphe.

Differences in the distance between the anus and the base of the genital tubercle (Fig. 18.14) are the most commonly used external feature to discriminate male from female fetuses. This disparity is first detectable in the 30-day (19-mm) dog or 42-day (27-mm) bovine embryo, after which time the anogenital distance remains constant in the female and increases in the male.

At the apex of the genital tubercle, where the **glans penis** is developing, a shallow invagination forms. From this a cord of epithelial cells grows into the tubercle then contacts and fuses with the urethral groove. Subsequently, this cord hollows out and remains patent, forming the distal portion of the penile urethra. In summary, the male urethra is derived from the endodermal urogenital sinus (pelvic urethra), the urogenital plate (penile urethra), and surface ectoderm of the glans penis (distal penile urethra).

The body of the penis is incorporated into the ventral abdominal wall of most domestic mammals, less so in the horse). In ungulate fetuses a circular band of muscles called the umbilical sphincter forms a sling that pulls the penis against the body wall.

Separation of a superficial ring of skin, the **prepuce**, from the distal body of the penis occurs secondarily (40-mm stage in the pig). A circular plate of ectodermal cells forms at the distal tip of the phallus and invaginates into the mesenchyme of the tubercle. Subsequently this ectodermal (glandopreputial) plate thickens and separates into two layers with a cleft, the **preputial cavity**, between them. The prepuce consists of the wall of tissue forming the external border of the cleft. The bovine preputial cavity is not completed until 4–9 months postnatally.

This ectodermal plate does not initially form a complete ring. There is a ventral connection, the **frenulum**, between the body of the penis and the prepuce. Normally this is the last structure to degenerate in completion of the preputial cavity, and loss of the frenulum is necessary for normal penile protrusion to occur. If a bull calf is castrated shortly after birth, preputial formation is incomplete and the frenulum often persists.

The genital swellings persist in the male and form the scrotum. In the dog, horse and ox they shift cranially, remaining closely apposed to the genital tubercle, while in the cat and pig they remain beneath the anus. In all cases these swellings initially overlie the gubernaculum and vaginal processes, which project from the inguinal canals.

MAMMARY GLANDS

In both sexes a pair of linear ectodermal thickenings, the **mammary ridges**, become visible on the ventrolateral surface of the trunk between the levels of the limbs (see Figure 10.4). These appear in most embryos of 12- to 16-mm length, slightly later in the horse, and the length of the ridge varies with the species. In carnivores and swine it reaches from the axilla to the inguinal region, but in ruminants and the horse it is limited to the inguinal region. Each mammary ridge undergoes a ventral displacement as the dorsal part of the trunk grows. Focal condensations of somatic mesoderm and thickening of overlying surface ectoderm occur at specific intervals along this ridge. At these sites the ectoderm invaginates into the mesenchyme, producing a series of cylindrical ingrowths called **mammary buds**, which indicate the sites of development of mammary glands.

Each mammary bud forms one or more epithelial diverticula (sprouts). These are initially solid cords extending into underlying somatic mesenchyme. They later become patent, forming **lactiferous ducts** that open onto the surface of the developing teat. The number of duct systems in one mammary gland varies among species of domestic animals (Table 18.4) from 1 to approximately 14.

In many species more mammary buds form than are found in the adult; these extra growths degenerate along with the intervening ridge. In cattle, extra mammary buds that persist caudal to or between the normal glands give rise to accessory mammary glands referred to as **supernumerary teats**. These often have glandular tissue associated with them. In sheep, the accessory glands typically occur cranial to the normal ones.

DESCENT OF THE GONADS

The mesonephric and paramesonephric ducts extend caudally from the level of the mesonephros to the urogenital sinus. They are located within mesenchyme in the mesothelial folds that project into the peritoneal cavity. As the mesonephros degenerates the mesenteries supporting the gonads and ducts remain attached to the wall of the peritoneal cavity. The site of attachment of these folds shifts from dorsolateral to ventrolateral as the ducts pass caudally.

The site on each side of the body where the ducts curve medially to fuse together (paramesonephric ducts) or enter the urogenital sinus (mesonephric ducts) is close to the position of the labioscrotal swellings. The somatic mesoderm in this region condenses, forming a mesenchymal cord, the **gubernaculum**, that extends from the labioscrotal swelling to the bend in the duct systems, and continues cranially to the gonad. In the male the bend in the duct system occurs at the junction of the tail of the epididymis and the deferent duct (Figs. 18.15 and 18.16). As the gubernacular mes-

Table 18.4.
Mammary glands and duct systems

Species	Glands	Duct systems per gland
Cat	8	5–7
Bitch	10	8–14
Sow	14	2
Cow	4	1
Ewe/Doe	2	1
Mare	2	2

enchyme located between the tail of the epididymis and the scrotal swellings enlarges, an outpocketing of the peritoneum, the **vaginal process**, grows ventrolaterally into the gubernaculum at the site of the future inguinal canal.

The process of testicular descent occurs in two stages. The first is a passive displacement of the testis caudally and ventrally to the site of the inguinal canal. This occurs largely as a result of growth and elongation of the body, with the testis remaining approximately the same distance from the urogenital sinus. In contrast, the metanephric kidneys remain attached to the dorsal axial tissues below the first few lumbar vertebrae as the caudal end of the embryo elongates. The gonad and its blood supply, the testicular vessels, remain at all times suspended by mesorchium.

Once the testis is positioned adjacent to the inguinal canal, changes must occur that reduce the size disparity between the canal and the gonad, and decrease resistance to the movement of the gonad through the canal.

These changes are provided by a swelling of the gubernaculum at the level of the inguinal canal (Fig. 18.15). This swelling is a result of mesenchymal cell proliferation and a large increase in the secretion of extracellular matrix materials, consisting mostly of hyaluronic acid. The accumulation of this extracellular secretion dilates the inguinal canal and causes the gubernaculum to become soft and jelly-like in consistency, decreasing its resistance to the descent of the gonad.

The process of descent is passive; there is no contractile tissue present in the gubernaculum to actively pull the gonad through the canal. During the process of descent, incorporation of the intra-abdominal (deep) gubernacular mesenchyme into the extra-abdominal component produces an absolute shortening of the gubernaculum. Simultaneously the extra-abdominal gubernacular mesenchyme continues to swell in the scrotal swelling. The gubernacular mesenchyme regresses after the testis descends through

the inguinal canal, producing an absolute decrease in its length.

The swelling of the extra-abdominal gubernaculum not only dilates the inguinal canal but also causes the lumen of the vaginal process to collapse. When the testis has passed through the inguinal canal its covering of visceral peritoneum is now called the **visceral vaginal tunic.** This is continuous with the mesorchium and is the lining of the peritoneum that forms one wall of the vaginal cavity. The other, outer, wall of the cavity becomes the **parietal vaginal tunic** (Figs. 18.15 and 18.16D). The mesenchyme surrounding the vaginal process forms the spermatic fascia, which is continuous with the connective tissues of abdominal wall muscles. The cremaster muscle is incorporated in this fascia outside the parietal vaginal tunic.

In the horse the vaginal process begins to grow into the gubernacular mesenchyme around 45 days of gestation. The testis does not reach the vaginal ring until 270 days of gestation. Also in this species the tail of the epididymis, where it joins the ductus deferens, extends into the gubernacular mesenchyme prior to the testis. This is a helpful landmark to locate in some cases of failure of the testis to descend (cryptorchidism).

The disparity in size between the fetal testis and inguinal canal is most remarkable in the equine fetus, in which the fetal testis grows to an extremely large size due to the proliferation of interstitial cells. Prior to descending into the scrotum, which normally occurs around birth, the testis regresses in size. At 150 days of gestation the equine fetal testis is 3 cm in diameter and weighs 20 g. By 250 days, it is 5 cm in diameter, weighing 50 g. However by 300 days it has elongated and softened and is 2.5 cm in diameter and weighs only 30 g. This size change and weight loss reflects a degeneration of fetal testicular interstitial cells. With this change in shape and size the testis is able to pass through the inguinal canal, as shown in Figure 18.16.

Descent of the testis through the inguinal canal normally occurs at 106 days of gesta-

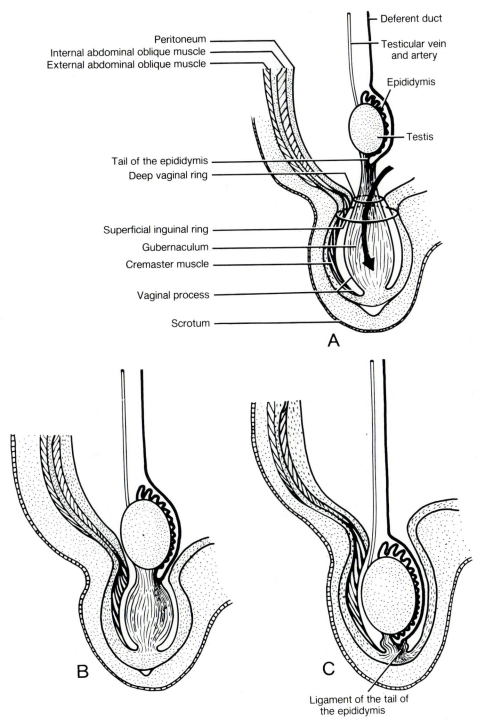

Peritoneum

Internal abdominal oblique muscle

External abdominal oblique muscle

Deferent duct

Testicular vein and artery

Epididymis

Testis

Tail of the epididymis

Deep vaginal ring

Superficial inguinal ring

Gubernaculum

Cremaster muscle

Vaginal process

Scrotum

A

B

C

Ligament of the tail of the epididymis

Figure 18.15. Descent of the canine testis. *A* and *B* illustrate the swelling of the gubernaculum to enlarge the inguinal canal (Redrawn from Wensing CJG: *Proceedings Konilklÿke Nederlandse Akademie van Wetenschappen: Series C* 74:373, 1973.)

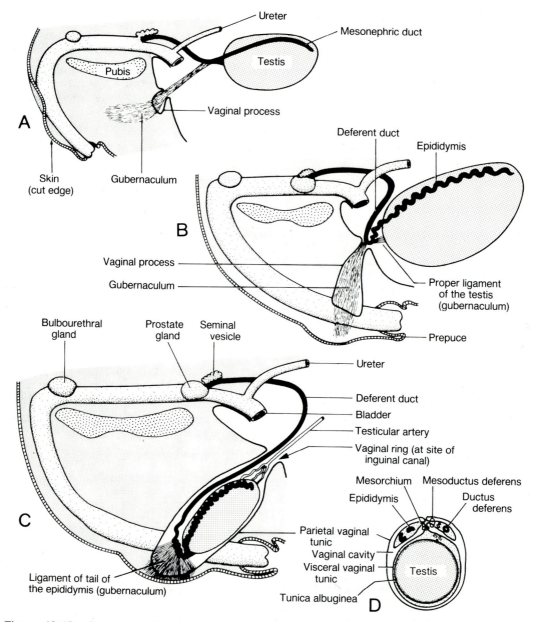

Figure 18.16. Descent of the testis in the horse, shown in schematic right lateral views of *A*, 75-day; *B*, 175-day; and *C*, term (330-day) fetuses. *D* is a transverse section through the descended testis to illustrate the medial location of the deferent duct and lateral epididymis, both of which are in folds of the visceral layer of the vaginal tunic. (Redrawn after Bergin WC, et al: *Biology of Reproduction* 3:82–92, 1970.)

tion in the bull, 70 days in the boar, at or near birth in the horse and 3–4 days postnatally in the dog. However, it is not until 35 days postpartum that the canine testis reaches its scrotal location. This final descent into the scrotum is related to regression of the gubernaculum, which commences as the testis is passing through the inguinal canal.

The gubernaculum is essential for normal descent of the testis and its swelling, elongation and regression are controlled by testicular secretions. Therefore the testis governs its own descent. This gubernacular outgrowth is stimulated by a nonandrogenic testicular factor that is enhanced by testosterone from the testis. Gubernacular regression is induced by testosterone.

MESENTERIES OF THE REPRODUCTIVE ORGANS

The mesothelial folds that developed in the embryo to suspend the mesonephros, gonad, and duct systems persist in the adult but support different organs in each sex, as summarized in Table 18.5. Regression of the gubernaculum converts a large mucoid-rich tissue into a small fibrous structure. This regression, which is primarily a result of loss of intercellular substance, results in "ligamentous" remnants that are observed in the gross dissection. As illustrated in Figure 18.16B, the gubernacular mesenchyme between the caudal pole of the testis and the bend in the mesonephric duct forms the **proper ligament of the testis**. This is covered by a fold of peritoneum continuous cranially with the mesorchium of the testis. Caudally the gubernaculum forms a mesenchymal cord, the **ligament of the tail of the epididymis**, located between the bend in the mesonephric duct and the scrotal swelling.

In the pig and ruminants the fetal ovary shifts caudally towards the pelvic inlet. In all other female domestic animals it retains a midabdominal position that approximates the site of its development. The gubernaculum in the female becomes the **proper ligament of the ovary** in the free edge of the mesometrium between the ovary and the uterine horn. Caudally, the gubernaculum forms the **round ligament of the uterus**, which extends from the proper ligament to the inguinal canal in the free edge of a ventrolateral fold of mesometrium. In the bitch it usually passes through the inguinal canal with the vaginal process.

A longitudinal groove forms between the gonadal ridge and the degenerating mesonephros (Figure 18.8), and the mesothelial (peritoneal) layer covering the gonad is reduced to a thin mesenchymal sheet at the site of this groove. This, together with the mesothelial remnants of the degenerated mesonephros, will become the attachment of the gonad to the body wall. In the male this forms the **mesorchium** and in the female, the **mesovarium**. These lateral mesenteries also support the gonadal vessels. In the male, the mesorchium and the testicular artery and vein that it suspends are continuous from the dorsolateral abdominal wall to the testis in the scrotum.

ABNORMAL DEVELOPMENT OF GERM CELLS

Deficits in the number of gametes usually are either the result of chromosomal abnor-

Table 18.5.
Mesenteries and ligaments of reproductive organs

Connective tissue remnants of the gubernaculum		
	Male	Female
Gonad to duct	(Junction of epididymis and ductus deferens)	(Junction of uterine horn and tube)
	Proper ligament of the testis	Proper ligament of the ovary
Duct to vaginal process	Ligament of tail of epididymis	Round ligament of uterus
Derivatives of the mesothelial covering of the mesonephros		
	Male	Female
Cranial to gonad	Mesorchium	Suspensory ligament
At the gonad	Mesorchium	Mesovarium[a]
Caudal to gonad	Mesepididymis	Mesosalpinx[a]
	Mesoductus deferens	Mesometrium[a]

[a] Components of the broad ligament.

malities that preclude normal tetrad formation during meiosis or are secondary to malformations of the gonads. Abnormal or ectopic embryogenesis from a germ cell results in the formation of a **teratoma**. This is a neoplasm composed of many types of tissue, including bone, hair, teeth, muscle, and neural tissues, all of which are randomly arranged. These neoplasms are rare in domestic animals and are usually benign, but can be malignant if pluripotential stem cells are present. Teratomas are most frequently found in testes and ovaries, and have been shown in mice to originate from germ cells. It is believed that teratomas in other locations are derived from germ cells that settled in ectopic positions.

STRUCTURAL MALFORMATIONS OF THE REPRODUCTIVE ORGANS*

Gonads

Hypoplasia of the gonad results in a small organ that usually lacks germ cells. Hypoplasia can be unilateral or bilateral and has been reported as hereditary in cattle. This condition is often accompanied by other structural or behavioral abnormalities, especially in the male, due to reduced gonadal secretions.

Cryptorchidism is a failure of the normal descent of the testis. The testis may be located immediately outside the inguinal canal or intra-abdominally and as far cranially as the level of the kidneys. This condition may result from an abnormal site or direction of gubernacular development. Exaggerated intra-abdominal swelling of the gubernaculum does not expand the inguinal canal sufficiently to permit testicular descent.

Animals with bilateral cryptorchidism are usually infertile because spermatogenesis does not occur. This is due to injurious effects of normal body temperature on spermatocytes and spermatids. Mammals with internalized testes, including elephants and marine mammals, do not show this heat sensitivity. Cryptorchid testes have an in-

creased incidence of neoplasia, and in dogs can be associated with umbilical hernia, defects of the penis and prepuce, hip dysplasia, and patellar dislocation.

Although inheritance has been implicated as a factor in cryptorchidism in most species, few studies have been performed to better define this correlation. A multiple gene defect has been proposed in a colony of Miniature Schnauzers with a high incidence of cryptorchidism, but the wide breed distribution of this abnormality in dogs suggests that other factors are involved.

Urogenital Ducts

Persistent vestigial structures are remnants of undifferentiated embryonic ducts that persist, usually close to the gonads or in the wall of the urogenital sinus (see Table 18.2 and Fig. 18.7). These rarely interfere with normal function unless they become cystic and enlarged.

Mesonephric duct abnormalities include stenosis or aplasia of the epididymis or ductus deferens. This can occur as an isolated entity or in conjunction with renal aplasia.

Paramesonephric duct abnormalities include improper fusion and various patterns of stenosis or atresia. Improper fusion results in a duplex uterus when the left and right paramesonephric ducts fail to join and fuse, so that each enters the vagina separately. Alternatively, fusion may be partial, with a small common uterine chamber. Unilateral uterine aplasia (uterus unicornis) is the absence of one uterine tube and horn. This is often associated with unilateral renal agenesis.

Focal defects in the development of the paramesonephric duct result in **segmental aplasia** or **stenosis** of a uterine tube or horn. Atresia is often accompanied by the formation of cysts in the uterus. It is an hereditary disease of Short Horn cattle called **white heifer disease** because it occurs in conjunction with the inheritance of white coat color.

External Genitals

Hypospadius (spadius = to open) is the complete or partial failure of the urethral

---

* Malformations involving abnormal development of male and female-specific structures are described in Chapter 19.

folds to close in the male, leaving the mucosa of the penile urethra exposed caudally and ventrally. It is usually associated with the abnormal development of other gender-specific structures.

Epispadius is a rare condition in males in which the penis is shortened and the dorsal surface of the penile urethra is open. This defect is accompanied by a failure of the caudal ventral abdominal wall to develop properly, so that the dorsal wall of the bladder and pelvic urethra are exposed ventrally, a condition called **extroversion of the bladder**. This appears to be due to abnormal development of caudal lateral mesoderm. As a result, bladder and urethral endoderm come into direct apposition with ventral body wall ectoderm, which results in the local degeneration of both these epithelia.

Bibliography

NORMAL DEVELOPMENT

Aitken RNC: Observations on the development of the seminal vesicles, prostate and bulbourethral glands in the ram. *J Anat* 93:43–51, 1959.

Backhouse KM, Butler H: The gubernaculum testis of the pig. *J Anat* 94:107–120, 1960.

Baumens V, Dijkstra G, Wensing CJG: Testicular descent in the dog. *Zbl Vet Med C Anat Histol Embryol* 10:97–110, 1981.

Bok G, Drews V: The role of the Wolffian ducts in the formation of the sinus vagina: an organ culture study. *J Embryol Exp Morphol* 73:275–295, 1983.

Bulmer D: The early stages of vaginal development in the sheep. *J Anat* 90:123–134, 1956.

Cole HH, Hart GH, Lyons WR, Catchpole HR: The development and hormonal content of fetal horse gonds. *Anat Rec* 56:275–293, 1931.

Forsberg J-G: On the development of the cloaca and perineum and the formation of the urethral plate in female rat embryos. *J Anat* 95:423–436, 1961.

Fujimoto T, Ukeshima A, Kiyofeyi R: The origin, migration and morphology of the primordial germ cells in the chick embryo. *Anat Rec* 185:139–154, 1976.

Fujimoto T, Miyayama Y, Fuyuta M: The origin, migration and fine morphology of human primordial germ cells. *Anat Rec* 188:315–330, 1977.

Glenister TW: The development of the penile urethra in the pig. *J Anat* 90:461–477, 1956.

Gropp A, Ohno S: The presence of a common embryonic blastema for ovarian and testicular parenchymal (follicular, interstitial, and tubular) cells in cattle, *Bos Taurus*. *Z Zellforsch Mikrosh Anat* 74:505–528, 1966.

Gunter G: Zur Entwicklung der auberen Genitalien des Kaninchens. I. Uber die Entwicklung des Penis beim Kaninchen. *Z Anat Entwicklungsgesch* 84:275–333, 1927.

Inomata T, Eguchi Y, Yamamoto M, Asari M, Kano Y, Mochizuki K: Development of the external genitalia in bovine fetuses. *Jap J Vet Sci* 44:489–496, 1982.

Johnson CA: The role of the fetal testicle in sexual differentiation. *Compend Cont Ed* 5:129–132, 1983.

Kanagasuntheram R, Anandaraja S: Development of the terminal urethra and prepuce in the dog. *J Anat* 949:121–129, 1960.

Nieuwkoop PD, Sutasurya LA: *Primordial Germ Cells in the Chordates*. Cambridge, Cambridge University Press, 1979.

Pelliniemi LJ: Ultrastructure of gonadal ridge in male and female pig embryos. *Anat Embryol* 147:19–34, 1975.

Pelliniemi LJ: Ultrastructure of the early ovary and testis in pig embryos. *Am J Anat* 144:89–112, 1975.

Pelliniemi LJ: Ultrastructure of the indifferent gonad in male and female pig embryos. *Tissue Cell* 8:163–174.

Price JM, Donahoe PK, Ito Y, Hendren III WH: Programmed cell death in the Mullerian duct induced by Mullerian inhibiting substance. *Am J Anat* 149:353–376, 1977.

Torrey TW: The development of the urogenital system of the albino rat. I. The kidney and its ducts. *Am J Anat* 72:113–144, 1943.

Torrey TW: The development of the urogenital system of the albino rat. III. The urogenital union. *Am J Anat* 81:139–153, 1947.

Vigier B, Prepin J, Jost A: Chronologie du developpement de l'appareil genital du foetus de veau. *Arch Anat Microsc Morphol Exp* 65:77–102, 1976.

Wartenberg H: The influence of the mesonephric blastema on gonadal development and sexual differentiation. In Byskov AG, Peters H, (eds): *Development and Function of Reproductive Organs.* Excerpta Medica, International Congress Series Amsterdam, 1981, pp 3–12.

Wensing CJG: Testicular descent in some domestic mammals. 1. Anatomical aspect of testicular descent. *Proc Ned Akad Wet* 71:423–434, 1968.

Wensing CJG: Testicular descent in some domestic mammals. The nature of the gubernacular change during the process of testicular descent in the pig. *Proc Ned Akad Wet* 76:190–202, 1973.

Zamboni L, Bezard J, Mauleon P: The role of the mesonephros in the development of the sheep fetal ovary. *Ann Biol Anim Biochim Biophys* 19:1153–1178, 1979.

Zamboni L, Upadhyay S: The contribution of the mesonephros to the development of the sheep fetal testis. *Am J Anat* 165:339–356, 1982.

MALFORMATIONS

Ashdown RR: Persistence of the penile frenulum in young bulls. *Vet Rec* 74:1464–1468, 1962.

Bennett RC, Olds D, Deaton OW, Thrift FA: Nature of white heifer disease (partial genital aplasia) and its mode of inheritance. *Am J Vet Res* 34:13–20, 1973.

Bergin WC, Gier HT, Marion GB, Coffman JR: A developmental concept of equine cryptorchidism. *Biol. Reprod* 3:82–92, 1970.

Cox JE, Edwards GB, Neal PA: An analysis of 500 cases of equine cryptorchidism. *Equine Vet J* 11:113–116, 1979.

Cox VS, Wallace LJ, Jensen CR: An anatomic and genetic study of canine cryptorchidism *Teratology* 18:233–240, 1978.

Pendergrass TW, Hayes Jr HM: Cryptorchidism and related defects in dogs: epidemiologic comparisons with man. *Teratology* 12:51–56, 1975.

Stevens LC: Teratomas derived from germ cells and embryos. In Austin CR, Edwards RG (eds): *Mechanisms of Sex Differentiation in Animals and Man.* New York, Academic Press, 1981, pp 301–328.

Stickle RL, Fessler JF; Retrospective study of 350 cases of equine cryptorchidism. *JAVMA* 172:343–346, 1978.

Wensing CJG: Abnormalities of testicular descent. *Proc Kon Ned Akad Wet* 76:373–385, 1973.

Wensing CJG: Developmental anomalies, including cryptorchidism. In Morrow DA (ed): *Current Therapy in Theriogenology: Diagnosis, Treatment and Prevention of Reproductive Diseases in Animals.* Philadelphia, Saunders, 1980.

Wykes PM, Soderberg SF: Congenital anomalies of the canine vagina and vulva. *J Am Anim Hosp Assoc* 19:995–1000, 1983.

Cytogenetics and Sex Determination

The study of chromosomes, especially their structure and role in heredity, is called **cytogenetics**.

Deviation from the normal number and composition of chromosomes in a gamete usually results in a malformation or death of the embryo to which it contributes. Single base pair additions and deletions, or substitutions and changes in the locations of nucleotide sequences can occur during any cell division, but are especially prevalent during meiosis. If the chromosome involved is a sex chromosome, the resulting organism will frequently develop an **intersex** condition. This describes any situation in which there is ambiguity in the structure of the gonads, reproductive tract or external genitals. Although most chromosomal aberrations are deleterious to the organism, occasionally they are beneficial and create diversity within a population, which is a necessary component of natural selection.

This chapter deals with the more gross of these genetic alterations. These involve either entire chromosomes or major parts of a chromosome that are translocated, in-serted into a different chromosome, or else deleted.

KARYOTYPING

Karyology is the study of the nucleus, more specifically the morphology of the chromosomes. Some chromosomal changes can be identified indirectly by clinical observation of the phenotype of the organism, but microscopic examination is required to document most of them. **Karyotyping** is the preparation of a systematized array of the chromosomes of a cell prepared by photographs. The resultant is a **karyogram** (Figs. 19.1 and 19.3).

In order to observe chromosomal morphology the cell to be studied must be in the metaphase stage of the mitotic cycle, when the chromosomes are condensed and visible using light microscopy. During metaphase the paired chromatids are contracted and joined by the centromere.

Some cells, such as white blood cells in a blood sample, have to be cultured to produce mitosis. Others (testis, bone marrow) are continually dividing and direct preparations can be made. White blood cells are the most frequently studied. When cultured with a mitosis-stimulating agent (**mitogen**) such as phytohemagglutinin for 1–3 days, these cells will divide. Exposure of the dividing cells in culture to colchicine will arrest mitosis at metaphase because the drug interferes with spindle formation. Finally, treating with a hypotonic solution causes swelling of the metaphase cells, after which they are squashed on a slide and stained, usually with Giemsa, to delineate the chromosomal structure. The chromosomes are photographed and a composite of the photo-

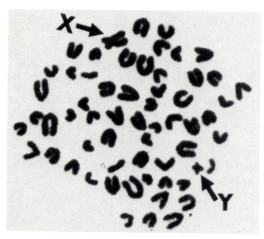

Figure 19.1. Metaphase-arrested chromosomes of a normal male ox (60XY). Note the size disparity between the X and Y chromosomes, and the acrocentric morphology of the autosomes. (From Dunn HO, et al: *Cornell Vet* 71:2, 1981.)

graphed chromosomes is prepared organizing the chromosomes by homologous pairs based on the length of the chromatids and the position of the centromere between the chromatids.

Chromosomes are categorized grossly by the position of the centromere. **Metacentric** indicates it is midway between the ends, **acrocentric** or telocentric if near or at one end, and **submetacentric** if the centromere is located between the middle and one end. In many cases the differences between some pairs are too subtle to allow exact identification. Table 19.1 gives the total number of chromosomes for each species and the kind of morphology characteristic for the species.

ALTERATIONS IN CHROMOSOME NUMBER

Ploidy refers to the number of chromosomes within a cell. **Haploid** (N) is the number in the gamete, while **diploid** (2N) is the normal number in a somatic cell (see Fig. 2.1 for details).

Polyploidy is a condition in which the number of chromosomes in a cell is increased by an exact multiple of the haploid state. For example, tetraploidy (4N) is common in liver cells and in some large neurons

in the central nervous system, including Purkinje cells. This could be due to interference with karyokinesis prior to anaphase resulting in the inclusion of the duplicated chromosomes within a nuclear membrane in the original cell. It could also occur if the nuclear membrane failed to disintegrate during prophase.

Aneuploidy is an increase or decrease in the number of one or more chromosomes, but not an entire haploid number. It usually refers to an increase or decrease of one chromosome. One extra chromosome added to a homologous pair is called **trisomy**, a loss of one from a homologous pair is **monosomy**. These changes result from **nondisjunction** of chromosomal material during mitosis or meiosis. Nondisjunction can occur in somatic or sex chromosomes within somatic or germ cells. In mitosis it results from failure of a centromere to separate; thus, one daughter cell obtains an extra chromosome (trisomy) and the other loses one (monosomy).

Meiotic nondisjunction can occur in either maturation division (Fig. 19.2). In the first maturation division a homologous pair of replicated chromosomes fails to separate and both enter one of the secondary germ cells. Nondisjunction during the second maturation division is similar to that which occurs during mitosis in that the centromere between 2 chromatids fails to separate.

ANEUPLOIDY IN SOMATIC CELLS

Somatic cell aneuploidy most commonly occurs in neoplasms and is restricted to the neoplastic cells; it is probably a result rather than a cause of the neoplasia. In dogs the transmissible venereal neoplasm contains cells with 59 and 60 chromosomes instead of 78. The presence of numerous metacentric somatic chromosomes in these cells suggests that several pairs of acrocentric chromosomes fused to form metacentrics, thereby decreasing the total number.

ANEUPLOIDY IN GERM CELLS

The effects of a chromosomal abnormality that arises during gametogenesis are usually

Table 19.1.
Karyotypes of domestic animals and man

Species	Diploid number	Composition	
Dog	78	76 Acrocentric	2 Metacentric (sex)
Horse	64	38 Acrocentric	26 Metacentric
Cattle	60	58 Acrocentric	2 Submetacentric (sex)
Goat	60	58 Acrocentric	2 Metacentric
Sheep	54	48 Acrocentric	6 Metacentric
Man	46	11 Acrocentric	35 Metacentric
Pig	38	12 Acrocentric	26 Metacentric
Cat	38	5 Acrocentric	33 Metacentric

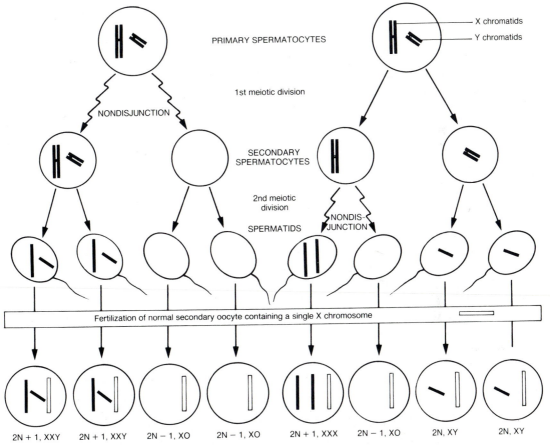

Figure 19.2. Schematic representation of the effects of nondisjunction of the sex chromosomes at either the first (left side) or second (right side) meiotic divisions during spermatogenesis. The bottom row shows the results of fertilizing a normal ovum with each of the sperm produced.

observed in many body systems since the malformation will be passed to all the cells of the body and influence organ formation from these cells. Most embryos with aneuploidy die in utero, and this is believed to be the most prevalent cause of early embryonic death.

Affecting Somatic Chromosomes

Trisomy 16 is the most common aneuploidy in humans, but it is always lethal to the embryo. Down's syndrome (mongoloid defects) is an example of trisomy in the 21st pair of chromosomes in humans. Instead of the normal 46 chromosomes, all cells of the body contain 47, with the extra one (trisomy) matching those in the 21st pair. This is the result of meiotic nondisjunction during oogenesis, and results in malformations in many body systems, including the face, hands, heart and, often, brain.

Trisomy 13 or trisomy 18 appear in 1 of every 8000 children and cause malformations in many body systems. These conditions can now be diagnosed during gestation by performing a karyogram on cells drawn from amniotic fluid.

Aneuploidy of somatic chromosomes is rare in domestic animals, probably because it is lethal. Trisomy 23 has been linked with congenital dwarfness in cattle, and stillborn brachygnathic cattle with a 61XY karyotype have been described. There are no known viable somatic chromosomal monosomies.

Affecting Sex Chromosomes

The aneuploid conditions which appear most frequently in domestic animals are those involving the sex chromosomes of the germ cells. In terms of chromosome distribution, the results of nondisjunctive meiosis on sex chromosomes are the same as for somatic chromosomes, as shown in Figure 19.2. Table 19.2 summarizes the genetic composition of domestic mammals derived from gametes having trisomy or monosomy of the sex chromosomes.

The **XO** genotype, which is most prevalent in horses, pigs and cats, results in an infertile, usually anestrus female with hypoplastic ovaries. These animals may have a small uterus and underdeveloped external genitals. In humans, this monosomy is called **Turner's syndrome**, and deafness and lowered mentality may occur. **YO** is usually lethal and no development occurs. Apparently the genes on at least one female sex chromosome must be present to keep the organism viable.

XXY (Figure 19.3) which is referred to as **Klinefelter's syndrome** in humans, produces males with infertility due to hypoplastic or aplastic testes. The presence of the Y chromosome allows the male determining genes to influence development to produce a male

Table 19.2.
Reported abnormal karyotypes due to sex chromosome nondisjunction

Species (2N)	Karyotype	Description
Ox (60)	61XXY	Hypoplastic testes, infertile
	61XXX	Hypoplastic ovaries, infertile
Horse (64)	63X0	Infertile
	65XXY	Hypoplastic ovaries, infertile
	65XXX	Intersex, infertile
	66XXXY	
Pig (38)	37X0	Infertile, short legs, small external genitals
	39XXY	Hypoplastic testes, infertile
Goat (60)	61XXY	Hypoplastic testes, infertile
	62XXXY	
Dog (78)	79XXY	Hypoplastic testes, infertile
Cat (38)	37X0	Intersex, infertile
	39XXY	
	40XXYY	

individual. The extra female sex chromosome interferes with the male gonad development so that spermatogenesis is incomplete. This is the most commonly reported sex chromosome trisomy.

The tortoiseshell and tricolor (calico) cats have provided a unique opportunity to study the XXY syndrome. The tortoiseshell cat has orange (yellow, cream) and black (grey, brown) patches; the calico (Fig. 19.4) has the same with varying amounts of white. The orange gene is a dominant sex-linked gene on the X chromosome. The black gene is either a codominant allele of the orange gene, or is autosomal and its function is masked by the orange gene. This nonallelic masking is called **epistasis**. The white genes are autosomal and are expressed independently of these other pigment genes.

Only one female sex chromosome is active in any cell. This **X chromosome inactivation** occurs in all embryonic cells except primordial germ cells shortly after the blastula or gastrula stages. X-inactivation is random so that in some cells the maternal X chromosome is active while in others it is the paternal X chromosome that is functioning. The

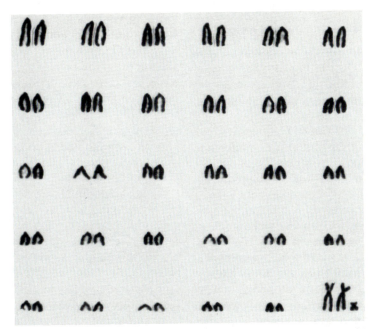

Figure 19.3. Karyogram of a 61XXY bovine cell. In this presentation the chromosomes have been arranged according to size for easier identification. Sex chromosomes are at the bottom right corner. (Courtesy of RH Johnson, Jr.)

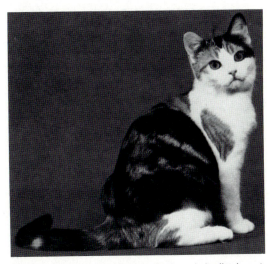

Figure 19.4. A female tricolored (calico) cat. (From Cat Fanciers Association, Inc. *Annual Yearbook*, 1983.)

reason for this inactivation is believed to be that the X chromosome is evolutionarily a double chromosome, and that if both X's were active it would be analogous to tetrasomy of a somatic chromosome.

In the epidermal pigment cells of the cat, if the active X chromosome carries the or-

ange gene, the hair will be orange color. An X chromosome expressing the black allele will cause deposition of black pigment granules in the hair. Thus, under normal conditions only a female tortoiseshell cat can exist, since two separate X chromosomes are required for orange and black pigmented spots to form.

However, about 1 in 3000 tortoiseshell cats are males. Cytogenetic analyses have revealed several different karyotypes in male tricolor cats, as summarized in Table 19.3. In all instances there are two female sex chromosomes in the animal and one male sex chromosome in at least some of the cells. Most of these toms are sterile, although occasionally they may be fertile. The reasons for the multiple genotypes listed below are explained in the section on Chimeric and Mosaic Animals.

HYBRIDS

A hybrid is an animal whose parents are of different species. The best known example is the mule, which results from the breeding of a female horse (*Equus caballus;* 2N = 64) with a male donkey, (*Equus asinus;* 2N =

Table 19.3.
Karyograms in calico cats (normal male = 38XY)

39XXY
38XX/38XY
38XY/38XY
38XY/39XXY
38XX/57XXY
38XY/57XXY
38XY/39XXY/40XXYY
38XX/38XY/39XXY
38XX/38XY/39XXY/40XXYY

62). The mule receives 32 chromosomes from the mare and 31 from the jackass. Thus the 2N number in the mule is 63. However, because donkey and horse chromosomes are not identical, a complete set of homologous pairs cannot form during prophase of the first meiotic maturation division. Meiosis stops and no gametes are formed; thus, the mule is sterile. However, the female mule is endocrinologically normal and is capable of carrying to term and delivering a horse fetus transferred to its uterus at the blastocyst stage.

Microscopic study of the male gonad of a different equine hybrid has confirmed the basis for hybrid sterility. The hybrid that results from the mating of a male donkey to a female Grant's zebra (*Equus burchelli boehmi;* 2N = 44) has a diploid number of chromosomes of 53 (31 + 22). In the seminiferous tubules of the testis of this hybrid there is no development beyond the primary spermatocyte stage of meiosis. The unlike complement of chromosomes from the two parents has prevented their pairing in prophase of the first maturation division and meiosis has ceased.

CHIMERIC AND MOSAIC ANIMALS

Chimeric and mosaic animals are those in which more than one genotype is represented in the population of cells constituting the organism. In a **mosaic** animal all the genotypes arise from a *single zygotic genotype* as a result of mitotic nondisjunction or chromosomal loss. For example, if a normal male feline zygote (38XY), were to undergo nondisjunction of the sex chromosomes at the first cleavage division, the resulting blas-

tomeres would be 39XXY and 37YO. The latter would degenerate and the individual would develop entirely from the 39XXY blastomere. However, if the nondisjunction were to occur later in development, then both normal (38XY) and trisomic (39XXY) cells would contribute to the developing mosaic embryo. The expression of the trisomic abnormalities depends upon when the nondisjunction occurs and where the affected cells are located.

A **chimeric** animal also has more than one genotype, but it is derived from *two or more zygotic genotypes.* For example, blood-borne cells may enter an embryo from its twin if placental **vascular anastomoses** occur between them. This occurs commonly in bovine twin fetuses, as can be demonstrated by the inability of one twin to reject tissue grafts from the other.

Chimeric animals also can be created by transplanting tissues from one embryo to another, for example the quail-chick chimeras described in Chapters 7, 9, 10 and 11, or by the mixing of blastomeres from different embryos (see Chapter 10, myogenesis). Recently the latter method has been extended to domestic animals. Blastomeres from 4- or 8-cell goat (*Capra hircus*) and sheep (*Ovis aries*) embryos were isolated and mixed together, placed inside an empty zona pellucida, and implanted into females of either species at the correct postestrous stage. Some of the offspring obtained can be proven to be chimeras by the appearance of both caprine hair and ovine fleece (Fig. 19.5), as well as by biochemical and serological analyses.

These chimeric animals are especially useful in analyses of placental function and maternal-fetal interactions. For example, the sheep placenta normally produces progesterone during gestation; that of the goat does not. Also, in preliminary studies the survival of these chimeras is best when the chorionic epithelium (trophoblast) is formed by cells of the same species as the foster mother, suggesting that there is a maternal reaction against tissues of a different species.

The most common naturally occurring bases for chimerism are believed to be the fusion of zygotes with fertilized polar bodies or fusion of two young (cleavage stage) embryos. The following are possible explanations for some of the feline genotypes listed in Table 19.3:

Example A: 38XX/57XXY
1. Normal sperm (19X) + egg (19X) → 38XX zygote
2. Normal sperm (19Y) + 1st polar body (38XX) → 57XXY zygote

These two embryos fuse during early development.

Example B: 38XX/57XXY
1. Two sperm (19X, 19Y) + egg (19X) → 57XXY
2. Normal sperm (19X) + 2nd polar body or egg (19X) → 38XX

This is an example of polyspermy, the incorporation of more than one sperm into the female gamete or polar body.

Example C: 38XX/38XY/39XXY
1. Normal sperm (19X) + egg (19X) → 38XX
2. Normal sperm (19Y) + 2nd polar body or egg (19X) → 38XY
3a. Normal sperm (19Y) + aneuploid egg (20XX) → 39XXY

OR

3b. 38XY blastomere → 39XXY + 37YO (nonviable) by mitotic nondisjunction

If the last of these occurs, the animal is both a chimera and a mosaic.

SEX DETERMINATION: GERM CELLS

Primordial germ cells are present in the gonadal ridge prior to overt testicular or ovarian development. However, they do not exert any known influence on these early stages of gonadogenesis. In animals whose primordial germ cells have been either surgically removed or killed using chemicals or irradiation, the gonads develop appropriate male or female characteristics. Males develop normally but are sterile; the female gonads are abnormal because estrogen-secreting follicular cells do not develop in the absence of oocytes.

In contrast, the phenotypic organization of the gonad dictates whether germ cells will become spermatogonia or oogonia. XY germ cells will form either male or female gametes depending upon their gonadal environment. However, for reasons that are not known, all XX germ cells degenerate in a testis soon after birth. This is seen, for example, in 6.5–8.4% of all genetically female polled goats. The polled gene (P) is an autosomal dominant for hornlessness. PP-XX goats have testes, but all their germ cells degenerate after forming primary spermatocytes. A similar condition has been reported in pigs and horses. These animals are phenotypically females, but may show a variable degree of masculinization (enlarged clitoris, increased anogenital distance).

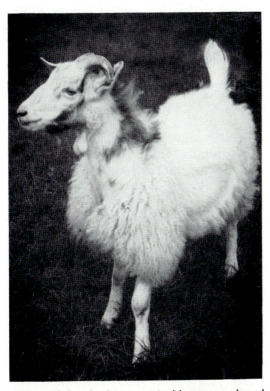

Figure 19.5. A sheep-goat chimera produced by mixing together blastomeres from each species at the 8-cell stage then implanting the chimeric embryo into a goat foster mother. (From Fehilly CB, et al: *Nature* 307:633–635, 1984.)

SEX DETERMINATION: GONADS

The first tissues to express unique male or female characteristics are those derived from the gonadal ridge in the mesonephros. This expression is not dependent upon an exogenous agent, but is due to tissue interactions between ridge tissues.

Testicular development is dependent upon the presence of a cell surface component found on intermediate mesodermal cells that have a Y chromosome. This cell surface protein is called the **H-Y factor.** Its name comes from experiments in which highly inbred male mice accepted female skin grafts but females rejected grafts of male skin. Graft rejection is due to antibody production in the female against a cell surface antigen on the male cells. This male histocompatibility antigen is normally determined or regulated by a gene on the Y chromosome; hence the name, H-Y factor (antigen). There is evidence that normal production of the H-Y factor requires activity of a gene on the X chromosome, also.

Several lines of investigation have shown that H-Y factor is present on and released by male gonadal somatic cells and is normally absent in those of the female. Male gonads grown *in vitro* in the presence of antibodies to H-Y, which effectively remove or block all H-Y antigen, develop as ovaries. Also, in chimeric gonads containing both XX and XY cells, H-Y produced by the latter cause the XX cells to form testicular ducts and other male-specific cell types. Finally, exposing a female indifferent-stage gonad to H-Y factor causes it to form a testis.

These experiments indicate that a Y-chromosome-dependent factor, H-Y, is an obligatory, primary component in transforming the indifferent gonad into a testis. This factor is bound to the cell surface, but can also act as a local, diffusible hormone upon nearby cells. The cells that release H-Y are the same as will form sustentacular (Sertoli) cells. In the absence of H-Y the gonad will form an ovary, regardless of the genotype of the cells.

The importance of the H-Y factor in gonadogenesis is well illustrated by animals that are genotypically XX but whose gonads develop as testes. For example, the polled XX goat is H-Y positive. In Cocker Spaniels, which have a high incidence of genital anomalies, a 78XX male has been described.

This animal was H-Y-positive, cryptorchid, and had a hypoplastic penis and small uterus. The mother of this dog was a 78XX female with one hypoplastic testis and an enlarged clitoris. She, too, was H-Y-positive. In these examples the H-Y-producing genes are either X-linked or autosomal. This raises the possibility that the Y chromosome normally serves to regulate X-Y factor-producing genes.

SEX DETERMINATION: REPRODUCTIVE TRACTS AND EXTERNAL GENITALS

There are two testicular products that regulate the patterns of differentiation of the mesonephric and paramesonephric ducts. **Testosterone,** secreted by interstitial (Leydig) cells, stimulates the mesonephric ducts to grow and differentiate into the male duct system, while a separate factor inhibits development of the paramesonephric duct and causes its degeneration.

The experiments that led to this two-factor hypothesis are summarized in Figure 19.6. Implanting a testis adjacent to the ovary in an immature female rabbit leads to retention of the mesonephric duct and degeneration of the paramesonephric duct near the implant. If an implant containing only testosterone is used, no regression of the paramesonephric duct occurs. Castration of a genetically male fetus similarly prevents degeneration of the female duct system. The testicular secretion responsible for degeneration of the paramesonephric ducts is a glycoprotein secreted by sustentacular (Sertoli) cells. It is called **paramesonephric duct inhibiting factor** (anti-müllerian factor).

Development of the urogenital sinus and external genitals is a testosterone-dependent process in the male. Mesenchymal cells in these tissues incorporate testosterone and convert it to dihydrotestosterone with the enzyme 5-α-reductase. Enlargement of the prostate gland and genital tubercle also occurs in response to testosterone, regardless of the sex genotype of the tissues. In rodents it has been documented that the anogenital distance of a female fetus located between two male fetuses is slightly longer than normal, presumably due to diffusion of slight

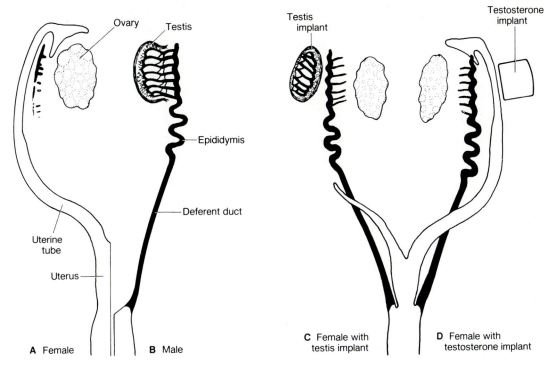

Figure 19.6. Hormonal control of reproductive tract development. *A* and *B* indicate the normal female and male structures. *C* shows the effects of implanting a piece of testicular tissue adjacent to the gonad of an XX fetus at the indifferent stage. In contrast, in *D*, only a pellet of testosterone was implanted. In this last situation the paramesonephric ducts continued to develop, indicating that testosterone is not the agent that normally causes their degeneration in the male.

amounts of testosterone across apposed chorions.

Testicular development in the ox is evident by about 36 days (17 mm) of gestation. Inhibition of paramesonephric duct development in the male normally commences between 40 and 48 days and the ducts normally disappear by 58 days (70 mm). Masculinization of the external genitals begins during the 7th week (36 mm), and stimulation of the mesonephric duct derivatives occurs after 60 days of development.

Thus, the differentiation of reproductive organs occurs in a highly integrated sequence, all based on the presence or absence of testicular secretions. Fertilization determines the **chromosomal sex** of the individual. Normally, the presence or absence of a Y chromosome in gonadal ridge mesenchymal cells determines the **gonadal sex**. This process is mediated by the H-Y factor, which influences cell-cell interactions resulting in the formation of seminiferous tubules and interstitial cells. Finally, the gonadal sex determines the pattern of reproductive duct and external genital development.

Testicular interstitial cells produce testosterone, that stimulates the mesonephric duct to form the deferent duct and epididymis. Sustentacular cells of the seminiferous tubules produce an inhibiting substance that causes paramesonephric ducts to degenerate. Circulating testosterone is converted to dihydrotestosterone in the mesodermal cells of the indifferent external genitals and induces elongation of the genital tubercle, hypertrophy and fusion of the urogenital folds and, later, the final stage of descent of the testes into the scrotum.

INTERSEX ANIMALS (HERMAPHRODITES)

The criteria for sex identification include:

1. Genetic (chromosomal) composition
2. Gonadal histology

3. Morphology of reproductive ducts
4. Appearance of external genitals.

An **intersex** animal or **hermaphrodite** is an animal in which one or more of these criteria are inconsistent with the others. Intersex conditions are classified as being hormonal or chromosomal in origin, a distinction based on whether or not the condition is due to chromosomal abnormalities in the embryonic reproductive tissues.

By established definition a false or **pseudohermaphrodite** has the gonads of one sex only and alteration of one or more of the other criteria for sex diagnosis. A true **hermaphrodite** has gonadal tissue of both sexes. A **lateral hermaphrodite** has an ovary on one side and a testis on the opposite side. A **unilateral hermaphrodite** has an ovotestis on one side and either an ovary or testis on the opposite side. A **bilateral hermaphrodite** has an ovotestis on both sides.

Any increase in the level of circulating androgens within the pregnant dam can severely affect the development of the fetus. For example if the dam is treated with androgens during gestation and later delivers a genetically female fetus, the neonate may have a masculinized duct system and external genitals along with a female duct system and ovaries. This is a **female pseudohermaphrodite**. A similar result will occur if the mother has a neoplasm of the adrenal cortex, which leads to excess synthesis of adrenocortical steroids, including androgens.

Alternatively, the fetal adrenal gland may produce abnormally high concentrations of androgens. This situation, which can be inherited in humans, is called the **adrenogenital syndrome**. In this disease an enzyme necessary to cortisol production is abnormal. In response to reduced cortisol levels, additional adrenocorticotrophic hormone (ACTH) is released by the adenohypophysis, which elevates the levels of production of other, normally minor adrenocortical products, including androgens.

The most common example of hormonally-altered sex differentation is the **freemartin,** * which is a sterile intersex female born twin to a normal male. Its gonadal tissues are XX but they display varying degrees of testicular organization. This situation occurs most commonly in cattle, and affects greater than 90% of the dizygotic twins of mixed sex (twinning occurs in 0.2–3.0% of bovine pregnancies, depending upon the breed).

Early in this century it was discovered that the extraembryonic chorioallantoic blood vessels of bovine twins become anastomosed (Fig. 19.7) at least a week before the initial appearance of unique male or female structures. In addition to serum components, including fetal hormones, cells in the blood can cross from one fetus to the other. White blood cells drawn from bovine twins of unlike sex routinely include both 60XX and 60XY leukocytes from each animal, although the ratios vary considerably. A few circulating primary germ cells from each embryo may become localized in the gonads of the other twin, but there is no cytogenetic evidence that any of these form viable gametes. Seminiferous tubules develop in these genetically female testes, but spermatogenesis does not occur, presumably because XX germ cells cannot form spermatocytes.

This gonadal sex reversal is due to the passage of a testicular-promoting substance from the developing male twin. H-Y antigen has been found in the gonads of the freemartin and is assumed to be the critical circulating inductor substance, although some researchers question whether the small amounts of circulating H-Y factor are sufficient to cause so profound a change in the gonad of the female twin. This change in gonadal development in the female twin occurs between 49 and 52 days of gestation, which is several days after testicular formation begins in the male twin.

Usually, the external genitals of the free-

---

* The term freemartin is derived from Scottish and Gaelic words meaning farrow mart (sterile cow). In the 17th century these animals were sacrificed on St. Martinmas Day.

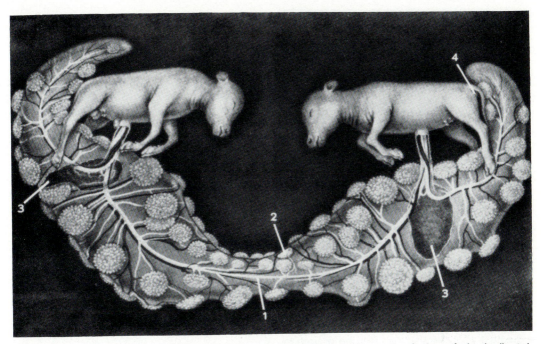

Figure 19.7.   This illustration from FR Lillie's 1917 publication shows the fusion of chorioallantoic blood vessels (*1*) between adjacent twin bovine embryos, as proven by injecting dye into the vessels of one twin. *2*, a cotyledon; *3*, openings cut in the chorioallantois; and *4*, the masculinized female fetus (freemartin).

martin calf are predominately female with a vulva, enlarged clitoris and increased anogenital distance. The slight male characteristics are due to circulating androgens from either the bull twin or the testis-like gonad of the freemartin.

The internal duct system is variable with respect to degrees of inhibition of the paramesonephric duct and development of the mesonephric duct (Fig. 19.8). The male duct system is most evident in the region nearest to the gonad. This is due to androgen production from the interstitial cells of the sex-reversed freemartin gonad.

The freemartin condition is less common in other domestic animals because of the infrequency of anastomosis of chorioallantoic blood vessels, although it has been reported in sheep, goats and pigs. Chimerism due to vascular anastomosis occurs routinely in marmosets and occasionally in humans. However, neither of these species has shown any abnormalities of reproductive tissues.

Male pseudohermaphroditism occurs also in Miniature Schnauzers. These dogs are characterized by undescended testes and a female duct system that persists along with the male duct system. The external genitals are male, and karyotyping reveals that all cells are 78XY (one dog was 79XXY).

It is assumed that this results from either a failure of fetal testicular sustentacular cells to produce paramesonephric duct-inhibiting substance or an inability of the paramesonephric ducts to respond to this secretion. A genetic basis for this disorder is suspected. These animals are presented clinically because of cryptorchidism and infertility, and they may show signs of sustentacular cell neoplasia in the cryptorchid testes. Alopecia (hair loss) and gynecomastia (enlarged mammary glands in a male) also occur in these dogs.

Intersex mosaic individuals produced by nondisjunctive mitosis involving a sex chromosome in the early stages of embryonic development have been reported. The male

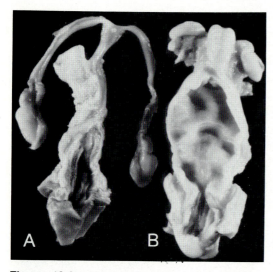

Figure 19.8. The reproductive tracts from 5-month bovine fetuses. *A* is a freemartin, *B* is a normal female. In both cases the vagina and vestibule have been opened. Note that the severity of the transformation of the XX freemartin is greatest near the gonads, and the urogenital sinus is less effected.

cat with one line of cells containing 39XXY chromosomes and a second line containing 38XY chromosomes is a probable example of such a mosaic. Testes form, but some degree of infertility usually is present.

An animal that has both male and female gonadal tissue is called a true hermaphrodite. This can result from the fusion of male and female zygotes or a zygote and fertilized polar body. In these chimeras the presence of both XX and XY cells in the gonadal ridges may result in a gonad with both female and male characteristics, an ovotestis, or in a lateral hermaphrodite. The development of the duct system and external genitalia will depend upon secretions by the testicular portion of the gonad.

This chimerism is exemplified by the results of cytogenetic analysis performed on two phenotypically similar intersex cattle. Each appeared externally as a male, with a penis and a scrotum lacking testes. Internally each had an ovotestis on one side and an ovary on the opposite side. A vagina opened into the pelvic urethra and communicated cranially with a normal bicornuate uterus. On the side with the ovotestis an epididymis and ductus deferens replaced the uterine tubule and connected to the uterine horn.

Chromosomal studies of these intersex animals revealed two cell lines in each. One animal had 60XX and 60XY leukocytes, with the former predominating; the other had mostly 60XX cells plus a few with a 90XXY karyotype. The latter animal may have resulted from dispermic fertilization of an oocyte (90XXY) which joined with another normally fertilized oocyte (60XX).

It is possible to have heritable intersex conditions in which the genetic basis cannot be recognized using cytogenetic methods. One such anomaly is the **testicular feminization syndrome**. All of the cells of the individual contain XY sex chromosomes and the testes appear normal. The duct systems and external genitalia are nonmasculinized and female in appearance. This male pseudohermaphrodite is thought to result either from failure of androgens to be produced by the male gonad or failure of the target organs to react to the androgens. The neutral condition, female, therefore predominates. This situation is especially prevalent in pigs, where it occurs in up to 0.4% of the members in some populations.

Bibliography

Reviews

Austin CR, Short RV: *Reproduction in Mammals. Vol 1: Germ Cells and Fertilization. Vol 2: Embryonic and Fetal Development.* Cambridge, Cambridge University Press, 1982.

Benirschke K: *Comparative Mammalian Cytogenetics.* New York, Springer-Verlag, 1969.

Benirschke K: Hermaphrodites, freemartins, mosaics and chimeras in animals. In Austin CR, Edwards RG, (eds): *Mechanisms of Sex Differentiation in Animals and Man.* New York, Academic Press, 1981, pp 421–463.

Byskov AG: Gonadal sex and germ cell differentiation. In Austin CR, Edwards RG, (eds): *Mechanisms of Sex Differentiation in Animals and Man.* New York, Academic Press, 1981, pp 145–164.

Hare WCD: Cytogenetics. In Morrow DA, (ed): *Current Therapy in Theriogenology: Diagnosis, Treatment and Prevention of Reproductive Diseases in Animals.* Philadelphia, Saunders, 1980, pp 119–142.

Josso N: Differentiation of the genital tract: stimulators and inhibitors. In Austin CR, Edwards RG, (eds): *Mechanisms of Sex Differentiation in Animals and Man.* New York, Academic Press, 1981, pp 165–203.

Rossant J, Croy BA, Chapman VM, Siracusa L, Clark DA: Interspecific chimeras in mammals: a new experimental system. *J Anim Sci* 55:1241–1248, 1981.

Wachtel, SS: Development of the heterogametic gonad: a model system for embryonic induction. *Curr Top Devel Biol* 18:189–216, 1983.

CYTOGENETICS AND SEX DETERMINATION

Dunn HO, Johnson RH Jr, Quaas RL: Sample size for detection of Y-chromosomes in lymphocytes of possible freemartins. *Cornell Vet.* 71:297–304, 1981.

Fehilly CB, Willadsen SM, Tucker EM: Interspecific chimerism between sheep and goat. *Nature* 307:633–635, 1984.

Johnson CA: The role of the fetal testicle in sexual differentiation. *Compend Cont Ed* 5:129–132, 1983.

Jones TC: Anomalies of sex chromosomes in tortoise-shell male cats. In Benirschke K (ed): *Comparative Mammalian Cytogenetics.* New York, Springer-Verlag, 1969, pp 414–433.

Ohno S, Christian LC: Hormone-like role of H-Y antigen in bovine freemartin gonad. *Nature* 261:597–598, 1976.

Pechan P, et al: H-Y antigen in the teleost. *Differentiation* 14;189–192, 1979.

Silvers WK, Wachtel SS: H-Y antigen: behavior and function. *Science* 195:956–960, 1977.

Wachtel SS: H-Y antigen and the genetics of sex determination. *Science* 198:797–799, 1977.

Wachtel SS: *H-Y Antigen and the Biology of Sex Determination.* New York, Grune & Stratton, 1983.

Wachtel SS, Koo GC: H-Y antigen and gonadal differentiation. In Austin CR, Edwards RG, (eds): *Mechanisms of Sex Differentiation in Animals and Man.* New York, Academic Press, 1981, pp 255–299.

Wilson JD: Sexual differentiation, *Annu Rev Physiol* 40:279–306, 1978.

Zaborski P, et al: H-Y antigen in ovariectomized chicks: disappearance of its expression during the transformation of the right gonad into a testis. *Biol Cell* 39:391–394, 1980.

INTERSEX CONDITIONS

Bennett RC, Olds D, Deaton OW, Thrift FA: Nature of white heifer disease (partial genital aplasia) and its mode of inheritance. *Am J Vet Res* 34:13–20, 1973.

Blue MG, Bruere AN, Dewes HF: The significance of the XO syndrome in infertility of the mare. *NZ Vet J* 26:137–141, 1978.

Bosu WTK, Chick BF, Basrur PK: Clinical, pathological and cytogenetic observations on two intersex dogs. *Cornell Vet* 68:376–390, 1978.

Bouters R, Vandeplassche M, de Moor A: An intersex (male pseudohermaphrodite) horse with 64XX/65XXY mosaicism. *Equine Vet J* 4:150–153, 1972.

Brown TT, Burek JD, McEntee KD: Male pseudohermaphroditism, cryptorchism, and Sertoli cell neoplasia in three Miniature Schnauzers. *JAVMA* 169:821–825, 1976.

Bruere AN, Marshall RB, Ward, DPJ: Testicular hypoplasia and XXY set chromosome complement in two rams: the ovine counterpart of Klinefelter's syndrome in man. *J Reprod Physiol* 19:103–108, 1969.

Buoen LC, Eilts BE, Rushmer A, Weber AF: Sterility associated with an XO karyotype in a Belgian mare. *JAVMA* 182:1120–1121, 1983.

Centerwall WR, Benirschke K: Male tortoiseshell and calico (T-C) cats. *J Hered* 64:272–278, 1973.

Centerwall WR, Benirschke K: An animal model for the XXY Klinefelter's syndrome in man: tortoiseshell and calico male cats. *Am J Vet Res* 36:1275–1280, 1975.

Dunn HO, Kenney RM, Lein RH: XX/XY chimerism in a bovine true hermaphrodite: an insight into the understanding of freemartinism. *Cytogenetics* 7:390–402, 1968.

Dunn HO, McEntee K, Hansel W: Diploid-triploid chimerism in a bovine true hermaphrodite. *Cytogenetics* 9:245–259, 1970.

Dunn HO, Johnson RH Jr: A 61XY cell line in a calf with extreme brachygnathia. *J Dairy Sci* 55:524–526, 1972.

Dunn HO, Vaughan JT, McEntee K: Bilateral cryptorchid stallion with female karyotype. *Cornell Vet* 64:265–275, 1974.

Dunn HO, Lein DH, McEntee K: Testicular hypoplasia in a hereford bull with 61XXY karyotype: the bovine counterpart of human Klinefelter's syndrome. *Cornell Vet* 70:137–146, 1980.

Dunn HO, McEntee K, Hall CE, Johnson RH Jr, Stone WH: Cytogenetic and reproductive studies of bulls born co-twin with freemartins. *J Reprod Fertil* 57:21–30, 1979.

Dunn HO, Smiley D, Duncan JR, McEntee K: Two equine true hermaphrodites with 64XX/64XY and 63XO/64XY chimerism. *Cornell Vet* 71:2, 1981.

Felts JA, Randall MG, Green RW, Scott RW: Hermaphroditism in a cat. *JAVMA* 181:925–926, 1982.

Hare WCD, McFeeley RA, Kelly DF: Familial 78XX male pseudohermaphroditism in three dogs. *J Reprod Fertil* 36:207–210, 1974.

Johnston SD, Buoen LC, Madl JE, Weber AF, Smith FO: X-chromosome monosomy (37XO) in a Burmese cat with gonadal dysgenesis. *JAVMA* 182:985–989, 1983.

Jost A, Vigier B, Prepin J: Freemartins in cattle: the first steps of sexual organogenesis. *J Reprod Fertil* 29:349–379, 1972.

McFeeley RA: Chromosomes and infertility. *JAVMA* 153:1672–1675, 1968.

McFeeley RA, Kresley LR: Intersexuality: In Hafez EGE (ed): *Reproduction in Farm Animals*, ed 4. Philadelphia, Lea & Febiger, 1980, pp 494–502.

Malouf N, Benirschke K, Hoefnagel D: XX/XY chimerism in a tricolored male cat. *Cytogenetics* 6:228–241, 1967.

Miyake Y-I, Inoue T, Kanagawa H, Satoh H, Ishikawa T: Four cases of anomalies of genital organs in horses. *Zbl Vet Med A* 29:602–608, 1982.

Marshall LS, Oewhlert ML, Haskins ME, Selden JR, Patterson DF: Persistent Mullerian duct syndrome in Miniature Schnauzers. *JAVMA* 181:798–800, 1982.

Monji Y, Yokoyama M, Ohsawa A, et al: A study on the external genital organs and chromosome constitution of intersex pigs. *Jpn J Swine Husb Res* 16:158–164, 1979.

Murti GS, et al: Canine intersex states. *JAVMA* 149:1183–1185, 1966.

Neuman F, Elger W, Steinbeck H: Drug-induced intersexuality in mammals. *J Reprod Fertil Suppl* 7:9–24, 1969.

Pakes SP, Griesemer RA: Current status of chromosome analysis in veterinary medicine. *JAVMA* 146:138–145, 1965.

Selden JR, Wachtel SS, Koo GC, Haskins ME, Patterson DG: Genetic bases of XX male syndrome and XX true hermaphroditism: evidence in the dog. *Science* 201:644–646, 1978.

Sharp AJ, Wachtel SS, Benirschke K: H-Y antigen in a fertile XY female horse. *J Reprod Fertil* 58:157–160,

1979.

Short RV: Cytogenetic and endocrine studies of freemartin heifer and its bull co-twin. *Cytogenetics* 8:369–388, 1969.

Smith MC, Dunn HO: Freemartin condition in a goat. *JAVMA* 178:735–737, 1981.

Stewart RW, et al: Canine intersexuality in a pug breeding kennel. *Cornell Vet* 62:464–473, 1972.

Tangner CH, Breider MA, Amoss MS: Lateral hermaphroditism in a dog. *JAVMA* 181:70–71, 1982.

Todoroff R: Congenital urogenital anomalies. *Compend Cont Ed* 1:780–787, 1979.

Wilkes PR, Wijeratne WVS, Munro IB: Reproductive anatomy and cytogenetics of freemartin heifers. *Vet Rec* 108:3499–3503, 1981.

Index

Words in CAPITALS indicate congenital MALFORMATIONS; *italicized* pages indicate location of illustrations.